Gabriele Doblhammer · Jordi Gumà
Editors

A Demographic Perspective on Gender, Family and Health in Europe

Editors
Gabriele Doblhammer
Institute for Sociology and Demography
University of Rostock
Rostock
Germany

and

German Center for Neurodegenerative Disease (DZNE)
Bonn
Germany

and

Rostock Center for the Study of Demographic Change
Rostock
Germany

Jordi Gumà
Department of Political and Social Sciences
University Pompeu Fabra
Barcelona
Spain

https://doi.org/10.1007/978-3-319-72356-3

Contents

Contributors

Isabella Buber-Ennser Wittgenstein Centre (IIASA, VID/ÖAW, WU), Vienna Institute of Demography/Austrian Academy of Sciences, Vienna, Austria

Giorgio Di Gessa Department of Global Health & Social Medicine, King's College London, London, UK

Gabriele Doblhammer German Center for Neurodegenerative Disease (DZNE), Bonn, Germany; Faculty of Economics and Social Sciences, Institute for Sociology and Demography, University of Rostock, Rostock, Germany; Rostock Center for the Study of Demographic Change, Rostock, Germany; Max Planck Institute for Demographic Research, Rostock, Germany

Viviana Egidi Department of Statistics, Sapienza University of Rome, Rome, Italy

Daniela Georges Institute for Sociology and Demography, University of Rostock, Rostock, Germany; Rostock Center for the Study of Demographic Change, Rostock, Germany

Patrizia Giannantoni La Sapienza University of Rome, Rome, Italy

Jordi Gumà Department of Political and Social Sciences, University Pompeu Fabra, Barcelona, Spain

Doris Hanappi University of California, Berkeley, Berkeley, USA; Austrian Academy of Sciences (ÖAW), Vienna, Austria

Karsten Hank Institute of Sociology and Social Psychology, University of Cologne, Cologne, Germany

Irena E. Kotowska Institute of Statistics and Demography, Warsaw School of Economics, Warsaw, Poland

Daniel Kreft Institute for Sociology and Demography, University of Rostock, Rostock, Germany; Rostock Center for the Study of Demographic Change, Rostock, Germany

Anna Oksuzyan Max Planck Institute for Demographic Research, Rostock, Germany

Livia Sz. Oláh Department of Sociology, Stockholm University, Stockholm, Sweden

Steffen Peters Rostock Center for the Study of Demographic Change, Rostock, Germany

Petra Rattay Robert Koch Institute, Berlin, Germany

Rudolf Richter Department of Sociology, University of Vienna, Vienna, Austria

Debora Rizzuto Department of Neurobiology, Care Sciences and Society, Karolinska Institutet, Aging Research Center, Stockholm, Sweden

Anja Steinbach Institute of Sociology, University of Duisburg-Essen, Duisburg, Germany

Cecilia Tomassini Department of Economics, University of Molise, Campobasso, Italy

Elena von der Lippe Robert Koch Institute, Berlin, Germany

Anna-Karin Welmer Department of Neurobiology, Care Sciences and Society, Karolinska Institutet, Aging Research Center, Stockholm, Sweden

Framework

Jordi Gumà and Gabriele Doblhammer

Family has been shown to be one of the most relevant socio-demographic factors in understanding health differences among individuals in Western countries. The difference in survival between the married and not married population was stated by William Farr as early as the 19th Century (Farr 1885). However, although the health advantages of those who live with a partner were already well known, the interest in this factor has increased among scholars in the past three decades. This increase has run parallel to two interrelated changes in traditional patterns which are contributing to reshape current European societies: diversification of family forms and the subsequent acceptance of the new forms among individuals; and the increase of female empowerment due to a progressive reduction of the gender gap.

The diversification of family forms has led to a more complex scenario that extends beyond merely comparing married and not-married individuals. At the same time, the traditional gender roles that men and women used to play within the context of the families in the past have also been modified. This family diversification and the process of gender balancing has not occurred with the same intensity and timing in all European countries. It has been stated that both processes have spread from the North and West to the South and East of the Continent (Surkyn and Lesthaeghe 2004). With these changes, family as a social determinant of health has become an ever more important factor of health, one which is rooted at the meso-level and extends beyond individual characteristics at the micro-level. Indeed, when one thinks about family, one figures a context where individuals provide

J. Gumà (✉)
Department of Political and Social Sciences, University Pompeu Fabra, Barcelona, Spain
e-mail: jordi.guma@upf.edu

G. Doblhammer
Institute for Sociology and Demography, University of Rostock, Rostock Germany
e-mail: gabriele.doblhammer@uni-rostock.de

G. Doblhammer and J. Gumà (eds.), *A Demographic Perspective on Gender, Family and Health in Europe*, https://doi.org/10.1007/978-3-319-72356-3_1

resources of different natures (economic, knowledge, social ties, etc.) and share these with the other members, thus compensating for or reinforcing existing individual advantages or disadvantages.

To understand the complex relationship of this triangle of family, gender, and health, one must understand patterns and trends in each of the three components separately, as well as their interdependencies. This book tries to expand upon the widely observable specialization in demographic research, which usually involves researchers studying either family or fertility processes or focusing on health and mortality. While both topics are commonly explored in the context of gender or sex, it is rare that a deeper understanding of health processes exists among researchers who deal with family processes. At the same time, researchers interested in health and mortality tend to lack insight into the structures of gendered processes in the family and the household. To overcome this lack of knowledge, this book compiles three keynote chapters that provide an overview about (1) the relationship between family and fertility characteristics and health, (2) the changing roles of men and women in the context of families and societies, and (3) sex and gender differences in health.

In addition to these keynote chapters, six country-specific case studies and one comparative study are presented in order to understand how different patterns in social change modify the link between family and health in women and men. The country-specific case studies range from the North of Europe (Sweden), to the Center (Germany and Austria) and the South (Italy). The comparative study explores twelve European countries from the North, Center, East and South of the Continent which are representative of different welfare states, gender models, household and family forms, and health profiles. Because this book's compilation of studies can provide only a small snapshot, we have tried to select country-specific case studies which focus on populations which have received less attention in the past, while presenting findings for other countries in the keynote chapter on the relationship between family, fertility, and health. We use the two keynote chapters on the new roles of men and women in family and society, and on sex differences in health as the basis for a joint framework, but we have abstained from harmonizing concepts in order to permit the authors to fully explore the data available in their countries. Hence, in the following we will briefly present the three keynote chapters and give a short overview about the different approaches to family, health, and gender that were used in these studies.

The Triangle Between Health, Gender, and Family

The three initial keynote chapters present the reader with a detailed background of the three sides of the triangle of family, health and gender. The first chapter by Hank and Steinbach offers a comprehensive summary of the main findings on the role of family relations in shaping individuals' health (and vice versa) or, in other words, the study of family as a social determinant of health as well as a source of selection into family transitions. This chapter covers the main literature about the influence of partnership and parenthood on an adult's health, as well as how a child's well-being varies according to different family structures and how these family circumstances shape health in later life. The authors extend their review to the link between intergenerational family relations and health, thereby including relations between relatives who likely do not live together in the same household. This chapter provides solid evidence of the relevance of family to shape individuals' health across the entire life-course: from early childhood, through adulthood, to very old-age.

The keynote chapter by Oláh, Richter, and Kotowska covers the second side of the triangle, the relationship between family and gender roles. Changes in family patterns have run parallel to the process of balancing gender inequalities (e.g. educational expansion of women, increase in female labour force participation, etc.). Therefore, family diversification cannot be understood completely without regarding the rise of female empowerment in Western societies. This keynote chapter first describes the increase in the diversity of family biographies. Second, linked to this higher family diversity, the authors describe the evolution of the main factors which help us understand the change of gender roles. Once both changes into family trajectories and gender roles are explained, the authors pinpoint the close bidirectional link between these two phenomena. The authors also discuss the recent research outcomes of family dynamics, especially regarding partnership transitions and parenthood and the organization of family life, and their association with changing gender roles.

The third keynote chapter by Oksuzyan, Gumà, and Doblhammer closes the triangle by revisiting the origins of health differences between men and women. First, the authors provide ample evidence of the existence of the sex gap in health, distinguishing between those which have been found based on objective and subjective measures of health. For objective measures the authors consider medical diagnoses, while subjective health measures are based on an individual's self-perception. Second, the authors provide a detailed literature review of the explanations for sex differences in health, dividing the section according to the nature of these explanations: biological, lifestyle behaviors, and social factors. The authors point out that, in the future, research in the social sciences cannot discard the biological root of the health differences between men and women, while health sciences cannot ignore the importance of the social context.

Different Approaches to the Concept of Family

Family can be conceptualized either in terms of ties between relatives who live together in the same household or independently of whether the individual members live together. In the first case, family is a synonym for household, e.g. the number of children refers to number of children living in the household, and partners are defined as living together. Depending on the survey design, the sample unit is either the individual or the household. If the individual is the sample unit, one usually has information about the characteristics of the respondent but not of the other members of the household. Many current surveys, however, take households as sample units and compile information on all their members. This permits researchers to address the study of family and health from two different viewpoints: individual characteristics and/or overall family characteristics and arrangements. In the second case, the notion of family extends beyond the household, most importantly when the number of children refers to ever born children. Sometimes information about the geographical distance between parents and children, and the frequency and quality of contacts is given, but there is rarely more information on the family member outside the survey household. Also, new forms of partnerships extend beyond the household such as living apart together (LAT).

This book provides examples of both approaches to the study of family, namely family confined to the household as well as family extending beyond the household. In addition, depending on the sample design, the studies explore the family effect based on individual information alone or, in the case of household samples, on characteristics of both the individual and the household.

Individual Level Characteristic

On the individual level, five case-studies explore the relationship between partnership, parenthood, and an individual's position within the household, as defined by the relationship of the household members, on health. The idea behind defining an individual's household position is to compile information about the partnership situation (married, consensual union, not partnered) with the information about children in the household and the relationship with the family nucleus. This approach allows us to study not only family arrangements but also the different levels of responsibilities related with being member of a household.

Doblhammer and Gumà apply the concept of household position in a comparative study of European countries representing different welfare state regimes. Buber-Ennser and Hanappi extend the basic concept of household position to include stepfamilies and new living arrangements such as LAT. The other studies use the categorizations of individuals according to their legal family status (von der Lippe and Rattay; Tomassini, Di Gessa, and Egidi) and partnership status (Doblhammer, Peters, and Welmer), to parenthood (children ever born yes/no, Doblhammer, Peters, and Welmer), fertility histories (Tomassini, Di Gessa, and Egidi), and children in the household (von der Lippe and Rattay).

Household Level Characteristics

Regarding the household level, two studies explore the impact of the household characteristics in addition to the individual characteristics. The study of Georges, Kreft, and Doblhammer explores the effect of the general household structure focusing on the composition of generations within the household. The rationale behind this approach is that in ethnically diverse populations the propensity to live in single-, one-, or multi-generational households as well as the number of children is stratified by ethnicity, which is also true for health. The other example is the study by Giannantoni and Egidi, who approach family from different characteristics at the household level such as socio-economic status, housing conditions, household size, and structure. Both chapters use multilevel methods in their analyses, with individuals as the first level, household as the second level, and, in the case of Giannantoni and Egidi, region as the third level.

In addition to exploring characteristics at the individual and meso-level, two of the studies also explore longitudinal information. Buber-Ennser and Hanappi use two waves of the Austrian Gender and Generation Study to analyze health among young and middle aged adults, while Doblhammer, Peters, Rizzuto and Welmer focus on the elderly using three waves of the Swedish National Study of Ageing and Care in Kungsholmen.

Different Approaches to the Concept of Health

The World Health Organization defined the concept of health in the preamble of its Constitution in 1946 as "a state of complete physical, mental and social well-being and not merely the absence of disease or infirmity". This holistic definition implies that it is almost impossible to summarize health in a single indicator and that it must be addressed by different approaches. Indeed, some of the studies chose more than one health indicator (e.g. Giannantoni and Egidi, and Tomassini, Di Gessa, and Egidi).

In this book, the most frequently studied health indicator is self-perceived (also called self-assessed) health, which compiles information about how individuals perceive their general health on a scale from very poor to very good. Apart from the capacity of this indicator to summarize the different dimensions of an individual's health in a single indicator, it can also inform us about how individuals perceive their evolution of health (Idler and Benyamini 1997). A more general health indicator explored in this book is derived from the question "Have you been ill or had an accidental injury within the last four weeks before the interview?" This indicator compiles information about long-lasting illnesses. The third health indicator analyzed which can be considered a measure of general health is functional limitations and personal independence through questions about Activities of Daily Living (ADL) (Katz et al. 1963) and the Instrumental Activities of Daily Living (IADL) scales (Lawton and Brody 1969).

Looking at more specific health indicators, mental health was analyzed through two different indicators, the depression score and the Mental Component Summary derived from the Short Form-12 Health Survey. Basically, both are synthetic indicators based on answers to a set of items related with depressive symptoms, such as feeling guilty or being irritable. In the case of physical performance, the indicators are walking speed and the Physical Component Summary derived from SF-12 Health Survey. The former is an objectively measured indicator which focuses on one aspect of physical performance, namely the speed of walking, although previous research has found a strong association with other health indicators and mortality. On the other hand, the physical component from SF-12 is another synthetic indicator derived from a set of questions about physical capacities of respondents.

Finally, healthy life-style is also analyzed based on smoking, alcohol consumption, diet, and physical activity. Exploring healthy-life style offers us a better understanding of the relationship between family and health because it is one of the intermediary behaviors that link family characteristics to health.

The Concept of Sex Versus the Concept of Gender

The book addresses the sometimes unclear difference between the concepts of sex differences and gender inequalities. It is relevant to make a distinction between the two concepts because their nature or origin is different. When talking about sex differences, one simply refers to differences in results between men and women that might have a diverse origin, whereas when talking about gender inequalities one refers to psychological, social, and cultural differences between males and females (e.g. distribution of roles within the household, different social behaviors assumed for men and women, etc.) (Giddens 2009). We can find a good example of this distinction in the keynote chapter about sex and health, in which the authors distinguish between biological sources of differences between men and women and social factors which originate in situations of gender inequality that affect an individual's health.

The use of the word "gender" in academic disciplines such as epidemiology and sociology also contributes to the confusion. The former generally employs this word to refer to studies where results of both sexes are compared, whereas the latter usually uses this concept to address differences rooted in social inequalities between men and women. In all the empirical chapters the authors compare male and female profiles and base their research questions, as well as their proposed explanations, on factors related to gender inequalities. In this direction, four of the chapters (Georges, Kreft, and Doblhammer; Doblhammer and Gumà; Buber-Ennser and Hanappi; Tomassini, Di Gessa, and Egidi) give a high relevance to the gendered distribution of roles within the context of the household, which are presented in detail in Oláh, Richter, and Kotowska.

Another argument related to gender inequalities is introduced by von der Lippe and Rattay and addresses the unequal level of social control to which men and women are exposed. This is also mentioned in the chapter of Oksuzyan, Gumà, and Doblhammer, and points to the fact that women bear a higher social control in terms of their life-style, which on the one hand protects them from unhealthy behaviors (i.e. smoking, drinking, etc.) though on the other hand exposes them to higher social sanctions in comparison with men in case of not avoiding these unhealthy behaviors.

References

Farr, W. (1885). Marriage and mortality. In *Vital statistics: A memorial volume of selections from the reports and writings of William Farr* (pp. 438–441). Sanitary Institute, London.

Giddens, A. (2009). Sociology (6th edition). Cambridge, UK.

Idler, E., & Benyamini, Y. (1997). Self-rated health and mortality: A review of twenty seven community studies. *Journal of Health and Social Behavior, 38,* 21–37.

Katz, S., Ford, A. B., Moskowitz, R. W., Jackson, B. A., & Jaffe, M. W. (1963). Studies of illness in the aged: The index of ADL: A standardized measure of biological and psychosocial function. *JAMA, 185*(12), 914–919.

Lawton, M. P., & Brody, E. M. (1969). Assessment of older people: Self-maintaining and instrumental activities of daily living. *The Gerontologist, 9*(3), 179–186.

Surkyn, J., & Lesthaeghe, R. (2004). Value orientations and the second demographic transition (SDT) in Northern, Western and Southern Europe. An update. *Demographic Research Special, 3*, 45–86. doi:https://doi.org/10.4054/DemRes.2004.S3.3.

Summary and Research Implications

Gabriele Doblhammer and Jordi Gumà

Despite considerable changes in family forms during the past decades, the influence of family on health is strong and persistent. All over Europe the elderly still live in more traditional family forms related to marriage and their family biographies are closely tied to the civil status of their partnership. On the other hand, new family forms have been emerging among the young, yet the prevalence and acceptance of these forms differs widely between societies. At a young age, the distribution of paid and unpaid work within the household is largely gendered, and in the case of families with children it is centred around the care provision for children; at old age, when paid work has ceased and income is secured by pension systems, the distribution of unpaid work is less of an issue, while the care provision for partners is at the heart of gendered family responsibilities.

Among the young and middle aged adults, where variability in health is low, little is known about new family and partnership forms, their relationship with health, and the pathways through which they act. The young population is heterogonous in terms of their ethnic background, and little is known whether the relationship between family forms and health is universal in a society or dependent on migration background and the respective values and norms. And little is known to what extent advantaged and disadvantaged family forms are universal in different welfare state regimes or whether they depend on the social and cultural context of a society.

Among the old, when different ageing trajectories result in an increasing variability in individual health, the health of the partner becomes even more important; in combination with an individual's own health there might be strong mutual

G. Doblhammer (✉)
Institute for Sociology and Demography, University of Rostock, Rostock, Germany
e-mail: gabriele.doblhammer@uni-rostock.de

J. Gumà
Department of Political and Social Sciences, University Pompeu Fabra, Barcelona, Spain
e-mail: jordi.guma@upf.edu

G. Doblhammer and J. Gumà (eds.), *A Demographic Perspective on Gender, Family and Health in Europe*, https://doi.org/10.1007/978-3-319-72356-3_2

influences. Thus, the present family situation and abrupt changes may become more important for an individual's health when compared to the lifelong family biography. Not much is known about if or how partners advancing in age start to resemble each other more closely in terms of health and how the health of the partner influences an individual's own health. Little is known about how geographical and emotional closeness or distance of family members affects health.

In the following we summarize and discuss the main findings of this book by touching on the issues mentioned above. While all these studies explore novel aspects in the triangle of health, family, and gender, they can provide only some insight into this wide-ranging topic. We will first focus on the relationship between traditional and new family forms and health among the young, then turn to the effect of partnership and parenthood among the old, then discuss some of the possible pathways, and end with future possible research directions. We try to give an encompassing view of all studies in this book but point out that the individual authors discuss their findings and future avenues of research in much more detail.

Traditional Family Forms, New Living Arrangements and Health Among the Young and Middle Aged

In all young and middle aged populations studied, the best health is found among the married and those living together with a partner, who have two or more children. This is true for all welfare state regimes (Doblhammer and Gumà) and, in the case of Germany, for both migrant and non-migrant groups (Georges, Kreft, and Doblhammer). This health advantage is larger for women than men and it is generally the case that women's health depends on household characteristics to a larger extent than does men's health (Doblhammer and Gumà).

While for women new family forms are by and large associated with a health disadvantage, the extent of this disadvantage differs between welfare state regimes. Most of the findings described below stem from cross-sectional perspectives; in the Austrian study (Buber-Ennser and Hanappi) they become even stronger in a longitudinal perspective when union dissolution and separation are studied, which generally result in worse health.

Consensual Unions and Stepfamilies

In Austria, women living in a stepfamily where at least one partner has a pre-union child, either living in the household or not, have worse health (Buber-Ennser and Hanappi). This finding is supported by the cross-country study for selected European countries where cohabiting women (with or without children) have worse health than the married (Doblhammer and Gumà). These effects seem to be largely the result of financial deprivation, because the inclusion of variables indicating the ability to financially make ends meet partly or fully attenuate the observed relations. Furthermore, poor health in complex stepfamilies is particularly prevalent among people with less education and is absent among the highly educated. In addition to financial aspects, another important influence appears to be a society's value climate towards new family forms. When the value climate is indirectly measured in terms of the proportion of a certain family form, the disadvantage of new family forms is smaller (or even disappears) in societies where they are comparatively more frequent.

Concerning stepfamilies and cohabitation, similar but much weaker health tendencies exist for men, which are statistically not significant. Financial difficulties are a less important mediator, and on the contrary cohabiting men seem to be better off in financial terms. Thus, there is a strongly gendered effect of the household structure on health.

Single Parents

Single mothers have worse health than the partnered in all countries studied and this is due largely to financial difficulties. While the negative effects of consensual unions disappear in societies where they are more frequent, this is not true for single mothers (Doblhammer and Gumà). The more frequent they are, the higher the disadvantage in terms of their health. Financial difficulties or deprivation partly explain this disadvantage. Single mothers are more prevalent in the Nordic Dual-Earner welfare states, where partners usually rely on two incomes, which makes it particularly difficult for single mothers to generate sufficient household income. Another important aspect may be the lack of a partner in daily childcare and household chores, a lack of general support by friends, family and society, and the burden of increased or even sole responsibilities for the child.

Living Apart Together

Another new living arrangement is living apart together (LAT) which has been studied in the Austrian context (Buber-Ennser and Hanappi). This is the only study among the young which did not confine family to the household and in which information about partners living outside the household was available. Both men and women in a LAT relationship experience better health, but for men the effect is larger than for women and statistically significant. When it comes to health, financial factors do not seem to play an important role.

Generational Household Composition Among Migrants and Non-migrants

While new family forms are negligible among the migrant groups studied in Germany, they differ markedly by their generational composition. Migrants from Turkey and Aussiedler, who primarily stem from countries of the former Soviet Union, more often live in a multi-generational household context than Germans (Georges, Kreft, and Doblhammer). These three groups also differ concerning their individual values, cultural norms, and their social backgrounds. Thus, one might expect differences in the effect of the household structure on individual health by migration background. The study, however, reveals (with few exceptions) a similar relationship in all three groups: individuals living in two generation households with multiple children, i.e. a couple with two or more children, have superior health compared to all other groups, and individuals living in a one generation household have the worst health. Living without a partner is negatively associated with health, and the extent of the effect is similar for all three groups. Furthermore, in all three groups women's health depends to a larger extent on the household form, but most importantly, the effect of a specific household form on health is equally gendered among migrants and native Germans. It is difficult to interpret this finding because it can imply two things. On the one hand, the social structure of German society, in the form of its welfare state, the health system, and the prevailing norms and values may simply overrule any differences in the relationship between household form and health that might result from different cultural backgrounds. On the other hand, Turkish migrants and Aussiedler in Germany, many of whom have spent extended periods in Germany, may have adopted norms and values of the majority populations with regards to family composition and health.

The Relationship Between Family and Health Among the Elderly

At young and middle ages the household composition influences women's health in particular and creates a disadvantage for all women who do not follow the traditional family norm of living in a marriage with two or more children. While similar tendencies do exist for men, the effects are much smaller. At old age this gendered response changes, with men's health becoming equally dependent on the household and family composition. Two country studies of Italy (Tomassini, Di Gessa, and Egidi) and Sweden (Doblhammer, Peters, Rizzuto, and Welmer) come to this conclusion, albeit by examining two populations with widely different welfare states, family values, and norms, and by using different health measures and study designs. In addition, a third Italian study (Giannantoni and Egidi) concludes that with advancing age the members of a household become more equal in their health outcome.

Children and Health

One of the two Italian studies investigates the relationships between fertility and late life health in a familialistic welfare state system where the family is at the centre of care provision, cohabitation between different generations is more frequent, and gender roles are more traditional (Tomassini, Di Gessa, and Egidi). In this context, the dependency between fertility and later life health for women may be even larger than in other populations for two reasons. First, health selection into fertility might be stronger due to social pressure into marriage and fertility, leaving the "unfit" more often unmarried and/or childless. Second, the negative consequences of having a large number of children might be stronger because the care burden of rearing the children has to be mainly covered by mothers (and grandmothers). On the other hand, large family networks might reduce stress related to child rearing by distributing care work on more (family) shoulders. The selection argument also holds for men, and large numbers of children would create additional pressure on fathers to provide economic resources. However, as this study focuses on elderly women and men, one might not expect such a large difference compared to other welfare state regimes, because the childbearing period of the cohorts observed usually took place before or at the beginning of the second demographic transition, at a time when welfare states, household compositions, and gender roles did not differ to such an extent as they do today.

At a first glance the Italian study reveals similar patterns to what was previously observed in other populations. Namely, health is best for mothers with one or two children; large numbers of children are detrimental to various health domains of mothers and also, to some extent, of fathers and the relationship is generally stronger among women than men. Most interestingly, the detrimental health effect is not modified by the quantity of contacts between mothers and children. Thus close relations with adult children might not be able to buffer the negative consequences of repeated pregnancies. These results are reflected in the Swedish study (Doblhammer, Peters, Rizzuto, and Welmer) insofar that having children is definitely beneficial for men's health but not necessarily for women's health. The Swedish study is set in a welfare state system in which the state is the centre of care provision, but in which more recently the family, and in particular the partner, has become more important in providing care. Cohabitation between old and middle aged generations is not frequent, and gender roles are more equal. While the Swedish study, due to sample size, was not able to look into the relationship by number of children, it was obvious that in terms of health men profited more from fatherhood than women do from motherhood.

In Italy, the childless do not suffer from worse health, which, given that health selection into childlessness does exist, might point towards the possibility that parenthood is also associated with negative social consequences that are avoided by being childless. On the other hand, only the fittest childless individuals might have survived until old age. The Swedish study permitted a somewhat deeper insight by differentiating between being childlessness while living with a partner and being childless without a partner. There it was interesting to see that the childless in partnerships had the fastest deterioration of health, which might be an indication of negative health selection having taken place.

The Italian study showed that social factors are able to modify possible biological effects of fertility on late life health. First, there was no effect of closely spaced children on any of the health domains late in life, which may point towards beneficial and stress reducing effects for parents rearing children in a closely knit family environment. In addition, having a child very early in life was positive for late life health among women in Southern Italy, while it was detrimental in Northern Italy, which may be related to a higher acceptance of early and high fertility in the South. Interestingly, indicators of marital history and early childhood circumstances did not influence the relationship between fertility and health, despite being significant themselves.

Partner and Health

In the above mentioned Italian study, present marital status was more predictive of health than the marital biography, and the presently married generally had better health. While the latter result was particularly strong and significant for self-rated health and limitations, it was also a tendency for ADL, IADL, and depressive symptoms. The Swedish study further extends these findings, by showing that in terms of walking speed as an indicator of health, living in a partnership is more beneficial for men than for women; for women it can even be detrimental. For men there is a positive relationship between walking speed and the number of possible resources of help in the family: the childless without a partner have the slowest walking speed, those with children and a partner have the fastest. For women no such relationship exists: children tend to be slightly positively related to walking speed, partners have a negative influence on walking speed.

In conclusion, the two studies provide strong evidence that biological factors partly underlie the relationship between fertility and late life health, particularly among women, but that this relationship is widely responsive to the social environment. In addition, living with a partner at old age can be beneficial, which is mainly seen for men. For women, however, it can also create an additional burden due to care giving which reflects negatively on their own health. Most interestingly, these findings appear to be independent of the welfare state regime.

The Effect of the Household Level on Health

The question whether the impact of the household situation on the health of its individual members differs in a familialistic welfare state regime is taken up in a different study (Giannantoni and Egidi). In the special context of Italy, dependent on the health indicator used, about 15–38% of the variability in health can be attributed to joint factors at the household level. These figures fall into the range reported by other studies, which, however, deal primarily with less developed countries. Figures reported for the US are between 9 and 15%. Most interestingly, the study reveals that the health of household members is more homogenous in small families and within couples, and that homogeneity increases with age, despite the fact that the variability in individual health increases with age. The authors attribute this increasing homogeneity not only to similar health determinants within a household, such as nutritional choices or prevention attitudes, but also to mutual influences, which they define in relation to the health outcome itself. In other words the good or poor health of one household member may influence the health outcomes of the other members. Whether this effect is stronger for men or for women cannot be answered based on the cross-sectional data the study uses, because a time reference for the deterioration of the health among partners is missing. Here, again, the Swedish study sheds some more light by showing that living in a partnership is not necessarily beneficial for the health of women, while it is definitely positive for men. Thus, as the authors of the Italian study hypothesize, the "contagion" of poor health from men to women might be stronger than from women to men. At the centre of this "contagion" is certainly the gender specific role of care provision in the context of lower life expectancy and earlier health deterioration among men. While there is strong evidence on the negative effects of the care giver burden, still more research is needed regarding to what extent this burden can be relieved by the health system in particular, the welfare state in general, as well as social attitudes in terms of formal and informal care provision. There is ample evidence that the care giver burden is particularly large when care is provided due to feelings of obligations rather than voluntarily. In addition, it is unclear to what extent the psychological effects of the poor health of a close family member exert a negative influence on the health and well-being of others independent of the burden of care giving.

Pathways

All studies in this book show that family type is correlated with social status measured, e.g. in terms of education, occupational status, and income, and that social status explains some of the differences in health by family status. However, much remains unexplained and other important pathways must exist additionally. Two pathways have been explored in detail in the individual country studies: financial difficulties and health behaviour.

Financial Difficulties

One important factor is financial difficulties measured in terms of the ability to make ends meet. This is a very powerful indicator that explains the disadvantaged health among women living in new family forms such as stepfamilies, consensual unions with or without children, and very importantly, of single mothers (Buber-Ennser and Hanappi). It accounts for many of the significant differences between women living in new family forms and married women with children. Interestingly, this is not the case for men because accounting for the presence of financial difficulties even increases the extent of male health differences by family status. This implies that financial responsibilities partly depress the health of married fathers, less so the health of men living in other family forms.

Financial deprivation is not only an important pathway in populations where new family forms are less frequent, such as the Familialistic and Transition Post-Socialist welfare states, but also in the countries of the Dual-Earner and the General Family Support regimes (Doblhammer and Gumà). However, the types of new family forms sensitive to financial deprivation differ. In the Nordic Dual-Earner welfare states, living in a consensual union has become an alternative to marriage even when children are present. These family types do not necessarily experience financial difficulties, and while women do suffer some disadvantage in health as compared to the married, the difference is rather small. In many of the other countries, however, consensual unions are often a transitory phase to marriage with probably little difference in the health outcome, but often they are also characterised by fragile living arrangements with low household income, instable and changing partnerships, and insufficient social support from family and friends. Women living in these types of consensual unions may indeed be very similar to single mothers, who are among the most disadvantaged groups in all welfare state regimes. Despite the high labour market involvement of single mothers (the latest OECD figures show that in all welfare states their labour participation reaches or even surpasses that of married women) they have a high risk of financial deprivation mainly due to part-time employment and the foregone income of a second adult household member.

Life-Style Factors

In addition to social status and financial deprivation, life style factors turn out to be an important pathway of differences in health by family status. Among German young and middle aged adults, those married with children follow better health behaviours in terms of diet, smoking, physical activity and alcohol consumption (von der Lippe and Rattay). Some of these differences, however, appear to be mediated by social status, e.g. the healthier diet of married women and men, while others such as the higher prevalence of smoking among the divorced and widowed are independent of social status. Here it is interesting to note that for both genders children have a genuine effect on better diet starting with the arrival of the first child, and smoking is less prevalent among parents with two or more children independent of social status.

As mentioned previously, single never married and divorced mothers are a particularly vulnerable group with the highest odds of smoking and at-risk alcohol consumption (although they do appear to be physically more active). This group is exposed to reinforcing risk factors of poor health, starting with financial deprivation and lack of social resources and appreciation, to unhealthy behaviour.

The number and ages of children are significant modulators of these associations. Having a higher number of children and living together with pre-school children usually leads to better health behaviour. While the German study is based on cross-sectional data, this finding hints at important life-course changes in health behaviour associated with the family biography.

Healthy behaviour appears to be linked with parenthood more closely among women than men and it has been suggested that this has to do with the social roles occupied by men and women. While the partnership status per se does not have a gendered influence on health behaviour in present day Germany, it did have a gendered impact in the past. One may speculate that this shall have to do with a disappearance of specific gender roles over time, with women being strongly involved in the labour force and men becoming more involved in household chores. However, the arrival of a first, and even more often, of a second child usually results in taking up more traditional social roles leading to gendered health behaviour of parents.

Biological Pathways

While the pathways described above are of social origin, some of the studies also pointed towards biological pathways, although we were not able to test these directly. Health selection into partnership status as well as into childlessness is to some extent certainly a biological phenomenon. More important, however, is the finding that among women high fertility may go together with worse health in the long-term. In the Italian study (Tomassini, Di Gessa, and Egidi), none of the indicators included in the partnership biography could explain the increase in poor health by repeated pregnancies, and frequency of contacts with children at old age also could not account for the negative strain. The biological origin of the health disadvantage is further strengthened by the absence of strong health patterns in relation to the number of children among men. The keynote chapter on gender and health discusses hormonal and genetic foundations of health differences between men and women (Oksuzyan, Gumà, and Doblhammer). These biological foundations may also be associated with fertility histories. Still, the societal context may be able to modify possible biological pathways, as pointed out by the keynote chapter on families and health.

Future Research Directions

Present research has widely documented the differences in health by family status between different populations at a specific point in time, different groups within population, for the young and middle aged, and the old.

The next step in understanding these differences must overcome the traditional characterization of family status by marital status, partnership status, or parenthood characteristics. Some of the studies in this book have started in this direction, but only first steps have been taken. One way to proceed further is to characterize fragile and non-fragile living arrangements. This categorization cannot only rely on the present family status but also has to include partnership and fertility biographies, in particular frequently changing and unstable partnerships as well as major disruptions such as the birth of a child, and the end of a partnership such as divorce or widowhood. The characterization of fragile family forms is of great importance among the young and middle aged where the new family forms have been emerging. However, they also need to be identified among the old, where it has probably more to do with geographical and emotional closeness or distance among family members not living in the same household.

This characterization could shed more light on the underlying pathways such as the immediate and long-lasting effects of financial deprivation, risky health behaviours, lack of social support, care obligations, etc. These pathways change over the course of family biographies, leading to periods of life with more or less positive health repercussions. These different periods may reinforce or counterbalance each other, and healthy or unhealthy behaviour during specific time periods or at specific family situations may have a particularly positive or negative outcome for immediate or long-lasting health.

When exploring sensible time periods and ages, not only the health of adult but also of child and adolescent members of a household should be investigated. This aspect was briefly touched upon in one of the keynote chapters of the book but was not taken further in the individual studies. Similar to other early-life influences, the question arises whether certain family situations do have an immediate or long-lasting effect on a young individual's health by initiating a certain pathway or by acting at a vulnerable age.

Another important step is to explore changes in health differences by family forms over time. With new family forms developing in the course of the second demographic transition and the emergence of new gender roles, the selection forces into specific family forms have also been changing and will continue to do so in future. Dependent on the social acceptance and, thus, on the social support of new family forms, one would expect a weakening (high acceptance) or strengthening (low acceptance) of the health advantage of the married (with children) with respective changes in gendered health behaviours, financial situation, and the distribution of paid and unpaid work.

In many European societies the baby boomer cohorts are among the forerunners of new family forms. They have been starting to approach young old age in recent years and will continue to do so in the near future. They will be the first cohorts in which new family forms at old age will become more prevalent and much may be learnt in studying their health profile in comparison with previous cohorts at the same age.

Over the last decades European societies have become more diverse due to migrant populations. These populations differ significantly in their family composition within households but also beyond the household. Earlier migrant cohorts are now approaching old age and little is known whether their relationships between family composition and health differ from those of the majority population. Other important migrant specific questions are whether family composition is related to re-migration and whether this is correlated with health, and whether life-course influences, such as age at migration, modify the relationship between family composition and health.

While working on this book it became ever more obvious that family demographers interested in the formation and dissolution of families, as well as the gendered distribution of tasks within families and demographers interested in morbidity and mortality, need to work together more closely. In order to gain a better understanding of the underlying processes in this wide-spread research area we will need to overcome the traditional boundaries in the field of demography.

But also boundaries between disciplines must be overcome to translate research findings into policy recommendations. Among others, demographers, health economists, political scientist and sociologists working on poverty and social inequality need to combine their research efforts to come up with ideas and suggestions for policies which can help battle poor health associated with certain family situations.

We close this summary of findings and ideas by observing that the relationship between health, family, and gender is a perfect example of the paradox that research leads to a better understanding, but even more, to unsolved puzzles. We hope that our contribution in the form of this book provides both new insights and new questions.

Part I
Keynote Chapters

Families and Health: A Review

Karsten Hank and Anja Steinbach

Introduction

Social scientists interested in individuals' health (and health inequalities) may take two—complementary—general perspectives: a *life-course* perspective (e.g., Kuh et al. 2003) and a *contextual* perspective (in which relevant social contexts may be defined at very different levels of aggregation, ranging from personal social networks to welfare states; e.g., Deindl et al. 2016). Arguably, the *family context* not only constitutes a core element of most individuals' social network structure, it also accompanies the individual across the entire life-course. Understanding the role of family in shaping individuals' health thus seems an important task, one which has received considerable attention in various social science disciplines (for recent reviews see Arránz Becker et al. 2017; Carr et al. 2014; Rapp and Klein 2015).

In this review, we basically follow the World Health Organization's definition of *health* as "a state of complete physical, mental and social well-being and not merely the absence of disease or infirmity", that is, health is conceptualized as a multidimensional outcome with objective and subjective components. The role of *family* in health is considered from the adult's perspective [focusing on partnership (Section "Partnership and Adult Health") and parenthood (Section "Parenthood and Adult Health")] as well as from the child's perspective [focusing on the consequences of parental separation and divorce (Section "Family Structure and Child

K. Hank (✉)
Institute of Sociology and Social Psychology, University of Cologne, Cologne, Germany
e-mail: hank@wiso.uni-koeln.de

A. Steinbach
Institute of Sociology, University of Duisburg-Essen, Duisburg, Germany
e-mail: anja.steinbach@uni-due.de

G. Doblhammer and J. Gumà (eds.), *A Demographic Perspective on Gender, Family and Health in Europe*, https://doi.org/10.1007/978-3-319-72356-3_3

Well-Being")]. We also review findings from research addressing the association of childhood circumstances (Section "Childhood Circumstances and Later Life Health") and intergenerational family relations (Section "Intergenerational Family Relations and Health") with health. This chapter concludes with a brief outlook on directions for future research (Section "Conclusions and Future Directions"). While our primary interest is on universal relationships between individuals' family context (histories, respectively) and different health outcomes, we are well aware of possible cross-national variations. Because in many cases the empirical evidence available is predominantly based on studies from the United States, we explicitly seek to include an overview of European research.

Partnership and Adult Health

Marriage has long been suggested to have a *protective effect* on health (including survival; for reviews see Koball et al. 2010; Rendall et al. 2011). Such a causal effect is said to result from both economic advantages and social support inherent in a marriage. Men in particular are purported to enjoy health benefits, as they tend to engage in healthier and less risky behaviors once married (e.g. drinking less alcohol and driving more carefully). However, caution is necessary: *First*, married people may overestimate their health, and the protective effect that marriage accords may diminish at the most severe levels of health (Zheng and Thomas 2013). *Second*, even more importantly, selection effects are likely to play a role here, as better health may affect one's chances to get (and remain) married. Healthier individuals may be more likely to possess characteristics such as a higher socio-economic status or greater physical attractiveness, making them more desirable (and more stable) marriage partners than those in poor health.

Even if selection is accounted for, a salutary effect of being married for a variety of physical and mental health outcomes has been demonstrated repeatedly (but see Kalmijn 2017). More recently, effects of changes in marital status and the consideration of *marital biographies* have received growing attention (e.g., Dupre and Meadows 2007; Hughes and Waite 2009). One important finding from this research is that dimensions of health which develop rather slowly, such as chronic conditions or mobility limitations, tend to be more strongly affected by marital history (pointing to the importance of time spent in a specific status), whereas others, such as depressive symptoms, seem to react more sensitively to current marital status.

Divorce has long been suggested to bring about negative short- and long-term effects on health, even among those who remarried (e.g., Lorenz et al. 2006). A recent European study, however, provides evidence for heterogeneous (that is, gendered) effects of union dissolution on self-assessed health: While for men separation more often leads to increases rather than decreases in health, women fare worse more often than well just after union dissolution (Monden and Uunk 2013). Gendered social pathways also seem to exist, if the reverse causal relationship is considered: Karraker and Latham (2015) found that only wives' onset of serious physical illness is associated with an elevated risk of divorce. There appear to be no gender differences, though, if the relationship between *widowhood* and health (specifically depression) is considered (e.g., Sasson and Umberson 2014; Schaan 2013). Across marital groups, the continuously married are better off compared to the widowed, whereas early (long-term) widowhood is associated with worse outcomes than late widowhood. Moreover, individuals reporting higher *marital quality* at baseline experience larger increases in the number of symptoms of depression after having entered widowhood than those with lower marital quality (see Walker and Luszcz 2009, for a review).

Along the same lines, Hank and Wagner (2013) found that having a partner does not contribute to greater psychological well-being per se: Only those reporting satisfaction with the extent of reciprocity in their relationship report lower numbers of depression symptoms than their unmarried counterparts. There is also evidence that marital strain accelerates the typical decline in self-rated health occurring over the life-course. This adverse effect has been shown to be similarly strong in men and women and to be greater at older ages (Umberson et al. 2006; also see Xu et al. 2016). Staying unhappily married may even be more detrimental to health than divorcing, as people in low-quality marriages were found to exhibit lower levels of overall well-being, largely independent of whether they remain unmarried or remarry (see Hawkins and Booth 2005).

Effects of marriage (marital history) on *mortality* have been investigated in the US (e.g., Henretta 2010; Rendall et al. 2011) as well as in a variety of European settings (e.g., Blomgren et al. 2012; Brockmann and Klein 2004). There is a consistent survival advantage of being married over unmarried both for women and—particularly—for men. Little evidence, however, is found for mortality differences between never-married, divorced/separated, and widowed statuses (see Shor et al. 2012a, b, for recent meta-analyses). Into an individual's current status, the marital biography has also been shown to be relevant: For example, multiple transitions into and out of marriage as well as a lower proportion of adult life spent married have been found to be associated with a higher hazard of dying after age 50 (also if current marital status is controlled for), even though the relationship tends to weaken at older ages.

Finally, although there appears to be some universality in the marriage-health-nexus reported above, it still seems important to situate marriage cohorts in their specific historical social contexts (cf. Newton et al. 2014; Schaan 2013). This also includes accounting properly for the growing complexity of *relationship* histories, that is, considering marriage alone is no longer sufficient to understand how living with (or without) a partner affects health (e.g., Schneider et al. 2014).

Parenthood and Adult Health[1]

Closely intertwined with individuals' partnership histories (and their association with adult health) is the reproductive history and the parenthood-health-nexus (cf. O'Flaherty et al. 2016; Kravdal et al. 2012). Two causal mechanisms have been suggested to drive the relationship between individuals' fertility and later life health outcomes including survival (see, for example, Grundy and Tomassini 2005; Mirowsky 2005; Henretta 2007). *First*, there is evidence for biological effects, that is, direct long-term physiological and psychological implications of women's reproductive history on particular diseases. Most notably, breast cancer as well as other cancers of the female reproductive system were shown to be associated with pregnancy, childbirth, and lactation (see Grundy and Kravdal 2010, for a recent analysis).

Second, childbearing has been proposed to be related to a variety of social factors that might have both positive and negative effects on women's and men's health in later years. Specifically, differences in socio-economic status, social relationships, and health behaviors across the life-course have been put forward as being potentially relevant in this regard (e.g., Grundy and Tomassini 2005; Henretta 2007; Kendig et al. 2007). Having children may lead to economic strain, and particularly early as well as non-marital childbearing are likely to be related to lower socio-economic status and poorer family functioning over the life course (cf. Mirowsky and Ross 2002; Koropeckyj-Cox et al. 2007). There also is considerable potential for role overload and stresses related to raising children, particularly among lone parents. This, however, is contrasted by potentially health enhancing aspects of parenthood, such as greater opportunities for community participation and social support by children in later life. Moreover, parenthood may be associated with incentives—and social pressures—to adopt healthier behaviors (e.g., Fletcher 2012; Perales et al. 2015). The net effect of these factors not only varies according to individuals' socio-economic circumstances, but also with particular fertility pathways (e.g. the timing of births).

The relative importance of these biological and social mechanisms in determining the childbearing-health-nexus is still poorly understood (cf. Grundy and Read 2015). Causal analysis is further complicated by a range of possible *selection effects*, that is, by factors affecting both fertility and health. For example, individuals with a poor initial health endowment may not only be less fecund than their healthier counterparts, but they are also less likely to marry; i.e., their opportunities to become a parent and to enjoy the health benefits of marriage are reduced as well (see Section "Partnership and Adult Health" for details).

Although there is empirical evidence for a differential effect of childbearing (particularly timing of births) on specific *physical health outcomes*, such as diabetes, cardiovascular disease, or cancer (e.g., Alonzo 2002; Henretta 2007), many studies have used composite health indices or other general health measures, such as individuals' self-rated health (e.g., Hank 2010; Mirowsky 2005; Sudha et al.

[1]This section draws heavily on Hank (2010: 277–278).

2006). Findings suggest that high parity (six or more children), early first birth, and the experience of infant death or pregnancy loss are associated with worse self-reported health at older ages. Early childbearing also bears a clear positive correlation with the prevalence of limitations in activities of daily living, whereas no significant effects of high parity were found. Looking at the presence of limiting long term illness, Grundy and Tomassini (2005) reported higher risks among older women with five or more children and those who had a teenage birth. Controlling for parity, mothers with short birth intervals were more likely to experience long term illness, whereas those who had a late birth (at age 40 or later) exhibited a reduced risk. Mirowsky (2005), however, reported a steep increase in later life general health problems among women who delayed their first birth beyond age 40.

Unlike other major social roles, a clear relationship between parenthood and *psychological well-being* (depression) could not be identified by previous research (e.g. Evenson and Simon 2005; Hank and Wagner 2013; Kruk and Reinhold 2014). Some studies suggest that older childless men and women exhibit lower levels of depressive symptoms than parents, particularly if they are compared to those who had their first child early (e.g. Henretta et al. 2008) or whose relationship with their offspring is of poor quality (e.g. Koropeckyj-Cox 2002). More recently, however, Huijts et al. (2013) found that being childless is associated with worse psychological well-being for men (but not for women). Also, Grundy et al. (2017) showed that in Eastern, but not Western, European countries childlessness and having one compared with two children were associated with more depressive symptoms.

Studies dealing with individuals' childbearing histories and *mortality* (for reviews see Högnäs et al. 2017; Hurt et al. 2006) generally suggest that early childbearing tends to be associated with a higher hazard of dying, whereas late children enhance women's longevity (e.g., Doblhammer 2000; Mirowsky 2005; Henretta 2007).[2] Grundy and Kravdal (2008), however, reported a positive association between earlier parenthood and later mortality as well as a reverse association with late age at last birth in Norway (with similar results for both men and women). Moreover, the authors found an overall negative association between higher parity and mortality, which is only partially consistent with Doblhammer (2000), for example, who showed for England/Wales and Austria that childless women *and* those with three or more children experienced excess mortality (also see Grundy and Tomassini 2005). Henretta (2007), however, did not find evidence for an effect of the number of children ever born on mortality. It seems important to keep in mind that even if the influence of reproductive history on longevity is statistically significant, it generally "is small compared to differences in longevity stemming from environmental factors such as level of education or family status" (Doblhammer 2000: 175; also see Hurt et al. 2006).

Recent evidence indicates that the fertility-health-nexus described above might vary across different *societal contexts* (e.g., Grundy 2009; Grundy and Foverskov 2016; Hank 2010). Along these lines, Grundy and Kravdal (2008) suggested that

---

[2]See Christiansen (2014) for an investigation of the association between *grand*parenthood and mortality.

'family friendly' policies—such as generous parental leave regulations (cf. Aitken et al. 2015; also see Guertzgen and Hank 2018)—may have resulted in long-term health benefits for parents.

Family Structure and Child Well-Being

In addition to child maltreatment (see Greenfield 2010; Oswald et al. 2010; Prosser and Corso 2007 for reviews), parental separation and divorce have been identified as major family-related threats to children's health or—more generally—well-being. Following Moore et al. (2014), four dimensions of child well-being may be distinguished: (a) *Physical well-being* refers to children's overall physical health. (b) *Psychological well-being* reflects how children think about themselves, their future, and how they manage their emotions and situational demands. Specific aspects of psychological well-being include internalizing and externalizing behavioral problems, prosocial behavior and depression, perception of stress, self-worth, perceived autonomy, and participation. (c) *Social well-being* is related to how comfortable children are with social relationships. Of foremost importance are parent-child relationships (involving both biological and step relations), especially positive communication and other elements of good relationship climate. It also includes, however, the quality of peer relations. (d) *Cognitive and educational well-being* encompasses children's learning abilities and their utilization of educational opportunities, which also bear a close association with (long-term) health outcomes. Increasingly, the focus has expanded from a deficit-oriented approach—involving, for example, deprivation, risk behaviors, and the absence of health—to positive quality of life outcomes from the child's perspective.

Empirical studies—primarily from the US—generally indicate that children with separated or divorced parents tend to score worse than children who live with both biological parents on measures of a range of behavioral, emotional, social, or cognitive outcomes (for overviews see Amato 2010; Jeynes 2006; Sweeney 2010) and the resulting inequalities have been shown to—potentially—last through adulthood (Kalmijn 2008, 2013; Klaus et al. 2012; Steinbach 2013). Because the majority of theoretical approaches employed to explain the differences in child well-being among nuclear, single-parent, and separated/divorced families rely at least in part upon concepts of stress, coping, risk and resilience, Amato (2000: 1271) suggested an integrating *'divorce-stress-adjustment perspective'*. From this perspective (which can easily be extended to include separation), the parents' divorce is not a singular event but rather a long-term developmental process that begins when the parents are still married and ends usually years after the legal act. In the underlying explanatory model of the divorce-stress-adjustment perspective, the divorce decree itself has minimal direct effects on children's well-being but the stressors und strains that accompany the divorce can indeed increase the likelihood of psychological, behavioral, and health problems for children. However, many factors moderate children's reactions and the speed of their adjustment to parental divorce.

The well-being of children with separated or divorced parents is at threat from *stressors* affecting parents and children (e.g., Amato 2010). Separated parents may experience stress from a decline of emotional support, increased frequency of conflict with the ex-partner or financial insecurity. Any number of other typical sources of parental stress can arise, such as multiple family transitions after the separation or divorce, a change of domicile, or a new job. For children, the decline of parental support and guidance, the reduction or the loss of contact with one parent, continuing conflicts between parents or economic decline can cause stress that undermines well-being. Other typical sources of post-separation stress also threaten children's well-being: a change of schools, a change of home, loss of friends, or the addition of a new stepparent.

Protective factors also influence separation and divorce outcomes. The action both of stressors and protective factors helps explain why children's reactions to separation and divorce are highly variable. Moreover, studies often use the selection perspective, which hypothesizes that some individuals carry traits that increase the likelihood that they will end up divorced or as single parents, to augment the divorce-stress-adjustment perspective (e.g., Amato 2000; Sweeney 2010). The well-being of children living in single-parent and stepfamilies is protected by factors that include available resources (individual, interpersonal, structural), the subjective meaning and normative connotation of separation and divorce as well as socio-demographic characteristics including the child's gender, the number of biological and stepsiblings, and the age of the child both at the time of parental separation and at the time when the stepfamily is established (e.g., Booth et al. 2010; Pryor 2008; Rodgers and Rose 2002; Turunen 2013). Other factors, for example a high degree of co-parenting among the adults involved or children's participation in decision making, can also serve to reduce post-separation stress and increase child well-being.

Finally, increasing attention has been paid to *residence and custody arrangements* among separated families and to the stressors and protective factors associated with them. In many cases, a separation or divorce leads to a significant reduction or loss of father-child contact (e.g., Smyth et al. 2004; Swiss and Le Bourdais 2009). This may reduce stress if it eliminates family conflict. Yet the loss of contact is also associated with a reduction of children's resources. Because paternal involvement in parenting has strongly increased overall during recent years (Williams 2008), fathers now more commonly maintain contact with their children after separation (Westphal et al. 2014). The number of working mothers who divide parenting responsibilities with the father, both before and after separation, has also increased. Together, these trends are leading to an increased number of post-separation, multi-household family structures, which bring about challenges of various kinds for all family members and are thus also likely to affect individuals' health and well-being.

Childhood Circumstances and Later Life Health

Next to the effects of family structure on child well-being described in the previous section, various aspects of individuals' childhood circumstances have been suggested to exhibit a lasting impact on adult health. On the one hand, adverse *macro-level* conditions during childhood, reflected by, for example, high infant mortality rates or economic recession seem to matter for later life health and mortality (e.g., Delaney et al. 2011; van den Berg et al. 2009). On the other hand, *micro-level* conditions closely related to the individual's family background—particularly early health and parental socio-economic status (SES)—have been shown to be important.[3]

These factors may affect later health directly or indirectly. On one hand, early nutritional deprivation, for example, might directly initiate negative health trajectories during the individual's childhood, which may persist or even aggravate during the ageing process, independent of adult SES ('latency model'; e.g., Huang et al. 2011; Zhang et al. 2008). On the other hand, poor health and economic deprivation in childhood might impact later life health indirectly through impaired adult socioeconomic attainment ('pathway model'; e.g., Case et al. 2005; Haas 2008).

Next to showing a consistently negative correlation between low early-life SES and self-rated health in adulthood, studies also revealed a significant relationship between *childhood SES* and older adults' risk of suffering from functional limitations (e.g., Haas 2008; Huang et al. 2011; Wen and Gu 2011), cognitive impairment (e.g., Wen and Gu 2011; Zhang et al. 2008), as well as chronic conditions and depressive symptoms (e.g., Luo and Waite 2005; Pavela and Latham 2016). Along the same lines, poor *childhood health* was shown to have long-term negative effects on, for example, individuals' functional status (e.g., Haas 2008; Huang et al. 2011) and chronic health conditions (e.g., Blackwell et al. 2001; Haas 2007). Despite being correlated with each other, early health and SES also appear to bear independent associations with adult health. Research by Case et al. (2005), for example, indicated that even if parents' income, education, and social class are controlled for, adults who suffered from poor childhood health exhibit significantly worse health outcomes than adults who did not experience poor health during their childhood (also see Blackwell et al. 2001; Haas 2007).

Intergenerational Family Relations and Health

Intergenerational family relations might impact individuals' health just as health might affect intergenerational relationships in the family. In the following, we consider both causal directions as well as different dimensions of 'intergenerational

[3]See Brandt et al. (2012) for a more comprehensive overview of the related literature and a joint empirical consideration of (contemporary) contextual and life-course (childhood) factors impacting later life health.

solidarity' (e.g., Bengtson and Roberts 1991) and well-being (physical and psychological health); also see Steinbach and Hank (2015).

The family social network constitutes, on the one hand, an important resource to protect individuals' health by, for example, reducing psychosocial stress and increasing one's overall well-being (e.g., Antonucci et al. 2007; Franks et al. 1992). Low relationship quality between parents and adult children (e.g., An and Cooney 2006; Koropeckyj-Cox 2002) or burdens associated with providing care to kin (e.g., Call et al. 1999; Sherwood et al. 2005), on the other hand, have been shown to result in health deterioration, especially if psychological well-being is considered. The individual's trust in the family network as a potential source of support and the emotional stability of family relations appear to be particularly important here. Some evidence suggests that the subjective perception of support might even be more relevant for individuals' health than the actual support one has (or has not) received (e.g., Antonucci 2001).

Whereas emotional closeness and relationship quality strongly influence the well-being of parents and adult children (e.g., Merz et al. 2009a, b), geographic proximity and frequency of contact appear to be unrelated to older parents' life satisfaction—at least if the exchange of instrumental support is controlled for (see Lowenstein et al. 2007). This latter finding underlines the importance of distinguishing between emotional support (including closeness and relationship quality) on the one hand, and instrumental support on the other hand. The former not only seems to be more beneficial for both generations in the family, but receipt of the latter may even reduce one's well-being (e.g., Merz and Consedine 2009; Merz et al. 2009b; also see Bordone 2015). This kind of adverse effect seems most likely in situations characterized by a strong imbalance in the exchange of intergenerational support (e.g., Lowenstein et al. 2007; Pillemer et al. 2007).

A large and growing number of empirical studies assess the impact of family relations on health beyond the parent-child-relationship, taking a three-generational perspective. Their results suggest a positive relationship between caring for one's grandchildren and a variety of physical and psychological health outcomes (Arpino and Bordone 2014; Di Gessa et al. 2016a, b; Hughes et al. 2007; Mahne and Huxhold 2015). Moreover, focusing on the role of the relationship to grandparents in the well-being of adolescent and young adult grandchildren, Ruiz and Silverstein (2007) showed that grandchildren benefit from a close relationship to their grandparents as well, especially if they are living in a non-traditional family context. This result is corroborated by a more general finding suggesting that grandparents are more likely to step in and provide help, if the middle generation's resources are limited, making grandparents support an all the more important resource for (grand-)children's health (e.g., Arránz Becker and Steinbach 2012; McIlvane et al. 2007).

Health, however, is not only affected by characteristics of intergenerational family relations, but is also a determinant of the latter. Good health may be an important resource to provide intergenerational support, whereas poor health might often trigger the need to establish an exchange of instrumental and/or financial support between generations in a family. It is therefore surprising that so far only relatively little empirical research has been conducted yet addressing this causal direction of the intergenerational relations and health nexus. Health outcomes are often merely treated as control variables in multivariate models, without much theoretical or thorough empirical consideration of possible underlying mechanisms. Longitudinal analyses in particular are missing—despite the obvious relevance of the question as to which extent changes in the individual's health status might affect various dimensions of intergenerational relationships.

Cross-sectional findings suggests that good (poor) health in both the parents' and the children's generation is positively (negatively) associated with reports of relationship quality (e.g., Rossi and Rossi 1990; Steinbach and Kopp 2010; Szydlik 2000). A longitudinal study by Merz et al. (2009a) supports the notion that the observed cross-sectional associations indeed reflect a causal effect of health on the intergenerational relationship. Stress has been put forward as a possible explanation for this: Health deterioration causes stress in parents and children, which eventually affects relationship quality in negative ways. Whereas changes in parents' health status appear to be unrelated to the frequency of contact with adult children (Ward et al. 2014), studies have found the expected changes in instrumental support: Those in poorer health—especially parents—are more likely to receive and less likely to provide help (e.g., Chan and Ermisch 2012; also see Ogg and Renaut 2013). Both parents and children are sensitive to the other generation's needs and variations across the life course (cf. Grundy 2005).

Conclusions and Future Directions

The evidence reviewed in the previous sections suggests that family matters greatly—and in various ways—for individuals' health across the entire life-course: from early childhood, through adulthood, to very old-age. Our review has also shown that the investigation of the multifaceted family-health-nexus is a flourishing field for empirical research in various social science disciplines (sociology, social epidemiology, demography, etc.). The increasing availability of high-quality international data sets providing detailed information on individuals' social (i.e. family) and health circumstances has spawned a plethora of studies beyond the US context. Even if many of the associations reported above appear to be fairly universal, it is still seems useful to corroborate these findings in a variety of societal settings. Europe—with its diversity of welfare, family, and other kinds of 'regimes'—has been fairly well-covered to date (except for many Eastern European countries) and our knowledge about the interrelationship between families and health in Asia (especially China) is also growing rapidly.

We conclude our review of the current state of the art with a (selective) outlook on what we consider to be some promising—and necessary—issues for future research:

- Partnership biographies and family structures have become increasingly complex. Empirical analyses should thus not only consider individuals' legal marital status and biological children, but they also need to account more generally for partnership or relationship status (e.g., Schneider et al. 2014) as well as for 'social' parenthood (e.g., Kravdal et al. 2012).
- Further investigations of biological risks (such as cardiovascular risk) and their associations with family circumstances (such as marital biography or marital quality; e.g., Liu and Waite 2014; McFarland et al. 2013) are likely to improve our understanding of the pathways to disease and disability.
- Although there is some evidence for spouses' concordance in health and well-being (see Walker and Luszcz 2009, for a review), relatively little attention has been paid so far to the various pathways through which other family members' health might be consequential for one's own health (e.g., Roth et al. 2015; Valle et al. 2013) or for other important outcomes, such as economic well-being (e.g., Heflin and Chiteji 2014).
- Last but not least, population aging draws our attention to the role of family ties in older people's health (e.g., Ryan and Willits 2007; Waite and Das 2010). This, however, should not ignore that the foundations for 'successful aging' are laid out very early in life and that family background (e.g. parental socio-economic status) is a crucial factor (e.g., Brandt et al. 2012; Schaan 2014).

References

Aitken, Z., Garrett, C. C., Hewitt, B., Keogh, L., Hocking, J. S., & Kavanagh, A. M. (2015). The maternal health outcomes of paid maternity leave: A systematic review. *Social Science and Medicine, 130,* 32–41.

Alonzo, A. A. (2002). Long-term health consequences of delayed childbirth: NHANES III. *Women's Health Issues, 12,* 37–45.

Amato, P. R. (2000). The consequences of divorce for adults and children. *Journal of Marriage and Family, 62,* 1269–1287.

Amato, P. R. (2010). Research on divorce: Continuing trends and new developments. *Journal of Marriage and Family, 72,* 650–666.

An, J. S., & Cooney, T. M. (2006). Psychological well-being in mid to late life: The role of generativity development and parent–child relationships across the lifespan. *International Journal of Behavioral Development, 30,* 410–421.

Antonucci, T. C. (2001). Social relations: An examination of social networks, social support and sense of control. In J. E. Birren & K. W. Schaie (Eds.), *Handbook of the psychology of aging* (5th ed., pp. 427–453). New York: Academic Press.

Antonucci, T. C., Jackson, J. S., & Biggs, S. (2007). Intergenerational relations: Theory, research, and policy. *Journal of Social Issues, 63,* 679–693.

Arránz Becker, O., Loter, K., & Becker, S. (2017). Familie und Gesundheit. Ein methodenkritischer Blick auf die aktuelle Forschung. In M. Jungbauer & P. Kriwy (Eds.), *Handbuch Gesundheitssoziologie* (pp. 1–27). Springer.

Arránz Becker, O., & Steinbach, A. (2012). Relations between grandparents and grandchildren in the context of the family system. *Comparative Population Studies—Zeitschrift für Bevölkerungswissenschaft, 37*, 543–566.

Arpino, B., & Bordone, V. (2014). Does grandparenting pay off? The effect of childcare on grandparents' cognitive functioning. *Journal of Marriage and Family, 76,* 337–351.

Bengtson, V. L., & Roberts, R. E. L. (1991). Intergenerational solidarity in aging families: An example of formal theory construction. *Journal of Marriage and the Family, 53,* 856–870.

Blackwell, D. L., Hayward, M. D., & Crimmins, E. M. (2001). Does childhood health affect chronic morbidity in later life? *Social Science and Medicine, 52,* 1269–1284.

Blomgren, J., Martikainen, P., Grundy, E., & Koskinen, S. (2012). Marital history 1971–1991 and mortality 1991–2004 in England & Wales and Finland. *Journal of Epidemiology and Community Health, 66,* 30–36.

Booth, A., Scott, M. E., & King, V. (2010). Father residence and adolescent problem behavior: Are youth always better off in two-parent families? *Journal of Family Issues, 31,* 585–605.

Bordone, V. (2015). Est modus in rebus: A longitudinal study of intergenerational solidarity and Locus of Control. *Ageing & Society, 35,* 1242–1277.

Brandt, M., Deindl, C., & Hank, K. (2012). Tracing the origins of successful aging: The role of childhood conditions and social inequality in later life health. *Social Science and Medicine, 74,* 1418–1425.

Brockmann, H., & Klein, T. (2004). Love and death in Germany: The marital biography and its effect on mortality. *Journal of Marriage and Family, 66,* 567–581.

Call, K. T., Finch, M. A., Huck, S. M., & Kane, R. A. (1999). Caregiver burden from a social exchange perspective: Caring for older people after hospital discharge. *Journal of Marriage and the Family, 61,* 688–699.

Carr, D., Springer, K. W., & Williams, K. (2014). Health and families. In J. Treas et al. (Eds.), *The Wiley Blackwell companion of to the sociology offamilies* (pp. 255–276). Hoboken, NJ: Wiley.

Case, A., Fertig, A., & Paxson, C. (2005). The lasting impact of childhood health and circumstance. *Journal of Health Economics, 24,* 365–389.

Chan, T. W., & Ermisch, J. (2012). Intergenerational exchange of instrumental support: Dynamic evidence from the British household panel survey. http://dosen.narotama.ac.id/wp-content/uploads/2012/03/Intergenerational-Exchange-of-Instrumental-Support-Dynamic-Evidence-from-the-British-Household-Panel-Survey.pdf.

Christiansen, S. G. (2014). The association between grandparenthood and mortality. *Social Science and Medicine, 118,* 89–96.

Deindl, C., Brandt, M., & Hank, K. (2016). Social networks, social cohesion, and later-life health. *Social Indicators Research, 126,* 1175–1187.

Delaney, L., McGovern, M., & Smith, J. P. (2011). From Angela's ashes to the Celtic Tiger: Early life conditions and adult health in Ireland. *Journal of Health Economics, 30,* 1–10.

Di Gessa, G., Glaser, K., & Tinker, A. (2016a). The impact of caring for grandchildren on the health of grandparents in Europe: A lifecourse approach. *Social Science and Medicine, 152,* 166–175.

Di Gessa, G., Glaser, K., & Tinker, A. (2016b). The health impact of intensive and nonintensive grandchild care in Europe: New evidence from SHARE. *Journal of Gerontology: Social Sciences, 71,* 867–879.

Dupre, M. E., & Meadows, S. O. (2007). Disaggregating the effects of marital trajectories on health. *Journal of Family Issues, 28,* 623–652.

Doblhammer, G. (2000). Reproductive history and mortality later in life: A comparative study of England and Wales and Austria. *Population Studies, 54,* 169–176.

Evenson, R. J., & Simon, R. W. (2005). Clarifying the relationship between parenthood and depression. *Journal of Health and Social Behavior, 46,* 341–358.

Fletcher, J. (2012). The effects of teenage childbearing on the short and long-term health behaviors of mothers. *Journal of Population Economics, 25,* 210–218.

Franks, P., Campbell, T. L., & Shields, C. G. (1992). Social relationships and health: The relative roles of family functioning and social support. *Social Science and Medicine, 34,* 779–788.

Greenfield, E. A. (2010). Child abuse as a life-course social determinant of adult health. *Maturitas, 66,* 51–55.

Grundy, E. (2005). Reciprocity in relationships: Socio-economic and health influences on intergenerational exchanges between third Age parents and their adult children in Great Britain. *The British Journal of Sociology, 56,* 233–255.

Grundy, E. (2009). Women's fertility and mortality in late mid-life: A comparison of three contemporary populations. *American Journal of Human Biology, 21,* 541–547.

Grundy, E., & Foverskov, E. (2016). Age at first birth and later life health in Western and Eastern Europe. *Population and Development Review, 42,* 245–269.

Grundy, E., & Kravdal, Ø. (2008). Reproductive history and mortality in late middle age among Norwegian men and women. *American Journal of Epidemiology, 167,* 271–279.

Grundy, E., & Kravdal, Ø. (2010). Fertility history and cause-specific mortality: A register-based analysis of complete cohorts of Norwegian women and men. *Social Science and Medicine, 70,* 1847–1857.

Grundy, E., & Read, S. (2015). Pathways from fertility history to later life health: Results from analyses of the english longitudinal study of ageing. *Demographic Research, 32,* 107–146.

Grundy, E., & Tomassini, C. (2005). Fertility history and health in later life: A record linkage study in England and Wales. *Social Science and Medicine, 61,* 217–228.

Grundy, E., van den Broek, T., & Keenan, K. (2017). Number of children, partnership status, and later-life depression in Eastern and Western Europe. *Journal of Gerontology: Social Sciences* [advance online access].

Guertzgen, N., & Hank, K. (2018). Maternity leave and mothers' long-term sickness absence—evidence from West Germany. *Demography* (forthcoming).

Haas, S. A. (2007). The long-term effects of poor childhood health: An assessment and application of retrospective reports. *Demography, 44,* 113–135.

Haas, S. A. (2008). Trajectories of functional health: The 'long arm' of childhood health and socioeconomic factors. *Social Science and Medicine, 66,* 849–861.

Hank, K. (2010). Childbearing history, later-life health, and mortality in Germany. *Population Studies, 64,* 275–291.

Hank, K., & Wagner, M. (2013). Parenthood, marital status, and well-being in later life: Evidence from SHARE. *Social Indicators Research, 114,* 639–653.

Hawkins, D. N., & Booth, A. (2005). Unhappily ever after: Effects of long-term, low-quality marriages on well-being. *Social Forces, 84,* 451–471.

Heflin, C. M., & Chiteji, N. (2014). My brother's keeper? The association between having siblings in poor health and wealth accumulation. *Journal of Family Issues, 35,* 358–383.

Henretta, J. C. (2007). Early childbearing, marital status, and women's health and mortality after age 50. *Journal of Health and Social Behavior, 48,* 154–266.

Henretta, J. C. (2010). Lifetime marital history and mortality after age 50. *Journal of Aging and Health, 22,* 1198–1212.

Henretta, J. C., Grundy, E., Okell, L. C., & Wadsworth, M. (2008). Early motherhood and mental health in midlife: A study of British and American cohorts. *Aging & Mental Health, 12,* 605–614.

Högnäs, R. S., Roelfs, D. J., Shor, E., Moore, C., & Reece, T. (2017). J-curve? A meta-analysis and meta-regression of parity and parental mortality. *Population Research and Policy Review, 36,* 273–308.

Huang, C., Soldo, B., & Elo, I. T. (2011). Do early-life conditions predict functional health status in adulthood? The case of Mexico. *Social Science and Medicine, 72,* 100–107.

Hughes, M. E., & Waite, L. J. (2009). Marital biography and health at mid-life. *Journal of Health and Social Behavior, 50,* 344–358.

Hughes, M. E., Waite, L. J., LaPierre, T. A., & Luo, Y. (2007). All in the family: The impact of caring for grandchildren on grandparents' health. *The Journals of Gerontology Series B: Psychological Sciences and Social Sciences, 62,* S108–S119.

Huijts, T., Kraaykamp, G., & Subramanian, S. V. (2013). Childlessness and psychological well-being in context: A multilevel study on 24 European countries. *European Sociological Review, 29,* 32–47.

Hurt, L. S., Ronsmans, C., & Thomas, S. L. (2006). The effect of number of births on women's mortality: Systematic review of the evidence for women who have completed their childbearing. *Population Studies, 60,* 55–71.

Jeynes, W. H. (2006). The impact of parental remarriage on children: A meta-analysis. *Marriage & Family Review, 40,* 75–98.

Kalmijn, M. (2008). The effects of separation and divorce on parent-child relationships in ten European countries. In C. Saraceno (Ed.), *Families, ageing and social policy. Intergenerational solidarity in European welfare states* (pp. 170–193). Cheltenham, Northampton, MA: Edward Elgar.

Kalmijn, M. (2013). Adult children's relationships with married parents, divorced parents, and stepparents: Biology, marriage, or residence? *Journal of Marriage and Family, 75,* 1181–1193.

Kalmijn, M. (2017). The ambiguous link between marriage and health: A dynamic reanalysis of loss and gain effects. *Social Forces* [advance online access].

Karraker, A., & Latham, K. (2015). In sickness and in health? Physical illness as a risk factor for marital dissolution in later life. *Journal of Health and Social Behavior, 56,* 420–435.

Kendig, H., Dykstra, P. A., van Gaalen, R. I., & Melkas, T. (2007). Health of aging parents and childless individuals. *Journal of Family Issues, 28,* 1457–1486.

Klaus, D., Nauck, B., & Steinbach, A. (2012). Relationships to stepfathers and biological fathers in adulthood: Complementary, substitutional, or neglected? *Advances in Life Course Research, 17,* 156–167.

Koball, H. L., Moiduddin, E., Henderson, J., Goesling, B., & Besculides, M. (2010). What do we know about the link between marriage and health? *Journal of Family Issues, 31,* 1019–1040.

Koropeckyj-Cox, T. (2002). Beyond parental status: Psychological well-being in middle and old age. *Journal of Marriage and Family, 64,* 957–971.

Koropeckyj-Cox, T., Pienta, A. M., & Brown, T. H. (2007). Women of the 1950s and the 'normative' life course: The implications of childlessness, fertility timing, and marital status for psychological well-being in late midlife. *International Journal of Aging and Human Development, 64,* 299–330.

Kravdal, Ø., Grundy, E., Lyngstad, T. H., & Wiik, K. A. (2012). Family life history and late mid-life mortality in Norway. *Population and Development Review, 38,* 237–257.

Kruk, E., & Reinhold, S. (2014). The effect of children on depression in old age. *Social Science and Medicine, 100,* 1–11.

Kuh, D., Ben-Shlomo, Y., Lynch, J., Hallqvist, J., & Power, C. (2003). Life course epidemiology. *Journal of Epidemiology and Community Health, 57,* 778–783.

Liu, H., & Waite, L. (2014). Bad marriage, broken heart? Age and gender differences in the link between marital quality and cardiovascular risks among older adults. *Journal of Health and Social Behavior, 55,* 403–423.

Lorenz, F. O., Wickrama, K. A. S., Conger, R. D., & Elder, G. H., Jr. (2006). The short-term and decade-long effects of divorce on women's midlife health. *Journal of Health and Social Behavior, 47,* 111–125.

Lowenstein, A., Katz, R., & Gur-Yaish, N. (2007). Reciprocity in parent–child exchange and life satisfaction among the elderly: A cross-national perspective. *Journal of Social Issues, 63,* 865–883.

Luo, Y., & Waite, L. J. (2005). The impact of childhood and adult SES on physical, mental, and cognitive well-being in later-life. *Journal of Gerontology: Social Sciences, 60B,* S93–S101.

Mahne, K., & Huxhold, O. (2015). Grandparenthood and subjective well-being: Moderating effects of educational level. *Journal of Gerontology: Social Sciences, 70,* 782–792.

McFarland, M. J., Hayward, M. D., & Brown, D. (2013). I've got you under my skin: Marital biography and biological risk. *Journal of Marriage and Family, 75,* 363–380.

McIlvane, J. M., Ajrouch, K. J., & Antonucci, T. C. (2007). Generational structure and social resources in mid-life: Influences on health and well-being. *Journal of Social Issues, 63,* 759–773.

Merz, E.-M., & Consedine, N. S. (2009). The association of family support and wellbeing in later life depends on adult attachment style. *Attachment & Human Development, 11,* 203–221.

Merz, E.-M., Schuengel, C., & Schulze, H.-J. (2009a). Intergenerational relations across 4 years: Well-being is affected by quality, not by support exchange. *The Gerontologist, 49,* 536–548.

Merz, E.-M., Consedine, N. S., Schulze, H.-J., & Schuengel, C. (2009b). Wellbeing of adult children and ageing parents: Associations with intergenerational support and relationship quality. *Ageing & Society, 29,* 783–802.

Mirowsky, J. (2005). Age at first birth, health, and mortality. *Journal of Health and Social Behavior, 46,* 32–50.

Mirowsky, J., & Ross, C. E. (2002). Depression, parenthood, and age at first birth. *Social Science and Medicine, 54,* 1281–1298.

Moonden, C. W. S., & Uunk, W. J. G. (2013). For better and for worse: The relationship between union dissolution and self-assessed health in European panel data. *European Journal of Population, 29,* 103–125.

Moore, K. A., Murphey, D., Bandy, T., & Lawner, E. (2014). Indices of child well-being and developmental contexts. In A. Ben-Arieh, F. Casas, I. Frønes, & J. E. Korbin (Eds.), *Handbook of child well-being. Theories, methods and policies in global perspective* (pp. 2807–2822). Dordrecht: Springer.

Newton, N. J., Ryan, L. H., King, R. T., & Smith, J. (2014). Cohort differences in the marriage-health relationship for midlife women. *Social Science and Medicine, 116,* 64–72.

O'Flaherty, M., Baxter, J., Haynes, M., & Turrell, G. (2016). The family life course and health: Partnership, fertility histories, and later-life physical health trajectories in Australia. *Demography, 53,* 777–804.

Ogg, J., & Renaut, S. (2013). Ageing and intergenerational support: The role of life course events. In A. Börsch-Supan, M. Brandt, H. Litwin, & G. Weber (Eds.), *Active aging and solidarity between generations in Europe* (pp. 379–389). Berlin, Boston: de Gruyter.

Oswald, S. H., Heil, K., & Goldbeck, L. (2010). History of maltreatment and mental health problems in foster children: A review of the literature. *Journal of Pediatric Psychology, 35,* 462–472.

Pavela, G., & Latham, K. (2016). Childhood conditions and multimorbidity among older adults. *Journal of Gerontology: Social Sciences, 71,* 889–901.

Perales, F., del Pozo-Cruz, J., & del Pozo-Cruz, B. (2015). Long-term dynamics in physical activity behavior across the transition to parenthood. *International Journal of Public Health, 60,* 301–308.

Pillemer, K., Suitor, J. J., Mock, S. E., Sabir, M., Pardo, T. B., & Sechrist, J. (2007). Capturing the complexity of intergenerational relations: Exploring ambivalence within later-life families. *Journal of Social Issues, 63,* 775–791.

Pryor, J. (2008). Children in stepfamilies: Relationships with nonresident parents. In J. Pryor (Ed.), *The international handbook of stepfamilies. Policy and practice in legal, research, and clinical environments* (pp. 345–368). Hoboken, NJ: Wiley.

Prosser, L. A., & Corso, P. S. (2007). Measuring health-related quality of life for child maltreatment: A systematic literature review. *Health and Quality of Life Outcomes, 5* (42).

Rapp, I., & Klein, T. (2015). Familie und Gesundheit. In P. Hill & J. Kopp (Eds.), *Handbuch Familiensoziologie* (pp. 775–790). Wiesbaden: Springer VS.

Rendall, M. S., Weden, M. M., Favreault, M. M., & Waldron, H. (2011). The protective effect of marriage for survival: A review and update. *Demography, 48,* 481–506.

Rodgers, K. B., & Rose, H. A. (2002). Risk and resiliency factors among adolescents who experience marital transitions. *Journal of Marriage and Family, 64,* 1024–1037.

Rossi, A. S., & Rossi, P. H. (1990). *Of human bounding. Parent-child relations across the life course.* New York: Aldine de Gruyter.

Roth, D. L., Fredman, L., & Haley, W. E. (2015). Informal caregiving and its impact on health: A reappraisal from population-based studies. *The Gerontologist, 55,* 309–319.

Ruiz, S. A., & Silverstein, M. (2007). Relationships with grandparents and the emotional well-being of late adolescent and young adult grandchildren. *Journal of Social Issues, 63,* 793–808.

Ryan, A. K., & Willits, F. K. (2007). Family ties, physical health, and psychological well-being. *Journal of Aging and Health, 19,* 907–920.

Sasson, I., & Umberson, D. J. (2014). Widowhood and depression: New light on gender differences, selection, and psychological adjustment. *Journal of Gerontology: Social Sciences, 69,* 135–145.

Schaan, B. (2013). Widowhood and depression among older Europeans—The role of gender, caregiving, marital quality, and regional context. *Journal of Gerontology: Social Sciences, 68,* 431–442.

Schaan, B. (2014). The interaction of family background and personal education on depressive symptoms in later life. *Social Science and Medicine, 102,* 94–102.

Schneider, B., Rapp, I., Klein, T., & Eckhardt, J. (2014). Relationship status and health: Does the use of different relationship indicators matter? *Global Public Health, 9,* 528–537.

Sherwood, P. R., Given, C. W., Given, B. A., & Von Eye, A. (2005). Caregiver burden and depressive symptoms analysis of common outcomes in caregivers of elderly patients. *Journal of Aging and Health, 17,* 125–147.

Shor, E., Roelfs, D. J., Bugyi, P., & Schwartz, J. E. (2012a). Meta-analysis of marital dissolution and mortality: Reevaluating the intersection of gender and age. *Social Science and Medicine, 75,* 46–59.

Shor, E., Roelfs, D. J., Curelli, M., Clemow, L., Burg, M. M., & Schwartz, J. E. (2012b). Widowhood and mortality: A meta-analysis and meta-regression. *Demography, 49,* 575–606.

Smyth, B., Caruana, C., & Ferro, A. (2004). Father-child contact after separation. Profiling five different patterns of care. *Family Matters, 67,* 20–27.

Steinbach, A. (2013). Family structure and parent-child contact: A comparison of native and migrant families. *Journal of Marriage and Family, 75,* 1114–1129.

Steinbach, A., & Hank, K. (2015). Familiale Generationenbeziehungen aus bevölkerungssoziologischer Perspektive. In Y. Niephaus, M. Kreyenfeld, & R. Sackmann (Eds.), *Handbuch Bevölkerungssoziologie* (pp. 367–392). Wiesbaden: Springer VS.

Steinbach, A., & Kopp, J. (2010). Determinanten der Beziehungszufriedenheit: Die Sicht erwachsener Kinder auf die Beziehungen zu ihren Eltern. In A. Ette, K. Ruckdeschel, & R. Unger (Eds.), *Potenziale intergenerationaler Beziehungen. Chancen und Herausforderungen für die Gestaltung des demografischen Wandels* (pp. 95–116). Würzburg: Ergon.

Sudha, S., Mutran, E. J., Williams, I. C., & Suchindran, C. (2006). Childbearing history and self-reported well-being in later life. *Research on Aging, 28,* 599–621.

Sweeney, M. M. (2010). Remarrige and stepfamilies: Strategic sites for family scholarship in the 21st century. *Journal of Marriage and Family, 72,* 667–684.

Swiss, L., & Le Bourdais, C. (2009). Father-child contact after separation: The influence of living arrangements. *Journal of Family Issues, 50,* 623–652.

Szydlik, M. (2000). *Lebenslange Solidarität? Generationenbeziehungen zwischen erwachsenen Kindern und Eltern.* Opladen: Leske + Budrich.

Turunen, J. (2013). Family structure, gender, and adolescent emotional well-being. *Journal of Divorce and Remarriage, 54,* 476–504.

Umberson, D., Williams, K., Powers, D. A., Liu, H., & Needham, B. (2006). You make me sick: Marital quality and health over the life course. *Journal of Health and Social Behavior, 47,* 1–16.

Valle, G., Weeks, J. A., Taylor, M. G., & Eberstein, I. W. (2013). Mental and physical health consequences of spousal health shocks among older adults. *Journal of Aging and Health, 25,* 1121–1142.

van den Berg, G. J., Lindeboom, M., & Lopez, M. (2009). Inequality in individual mortality and economic conditions earlier in life. *Social Science and Medicine, 69,* 1360–1367.

Waite, L., & Das, A. (2010). Families, social life, and well-being at older ages. *Demography, 47,* S87–S109.

Walker, R. B., & Luszcz, M. A. (2009). The health and relationship dynamics of late-life couples: A systematic review of the literature. *Ageing & Society, 29,* 455–480.

Ward, R., Deane, G., & Spitze, G. (2014). Life-course changes and parent–adult child contact. *Research on Aging, 36,* 568–602.

Wen, M., & Gu, D. (2011). The effects of childhood, adult, and community socioeconomic conditions on health and mortality among older adults in China. *Demography, 48,* 153–181.

Westphal, S. K., Poortman, A.-R., & Van der Lippe, T. (2014). Non-resident father–child contact across divorce cohorts: The role of father involvement during marriage. *European Sociological Review, 30,* 444–456.

Williams, S. (2008). What is fatherhood? Searching for the reflexive father. *Sociology, 42,* 487–502.

Xu, M., Thomas, P. A., & Umberson, D. (2016). Marital quality and cognitive limitations in late life. *Journal of Gerontology: Social Sciences, 71,* 165–176.

Zhang, Z., Gu, D., & Hayward, M. D. (2008). Early life influences on cognitive impairment among oldest old Chinese. *Journal of Gerontology: Social Sciences, 63B,* S25–S33.

Zheng, H., & Thomas, P. A. (2013). Marital status, self-rated health, and mortality: Overestimation of health or diminishing protection of marriage? *Journal of Health and Social Behavior, 54,* 128–143.

The New Roles of Men and Women and Implications for Families and Societies

Livia Sz. Oláh, Irena E. Kotowska and Rudolf Richter

Introduction

The major trends in family structures and their shifts across the industrialized world over the past decades are well known: fertility rates have declined below the level sufficient for the replacement of the population and childbearing occurs later and more often outside marriage. Marriage, too, is being postponed and is more often foregone, and couple relationships—both marital and non-marital ones—have become more fragile. These changes have led to increasingly complex family compositions and to a previously unprecedented diversity of family forms and relationships over the life course. The new family trends and patterns have been paralleled by changes in gender roles, especially an expansion of the female role to an economic provider for a family, and lately also transformation of men's role with more extensive involvement in family responsibilities, mainly care for children. In contemporary family scholarship there is an increasing awareness of gender and family changes being interconnected, and conceptualization of the gender revolution has gained terrain (Goldscheider 1990; Puur et al. 2008; Esping-Andersen 2009; England 2010). Developments related to women's new role are seen as weakening the family and have been attributed to the first phase of the gender

L. Sz.Oláh (✉)
Department of Sociology, Stockholm University, Stockholm, Sweden
e-mail: livia.olah@sociology.su.se

I. E. Kotowska
Institute of Statistics and Demography, Warsaw School of Economics, Warsaw, Poland
e-mail: iekoto@sgh.waw.pl

R. Richter
Department of Sociology, University of Vienna, Vienna, Austria
e-mail: rudolf.richter@univie.ac.at

G. Doblhammer and J. Gumà (eds.), *A Demographic Perspective on Gender, Family and Health in Europe*, https://doi.org/10.1007/978-3-319-72356-3_4

revolution, while more recent family changes and the emerging caring male role have been linked to the second phase (Goldscheider et al. 2015).

To understand the everyday realities of modern societies we need to recognize that the family is a dynamic entity, characterized by growing complexity with respect to decision-making processes regarding transitions over the family life course and organization of family life. Indeed, the family can no longer be described simply as a set of well-defined roles; it is negotiated on a daily basis, constructed by interactions between partners at the micro-level (Morgan 2011), and influenced by macro structures of the political and economic spheres. Work and family lives are increasingly influencing each other as both women and men engage in earning as well as caring activities, often reinforced by the labour market developments with specific skill demands, together with increasing employment instability and precariousness. Gender relations and related values and attitudes have become more fluid, changing dynamically over the life course in the context of blurring boundaries of family and work life. Also, different policy contexts affect new constructions of gender in doing family in various ways, impeding convergence to a singular pattern of family life courses across countries.

In this chapter we seek to shed more light on these complex developments in the European context. First we present the changes in family patterns over the past fifty years, before addressing the transition of gender roles and views on their interplay with the demographic developments. Next, we discuss new challenges related to transitions in and organizations of contemporary family life based on an overview of theoretical as well as empirical advances of research. A brief conclusion ends this chapter.

Increasingly Diverse Family Biographies

Family patterns in Europe have undergone extensive changes in the past half century. The early to mid-1960s marked the end of the "Golden Age of the Family" (Skolnick 1978; Sobotka 2011), with high marriage and birth rates at relatively young ages, few divorces, and a low prevalence of non-traditional family forms. By the late 20th century, fertility rates had declined well below the replacement level of 2.1 children per woman on average, while marriage and parenthood had been delayed to more mature ages, new forms of couple relationships emerged while the propensity to marry decreased, and family dissolution became quite frequent even among couples with children (Frejka et al. 2008). People are increasingly refraining from long-term commitments in respect of partnership formation and childbearing, which indicates a de-standardization of the family life course (Bruckner and Mayer 2005; Elzinga and Liefbroer 2007), but in the long run may lead to a re-standardization of family patterns (Huinink 2013). In any case, there is a considerable diversity in the extent of and the pace at which these new patterns emerged across Europe (Neyer 2013).

Acknowledging the importance of the social context for family dynamics as suggested in the literature (see e.g. Frejka et al. 2008; OECD 2011), we display the trends by welfare regime/policy configuration types (Esping-Andersen 1990; Korpi 2000), highlighting the details of changes in family patterns. We distinguish among the Dual-Earner policy configuration type or Social Democratic welfare regime with extensive policy provisions facilitating a work-life balance for both women and men; the Liberal or Market-Oriented regime with limited and usually means-tested state support to families and the dominance of market-based solutions regarding welfare provision; the General Family Support policy configuration type or Conservative welfare regime in which men's primacy in the labour market has not really been questioned while the range of state support to families and to women to combine paid work and family responsibilities varies greatly across countries; the Familialistic or Mediterranean welfare regime with nearly no or extremely limited policy provisions to families and pronounced gender role differentiation; and the Transition Post-Socialist cluster which represents a hybrid model and is also rather heterogeneous in terms of state support to families and to women to combine labour market participation and family life (Hobson and Oláh 2006; Saraceno 2008; Cerami and Vanhuysse 2009; Neyer 2013).

The de-standardization of the family life course in Europe that has led to increasingly diverse family biographies started with the decline in childbearing (Van de Kaa 1987; Lesthaeghe 2010). As shown in Fig. 1, the baby boom of the 1950s-early 1960s was followed by a dramatic decrease of period fertility rates, below the level necessary for the simple reproduction of a population. This occurred first in the Dual-Earner and the General Family Support clusters, in the early 1970s. Countries of the Familialistic regime entered the low fertility path in the early 1980s, followed by the Liberal regime and the Transition Post-Socialist cluster in the same decade. Fertility rates continued to decline in all but the Dual-Earner and the Liberal regimes to and even below the so-called critical level of low fertility, i.e., 1.5 children per woman on average, known to accelerate population ageing if sustained for a longer period (McDonald 2006). The German-speaking countries in the General Family Support policy configuration type also have shown very low levels of childbearing, though more or less counterbalanced by reasonably high fertility rates in other countries of that cluster. In the first years of the 21st century, the trends turned slightly upwards, generating hopes for a fertility recovery, but the increase has stopped and/or reversed in recent years, with childbearing at or somewhat below the critical level in the majority of European countries.

Period rates are, however, not seen as an optimal measure of fertility, as they are highly influenced by variations in timing and spacing of births (Sobotka and Lutz 2010); cohort fertility or completed family size is considered to be more reliable. As seen in Fig. 2, cohort fertility varies across countries as well as over female birth cohorts, that is, women born in the mid-1930s, 1940s, 1950s, 1960s and 1970s (the latter based on predicted cohort fertility). In all countries we find higher fertility levels for the older cohorts, in line with the decline seen for period fertility rates. Focusing on women born in the second half of the 20th century, the picture is more diverse. For the mid-1960 and -70 cohorts, fertility did not decline for countries of

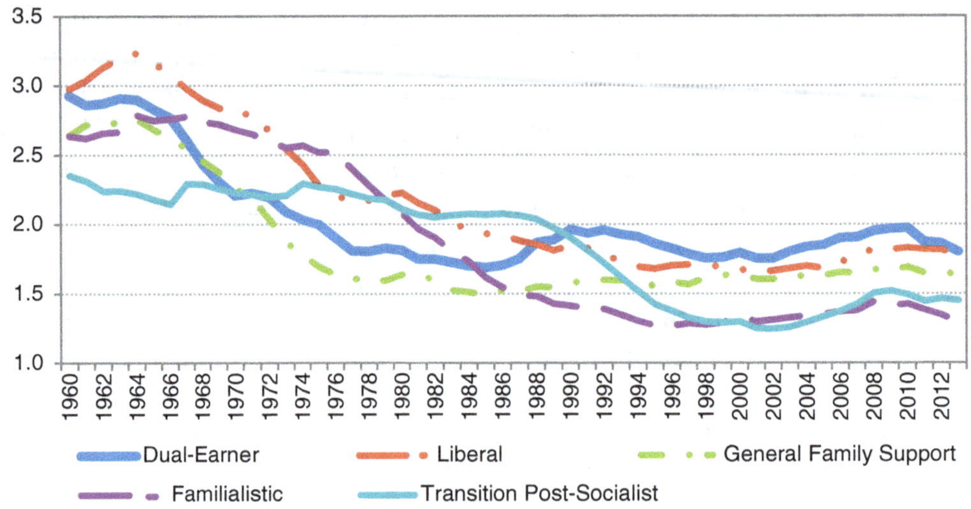

Fig. 1 Period total fertility rates (average number of children per woman) in different welfare regimes/policy configuration types, 1960–2013.
Source INED (2013) for the years 1960–2008; Eurostat (2015) for the years 2009–2013.
Note Means for each group. Countries are grouped as follows: Dual-Earner: Denmark, Finland, Iceland, Norway, and Sweden; Liberal: United Kingdom, Ireland, and Switzerland; General Family Support: Austria, Belgium, France, Germany [for the years 1960–1989 West Germany only], Luxembourg, and the Netherlands; Familialistic: Greece, Italy, Portugal, and Spain; Transition Post-Socialist: Bulgaria, Czech Republic, Estonia, East-Germany (1960–1989); Hungary, Latvia, Lithuania, Poland, Romania, Slovakia, and Slovenia

the Dual-Earner cluster, nor for France, Belgium, or the UK, where even the youngest cohorts display fertility levels of about two children per woman on average, unlike in other countries and clusters. In contrast, we see completed family sizes at or slightly above 1.5 for the 1965 and 1975 cohorts for Switzerland and the German-speaking countries, and for the 1975 cohort for the Familialistic cluster, along with Bulgaria, Poland, and Romania, and only somewhat higher levels for other countries in the Transition Post-Socialist cluster. Taken together, Figs. 1 and 2 thus indicate that the European policy agenda should continue to be concerned about demographic sustainability given these low fertility levels (see also Oláh and Fahlén 2013, for a more detailed discussion).

The decline of period fertility rates has been accompanied by the ageing of fertility, that is, a rising mean age at first birth (Frejka et al. 2008). In the 1960s and 1970s, women in Europe had their first child in their early to mid-twenties, with the youngest first-time mothers in the Transition Post-Socialist cluster and the oldest ones in the Familialistic cluster. The postponement of first births started during the 1980s in all but the Transition Post-Socialist policy configuration type, where such a trend first emerged in the early/mid-1990s. In the beginning of the 21st century, motherhood is entered at around age thirty in Liberal regime countries and at the late twenties in other clusters. Ages of first fatherhood are a few years above that of first motherhood, because men start their family careers later than women. In any case, as Figs. 1 and 2 suggest, early entry into parenthood, as in the Transition

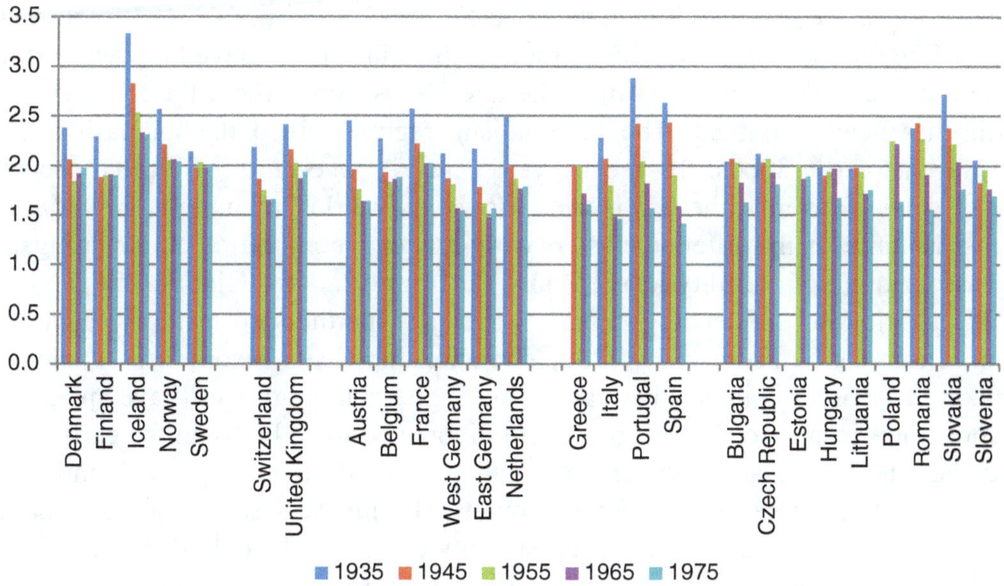

Fig. 2 Total completed cohort fertility (average number of children per woman) of selected birth cohorts.
Source INED (2013) for cohorts: 1935–1965; Myrskylä et al. (2013) for cohort 1975.
Note For Belgium the cohort 1960 is displayed instead of 1965, for Lithuania the cohort 1940 is displayed instead of 1935; for Poland the cohorts 1950 and 1960 are displayed instead of 1955 and 1965

Post-Socialist cluster, is not necessarily accompanied by high fertility levels, whereas a late start of childbearing may not be a hindrance for achieving reasonably high fertility rates, the latter seen in the Dual-Earner and the Liberal regimes.

When discussing changes in fertility behavior, an important dimension to be addressed is the upsurge of extramarital childbearing in connection with new partnership patterns. Indeed, marriage had nearly ceased to be the dominant form of couple relationships in the Dual-Earner, the General Family Support, and the Liberal clusters by the late 1970s, as non-marital cohabitation has become increasingly prevalent. The Familialistic regime joined the trend in the early 1980s, and the Transition Post-Socialist cluster followed from the early 1990s. In these latter groups, the decline in marriage rates was suggested to be strongly related to growing economic uncertainty and housing shortages (Sardon 1993; Philipov and Dorbritz 2003).

Independent of the cause, marriage formation has been increasingly postponed from the early-/mid-1980s in most regime types, and since the mid-1990s even in the Transition Post-Socialist cluster (Frejka et al. 2008). By the early 21st century, first marriage is entered around age thirty by women, but somewhat earlier in the Post-Socialist cluster. In fact, the mean age at first marriage has been above that of first parenthood in the past decades in the Dual-Earner policy configuration type as couples entered marriage after the birth of their first or second child. A similar pattern has also emerged lately in the Liberal and the General Family Support clusters.

As the propensity to marry declined, births have increasingly occurred in consensual relationships. In the early 1960s, when marriage rates were still high, the proportion of out-of-wedlock births was around 10% or less in European countries.

This share has increased rapidly in the Dual-Earner cluster since the 1970s, currently accounting for about half of all births there. Other clusters displayed moderate levels of non-marital childbearing up until the late 1980s. Since then, the share of such births has nearly doubled. The Familialistic regime joined the increasing trend during the early 2000s. In recent years, nearly one-third of births occurred out-of-wedlock even in these countries. However, we do find quite large variations across countries in the different clusters with respect to non-marital childbearing, and the association with fertility levels is also far from clear-cut (Oláh 2015).

In addition to influencing fertility, the new partnership patterns have had implications for family stability. Couple relationships have become less stable over time as consensual unions, which are more fragile than marriages, have spread and divorce rates increased. The propensity to divorce doubled between the early 1960s and the late 1990s, and divorce rates remained modest only in the Familialistic regime cluster, where it has increased mainly during the last decade (Spijker and Solsona 2012). Declining relationship stability can also affect childbearing. On the one hand, it can reduce fertility as the time people spend in couple relationships shortens, and as women and men may choose to have fewer children because of the prospect of either having to raise their children alone or not being able to be involved with the children because of separation or divorce (Lillard and Waite 1993). On the other hand, high rates of family dissolution can raise fertility rates as second and higher-order partnerships are increasingly formed during the reproductive ages, and couples may opt for joint offspring even if they already have children from previous relationships (Thomson 2004). In any case, the high and/or rising instability of partnerships contributes to the increasing diversity of family biographies in Europe.

Changing Gender Roles

The changes in family patterns outlined in the previous section, especially the decline of fertility rates to (far) below the replacement level, have been paralleled by a substantial increase in female labour force participation over time (Bernhardt 1993; OECD 2012). In Central-East European countries (i.e. the Transition Post-Socialist cluster), high female and maternal employment levels were common in the state-socialist period. In Western Europe, the upsurge of female economic activity and mothers' employment occurred first in the Nordic countries (i.e. the Dual-Earner cluster), where the new family patterns emerged first. These countries were also the first to experience a change in women's employment aspirations resulting in the new female work pattern, according to which women do not withdraw from the labour market upon marriage or motherhood, but remain employed until reaching retirement age (Gornick and Meyers 2003; Oláh and Fahlén 2013). Countries of the Liberal and the General Family Support clusters joined the trend during the late 1980s, followed by the Familialistic cluster in the mid-/late 1990s. Anomalously, the end of the state-socialist era brought a substantial decline in female labour force participation in the Transition Post-Socialist cluster imposed by the economic restructuring, followed by some increase in female economic activity as the countries' economic performance gradually improved. Nevertheless, cuts in family policy provisions, especially regarding childcare for the very youngest (i.e. children below age three), along with rigid labour market structures increased the difficulties with respect to work-family reconciliation (Matysiak 2011).

In any case, by the early 21st century gender differences in labour force participation in Europe had greatly diminished (see Fig. 3). The gender gap is rather small in the Dual-Earner cluster and has been quite limited in the Transition Post-Socialist regimes, even though there are lower activity rates for both men and women. More recently, the gender gap has also diminished greatly in the Liberal and the General Family Support regimes. The Familialistic cluster has been characterized by the largest activity gap, as gender role differentiation has been most pronounced there and traditional gender norms have had a strong hold (Lewis 2006; Plantenga et al. 2009). Women's increasing economic activities have also boosted their engagement in higher education (Blossfeld 1995). By the mid-1990s, female educational attainment surpassed that of men in the main childbearing ages in all regime clusters, and it reached the same level as men in the broader working age population (Oláh 2015). The new female educational advantage has been most

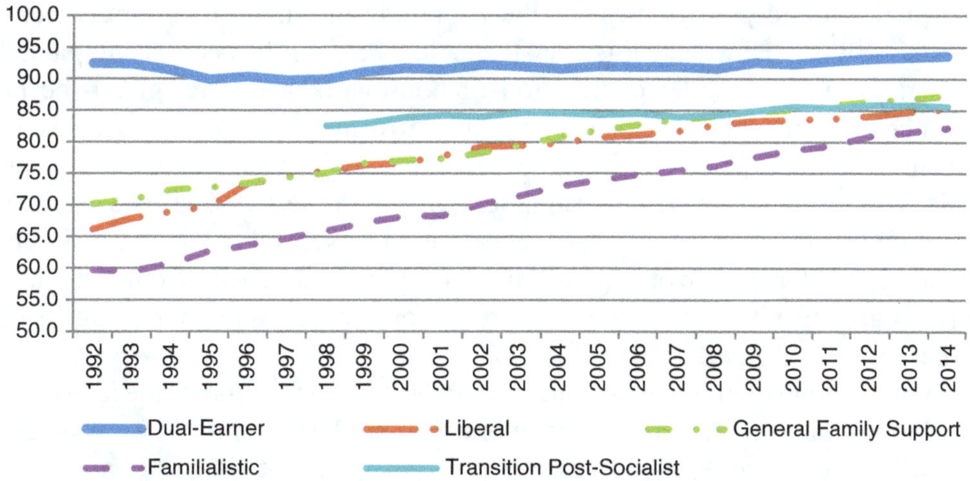

Fig. 3 Gender differences in labour market activity [women's activity rate in proportion of men's rate; ages 20–64] in different welfare regimes/policy configuration types, 1992–2014.
Source Eurostat (2016).
Note Means for each group. Countries are grouped as follows (years for missing data listed in brackets): Dual-Earner: Denmark, Finland, Iceland (1992–2002), Norway (1992–1999), and Sweden; Liberal: United Kingdom, Ireland, and Switzerland (1992–1995); General Family Support: Austria (1992–1993), Belgium, France, Germany, Luxembourg, and the Netherlands; Familialistic: Greece, Italy (1992), Portugal, and Spain; Transition Post-Socialist: Bulgaria (1992–1998), Czech Republic (1992–1997), Estonia (1992–1997), Hungary (1992–1995), Latvia (1992–1997), Lithuania (1992–1997), Poland (1992–1996), Romania (1992–1996), Slovakia (1992–1997), and Slovenia (1992–1995)

pronounced for the Familialistic cluster, despite female employment rates being lowest there.

The substantially reduced gender employment gap notwithstanding, women earn on average 16% less than men, and this difference is even larger among top earners, about 21% (OECD 2012). The female wage disadvantage is strongly related to their weaker position in the labour market, as women have continued to bear a disproportionately large share of family responsibilities despite their growing involvement in paid work. Hence, part-time work is much more common among women than men and is increasingly used. Currently, about 45% of employed women work part-time in the Liberal and the General Family Support clusters, and one-third in the Dual-Earner cluster, compared to 20 and 10% in the Familialistic regime and the Transition Post-Socialist countries, respectively (Oláh 2015), given more rigid labour market structures in the latter clusters. The share of male part-time work varies between 5 and 15% across regime types.

Gender differences are more modest for unemployment levels, which vary between 5 and 20%, with the highest rates displayed in the Familialistic and the Transition Post-Socialist clusters where economic problems have been pronounced since long before the recent economic crisis. Youth unemployment levels have been much higher though, which can hamper family building, especially among the less educated, men and women alike (Mills et al. 2005; Oláh and Fratczak 2013).

Taken together the trends suggest that the new female gender role has increasingly incorporated dimensions of economic independence and support responsibilities that until quite recently belonged to the male domain, and has promoted a redistribution of responsibilities for the economic provision to a family between men and women. However, this transformation has hardly been accompanied by new patterns in the gender distribution of housework and care, given the rather limited changes in sharing unpaid work among women and men in most countries (Bianchi et al. 2000; Anxo et al. 2011). Much of the decrease in the gender gap for unpaid work is due to women investing less time in domestic duties because of their greater involvement in paid work, than due to a substantial increase in men's household- and/or care work contribution (Sayer et al. 2004; Craig and Mullan 2011). It has resulted in a double burden for women and increasing tensions between work and family life.

Among younger cohorts, more and more fathers seem to embrace the idea of active parenting (Seward et al. 2006; Hobson and Fahlén 2009; Smith Koslowski 2011). Their efforts have received increasing policy support at both the national and European levels (Hobson 2002; Moss 2014). However, the company level, especially employers' and co-workers' attitude towards active fathers, is likely to be of particular importance for the transformation of the male gender role (Brandt and Kvande 2002; Haas and Hwang 2009; Behnke and Meuser 2012). Moreover, mothers need to accept fathers as their equals when it comes to parental care for children in order for the new male role to become established (Allen and Hawkins 1999). Until men's contribution to domestic tasks and care work can match that of women in paid work, the gender revolution will remain incomplete (Esping-Andersen 2009; Goldscheider et al. 2010).

Making Sense of the Interplay Between Family Complexity and Gender Role Changes

Contemporary scholarship of economics, demography, sociology, and gender studies has recognized for a long time that new family patterns and evolving gender roles are interlinked. Given declining fertility and nuptiality, increasing instability of couple relationships and a nearly simultaneous growth of female labour force participation, women's increasing economic independence has been seen as a main cause of family changes in economic theorizing, which identifies gender role specialization as one of its main paradigms (see Becker 1991). Labour market developments in the 1980s and 1990s, especially rising educational demands and greater flexibility along with higher levels of job uncertainty, made this paradigm increasingly contested. An influential argument, presented by Oppenheimer (1994, 1997), pointed out the benefits of collaboration among spouses/partners with respect to economic contributions to the family, as by pooling resources couples can better adapt to new challenges in the labour market. As women's educational attainment approaches that of men, they are also better prepared to share with their male partner the responsibilities of providing for the family (Blossfeld 1995; Blossfeld and Drobnic 2001).

In sociology in contrast, it has been argued that ideational changes, such as the spread of individualism and thus the greater emphasis on self-realization, together with changing aspirations for paid work, are the main driving forces behind the postponement of family formation (both marriage and childbearing) and the increasing fragility of couple relationships in modern societies (Bengtson et al. 2005; Steel et al. 2012). In this respect, the Second Demographic Transition (SDT) theory is of particular importance (Van de Kaa 1994; Lesthaeghe 2010). According to the SDT theory, the weakening of normative constraints in advanced societies in combination with access to effective contraception led to fundamental changes in sexual relations, loosening the links between marriage and childbearing. This in turn resulted in delayed marriage and births, rising childlessness, non-marital cohabitation, and partnership instability. Critics pointed out that even though the SDT conceptual framework included structural components of market economy and improving living conditions, labour market developments and the related increase in economic uncertainties were largely ignored when explaining family changes (Perelli-Harris et al. 2010). Moreover, the SDT lacks an explicit gender perspective, notwithstanding its acknowledgement of women's increasing educational attainment and economic activity as part of societal changes (Bernhardt 2004). These latter aspects seem to be crucial for contesting the explanatory power of the SDT framework, especially with respect to family changes of the last decades and their interplay with labour market developments, in particular women's employment.

Indeed, in more recent studies increasing attention has been paid to gender equality in the public sphere and gender equity with respect to family life seen as the main drivers of family change (McDonald 2000, 2006; Esping-Andersen 2009,

Neyer et al. 2013), linking back to the hypothesis on work-family incompatibility (Liefbroer and Corijn 1999; Brewster and Rindfuss 2000). These dimensions have been synthesized in new theoretical frameworks on multiple equilibrium (Esping-Andersen and Billari 2015) and the gender revolution (Goldscheider et al. 2015) aimed at explaining past trends as well as recent family changes from the point of view of the ongoing transformation of gender roles. Both concepts focus on the interplay between family related behaviour and shifts in women's and men's social roles reflected in their gendered responsibilities for economic provision and care in a family.

The multiple equilibrium framework addresses the evolution of the family from the male breadwinner model to the dual-earner—dual-carer model with special focus on the female revolution, following the transformation of gender roles on the path towards gender egalitarianism. Family related demographic behaviours are seen as strictly associated with transitions across family equilibria, aiming for consistency between people's evolving preferences and behaviours (Esping-Andersen and Billari 2015). In contrast, Goldscheider et al. (2015) distinguish between two phases of the transformation of gender roles. The first phase of the gender revolution is characterised by a strong rise in women's labor force participation and a gradual adaptation of the public sphere to this change towards increasing gender equality, while gender roles within the family remain unchanged. This stage includes transitions from the male breadwinner model to the modernised male breadwinner or dual earner-women's double burden model. The second phase of the gender revolution starts with increasing involvement of men in the family chores, marking the transition towards the dual-earner—dual-carer model. Both conceptual frameworks highlight the relevance of the transformation of gender roles outside and within the family, in line with McDonald's views on the importance of gender equality and gender equity for fertility change (McDonald 2000, 2006). In addition, they call for attention to men's situation, which until relatively recently has been quite neglected (for exceptions see Goldscheider and Kaufman 1996; Puur et al. 2008; Goldscheider et al. 2010), even though the decline in male wages and men's labour force activity along with growing labour market uncertainty have been recognized (Oppenheimer et al. 1997; Booth et al. 1999; Mills et al. 2005).

The role of social context in the interplay of gender and family changes has been addressed in the Capabilities approach, originated in Amartya Sen's (1993) framework of capabilities and their relation to the institutional environment. The approach has been applied focusing on gendered agency and capabilities to form and maintain stable relationships and have and care for children (Hobson and Oláh 2006; Hobson 2011). Studies on fertility and partnership changes and women's increasing labor market activities frequently rely on the policy regime framework, first presented by Esping-Andersen (1990), addressing the constraints and opportunities for individuals and families that affect the organization of paid and unpaid work and family formation. More recent welfare regime typologies (Lewis 2009; Thévenon 2011) and policy configuration approaches (Korpi 2000; Korpi et al. 2013) also highlight the linkages between variations of family, fertility and reconciliation policies.

In addition to theorizing about transitions over the family life course and their interlinkages with gender role changes, another major topic of scholarly attention has been the organization of family life. Studies of families and the division of work within households show that family members do gender as they do housework and childcare (Berk 1985; West and Fenstermaker 1995). Acts are performative in the sense that they construct, corroborate, and reconstruct identities in relation to jointly agreed-upon definitions. The performativity makes it possible to create and maintain an illusion of two essential and polar gender identities, at the same time enabling the reconstructions of gender (Butler 1990). This 'doing gender' approach emphasizes that we are assessed by and held accountable for based on gender in nearly everything we do (West and Zimmerman 1987; Jurczyk et al. 2014). This accountability, in turn, influences the social constructions of roles such as husbands and wives, mothers and fathers. Rooted in the concept of doing gender, the 'doing family' approach, looking at practices resulting in gender differences (Morgan 1999, 2011; Smart 2000; Nelson 2006), takes into account the fact that social habits are reproduced through everyday interactions. It argues that family life is not a given per se, but rather a social construction, because families embed their everyday family lives in internal daily routines, practices, and external social activities interlinked with changes in gender roles and family relationships.

Following upon the logic of the interplay between demographic changes and transformation of gender roles as outlined above, we will now address both transitions as well as the organization of family life. These are interpreted in the context of the de-standardized family life course and the growing complexity of family forms and relationships. In our overview of research, we focus first on women's new role and its implications for family dynamics, considering both women and men as main actors. Next we turn to the topic of gendered transition to parenthood, a borderline issue between family transitions and family life organization. The latter aspect is more thoroughly addressed in the discussion of new gender roles in doing families. Finally, we focus on coping strategies in family and work reconciliation under conditions of uncertainty and precariousness, an issue of growing importance for understanding transitions in family life.

New Challenges of Transitions in and Organization of Family Life

In this section we discuss recent research outcomes of family dynamics in a comparative perspective, especially regarding partnership transitions and parenthood and the organization of family life, and their association with changing gender roles. The results we present here refer to the main outcomes of Work Package 3 of the FamiliesAndSocieties project: The new roles of men and women and implications for families and societies. First, we focus on the reversal of the gender gap in education, a main driver of the transformation of gender roles, and its impacts on family patterns, especially on couple formation and fertility. New conceptual approaches are needed in order to study these processes. It is important to take into account both the more diverse ways of starting a family in modern societies compared to that of previous decades and the education-specific mating squeeze, resulting from the expansion of higher education, affecting women in particular. Next, we focus on the gendered transition to parenthood in Sweden, Switzerland, and Austria, countries with different institutional and gender systems and advancements in transformation of the family regarding economic provision and caring duties.

Men's involvement in family life can also be approached from the perspective of its organization. To illustrate how evolving gender roles are reflected in doing family, outcomes of two comparative studies are discussed addressing time spent by fathers with children and the gender gap in household work in different family types across Europe. Finally, coping strategies in family and work reconciliation under conditions of uncertainty and precariousness will be discussed.

Women's New Role and Its Implications for Family Dynamics

Women's new social role is closely connected to their educational attainment. Aggregated data show that women have outperformed men in formal education in the past decades, and consequently they now have increasingly as much or more education as their partners, unlike in the past. The reversal of the gender gap in education has far-reaching implications for family dynamics and needs to be taken into account not only in studying behaviours relevant for demographic development and social relations but also in applying an adequate analytical approach. Moreover, to account for the increasing importance of non-marital cohabitation as well as a growing proportion of children born in consensual unions instead of marriage, the conventional concept of the "marriage squeeze" should be extended to include this partnership type. Van Bavel (2012) proposed to address imbalances on the "mating market" instead of the "marriage market" only, and to pay attention to education accounting for an education-specific mating squeeze. Relying on data from the European Labour Force Survey (LFS) and Eurostat official statistics on population, his co-authored study demonstrates the importance of the mating squeeze for family formation in modern societies (De Hauw et al. 2014).

Indeed, the expansion of higher education among women and resulting patterns of assortative mating affect family formation, fertility, and divorce (Schwartz and Han 2014; Grow and Van Bavel 2015). Contrary to expectations, highly educated women are not more likely to remain single. Rather, they appear to partner more often with men with less education than themselves. How exactly this is related to the timing instead of the likelihood of partnership formation is, however, still an open question (De Hauw and Van Bavel 2016). The reversal of gender inequality has also resulted in remarkable shifts in educational pairing: educational hypergamy (women marrying up) is declining while homogamy and hypogamy (women marrying down) are becoming more prevalent (Esteve et al. 2012). In a study of Klesment and Van Bavel (2015), based on EU-SILC data, educationally homogamous couples constitute more than half of the sample and the share of hypogamous couples exceeds that of hypergamous couples (except for Austria, Germany, the Czech Republic, and Romania). Between 2007 and 2011 the proportion of highly educated homogamous couples increased similarly to the share of hypogamous partnerships with highly educated woman.

New patterns of educational pairings affect the decision-making processes related to fertility, as a comparative study based on the EU-SILC panel data on 17 countries reveals (Nitsche et al. 2015). Homogamous highly educated couples show a distinct childbearing behaviour in most societies studied. They tend to postpone the first birth longest, while transition rates to subsequent (second and third) births are highest for them compared to other educational pairings, especially to couples with a highly educated woman and a lower educated man. This suggests that homogamous highly educated couples recuperate their postponed transition to the first birth by progressing to second and/or third births faster. Moreover, differences in childbearing behaviour within the group of highly educated men are in contrast to what may be expected based on the conventional economic models of the family. Hypergamous couples with a highly educated man and a lower educated woman display significantly lower second and third birth transition rates than homogamous highly educated couples across the majority of countries. There is no country in which second or third birth transitions rates among this type of couples are higher than rates of homogamous highly educated couples. These findings are in line with Oppenheimer's (1994) hypothesis on pooling resources in a couple instead of Becker's (1991) economic model.

The Gendered Transition to Parenthood

In our research on the gendered transition to parenthood, country-specific studies based on both qualitative and quantitative approaches provide in-depth insights into combining parenthood with working careers. Leaves for child care are considered a crucial policy measure to support reconciliation of work and caring responsibilities. Especially fathers' entitlements and use of leave play an important role in reversing the asymmetry in the gendered impacts of parenthood on work performance of men and women. When becoming a father, men tend to strengthen their economic provision to the family, also by increasing their working hours, while women take leave from employment to care for a child and quite often either stay at home or switch to part-time work until the child starts day care. Below we discuss two country specific studies on leave practices in Sweden and Switzerland, countries with contrasting leave systems, different stages of family change and transformation of gender roles.

The study on Sweden, a Dual-Earner cluster country, explores how both men's and women's "new" roles are related to their time spent in paid work and in care, taking into account children-parents ties (Evertsson et al. 2015). By combining analyses of quantitative survey data (YAPS—Young Adult Panel Study, Sweden) and qualitative interviews conducted with middle-class first-time parents, new insights into the division of parental leave in Sweden are provided. The findings suggest that fathers' family orientation and willingness to share caring responsibilities are the main determinants of longer leaves of fathers. Reasons for couple's unequal leave use vary from mothers' preferences to stay home for a long period, and fathers' refusal to take leave, or work-related reasons, to the economic situation of the family. Father's work conditions are more important for his leave duration than the work conditions of mother for her leave length; and income difference is sometimes used as a motive for a father to take a short leave irrespective of who earns the most. In any case, the duration of the father's parental leave significantly affects his contribution to child care even when both parents resume paid work, i.e. the longer the father's leave, the more likely child care is to be equally divided in the long-term. These qualitative findings indicate that traditional norms and ideals about the mother as primary care taker hinder an equal sharing of the leave during the child's first year, despite ideals of gender equality and equal parenting being highly regarded by the parents interviewed. Thus family income and factors related to the parents' work conditions seem to interact with norms and ideals, and they produce different outcomes across couples. The study also suggests several mechanisms through which fathers' parental leave uptake may causally influence the share of care between parents when a child is older. Fathers' parental leave uptake is linked to a closer relationship between the father and the child and also contributes to a greater understanding between the parents, both when it comes to sharing home tasks when a child is small and to combining paid work with unpaid work, including care.

The institutional context in Switzerland, a Liberal regime country, is completely different from that of Sweden: employed men do not have access to any statutory leave when they become fathers. However, companies may implement their own regulations on leaves. The case study of a public administration organization that implemented a one-month paternity leave to be taken over one year, based also on mixed methods, shows limited gender equality effects in terms of gender roles perceptions and participation in care and domestic duties and uptake of paternity leave (Valarino 2014; Valarino and Gauthier 2016). The opportunity of a one-month paid paternity leave did not substantially change men's employment patterns or a division of family work but it did enable fathers to strengthen their sense of competence regarding care obligations and appropriation of their new father identity. However, the traditional idea of different abilities of men and women in relation to the newborn prevailed. Also, the important role of the workplace and job characteristics was confirmed. The limited effects of implementation of paternity leave at the company level in Switzerland seem to strengthen arguments that national efforts are necessary for progress in transformation of gender roles at both societal and family levels.

A crucial role of men's perception about parenting in relation to take-up of parental leave was also confirmed by the in-depth analysis of the transition to parenthood in Austria, a country of the General Family Support cluster. The decision for sharing parental leave, even if displayed as a joint decision, was father-centred as the decision was oriented towards the father's wish and willingness, in close connection to the perceived organizational necessities. The decision for the father's leave was expected to be as beneficial as possible for him, and both partners valued the father's leave higher than the mother's (Schmidt et al. 2015). More attention was given to his work situation, while mothers' leave seemed rather to be self-evident. Regardless of the parental leave arrangement, masculinity remained hegemonic in being superior to femininity, even if feminine aspects of caring were incorporated due to following findings: (i) only the man was deemed to be in the position to agree to the interruption of his career; (ii) the woman supported her partner‘s claims for external recognition or gratefully presented him as an exceptional example of a good father; (iii) as taking up parental leave and doing care work contradict hegemonic masculinity, this was compensated for by the construction of a father's leave taking as a highly masculine act of being courageous.

New Gender Roles in Doing Families

As discussed earlier, on-going transformation of gender roles, reflected predominantly in shifts of women's position in the social sphere and within the family, imposed changes in the gendered economic provision for a family and organization of family life. Women's increasing employment was not accompanied by a reduction in women's household chores and care responsibilities, nor by substantial engagement of men in household duties or care. More and more scholars indicate that a redefinition of men's role within the family is crucial for progressing in transformation of gender roles (see e.g. Esping-Andersen and Billari 2015; Goldscheider et al. 2015). Along with empowering mothers as economic providers, the new role of fathers should be strengthened. New fatherhood is generally defined as a present, more involved and caring father (Tanturri et al. 2016). There is some evidence that fatherhood is in transition in Europe in terms of both social norms and practices, however that process is strongly diversified across countries (Goldscheider et al. 2015). The transition from the male breadwinner model to the dual-earner—dual-carer model is more advanced in the Dual-Earner cluster (i.e. Nordic countries), while more traditional perception of fatherhood still prevails in the Familialistic and Transition Post-Socialist clusters (i.e. the Mediterranean and in Central-Eastern Europe).

Assuming that fathers' time with children reflects how the country is progressing in new fatherhood, Tanturri et al. (2016) relied on Time Use Survey data to examine fathers' involvement in the family in Sweden, Italy, France, and the United Kingdom, that is in countries of various welfare regimes and with a range of policies on work-family reconciliation. Three indicators were used: the total time of fathers spent with their children, the time spent alone with children, and the time fathers allocated to childcare. The results show that the Dual-Earner cluster (Sweden) progressed most in the transition to involved fatherhood, followed by the Liberal cluster (United Kingdom). Fewer advances were seen for the Familialistic and the General Family Support clusters, respectively. Italian fathers spend more total time with children than did fathers in France, while the opposite holds for the time spent alone with children. French fathers allocate a similar quantity of time to child care as fathers in the UK and in Italy, however the share of time for caring alone is visibly higher in France. In searching for factors that matter most for fathers' involvement with children, it was found that the most involved fathers are those with a high school certificate. Hence, the increasing number of more highly educated men may strengthen the progress of new fatherhood. Another stimulating factor seems to be the growing prevalence of dual earner couples—men are more engaged with their children especially when their partner works full time, compared to male breadwinner families. Also, more favourable working conditions (being a clerk or working less than 35 hours a week) increase fathers' involvement in family life, while working long hours diminished fathers' time dedicated to children.

Another aspect of the interrelationship between changing gender roles and doing families refers to patterns of housework division between men and women in different family models by their labour market involvement. A comparative study of ten European countries, relying on data from the European Social Survey, investigated how housework is divided between men and women across various family models and how the patterns vary across welfare regimes with different work-family reconciliation policies and gender norms (Fahlén 2015). The results suggest the importance of occupational position within the couple to understand how time is allocated to cope with work and home demands: dual-career couples (both partners are at the higher occupational levels), female-career couples and female single-earner couples divide the housework more equally than do dual-earner couples. However, this result can be attributed to the fact that women do less housework when being more engaged in paid work but not to increased housework by their partner. Moreover, outcomes on men's and women's actual housework hours suggest that occupational position matters more for women than for men. Smaller gender differences in the division of housework were shown in Dual-Earner cluster countries, with more institutional support for work-family reconciliation and less traditional gender norms. Moreover, the results suggest that dual-earner families and dual-career families are confronted with different challenges to combine work and home duties. They also have different capabilities to cope with these challenges, especially in countries with weaker support for work-family reconciliation. The gender gap in doing housework is largest in countries with more traditional gender norms for both dual-earner and dual-career couples, especially so in the Transition Post-Socialist cluster (i.e. Central-Eastern Europe).

Coping Strategies in Family and Work Reconciliation Under Conditions of Uncertainty and Precariousness, and Impacts on Fertility

Low fertility is a major concern in Europe, strongly influenced by career expectations, couples' education, and possibilities of combining work and family life.

The labour market prospects, especially job uncertainty and instability are being broadly voiced as crucial factors for becoming a parent and/or having subsequent children, despite significant cross-country differences with respect to fertility and the labour market situation. Hence, we focus here on coping strategies of families as expressed in the fertility intentions of both women and men, reducing the knowledge gap of especially men's responses to economic uncertainty.

The comparative study by Fahlén and Oláh (2015) on the interplay between societal economic conditions, individual economic uncertainty, and short-term childbearing intentions in ten European countries representing different welfare regimes made use of the data from the European Social Survey (2004/05 and 2010/11). The aggregated short-term childbearing intentions of childless people and of one-child parents were analysed in relation to changes in unemployment and employment protection. In addition, the micro-level association between childbearing intentions and perceived economic uncertainty was addressed. The study reveals that economic uncertainty impacts short-term childbearing intentions across welfare states, but the association varies by gender and parity. Childless men and one-child fathers are those responding most to changes in unemployment risks, while job protection is important mainly for the childbearing plans of one-child mothers and childless men. Also the micro-level findings confirm that perceived economic uncertainty is an important factor for childbearing plans, however this impact again varies by gender, age, parenthood status, and the institutional context. Especially, the low intentions among fathers in the Transition Post-Socialist cluster (Central-Eastern Europe) indicate that in institutional contexts that promote a more traditional gender division of work and care, a highly uncertain economic situation in terms of employment-, income security and unemployment risks substantially reduces fathers' intentions to have a second child. This offers additional arguments in favour of supporting women's employment and gender equality to counteract negative impacts of economic uncertainty on the family economic situation and consequently, on fathers' plans to have more children.

Research on childbearing decisions seen as outcomes of coping strategies in work and family reconciliation under economic uncertainty and precariousness in Switzerland, a Liberal cluster country, goes beyond the approach usually applied to examine the relationship between employment and fertility, in which only women's job characteristics (e.g. employment status, work hours) are focused on (Hanappi et al. 2014). To understand more clearly the linkages between the institutional context, employment uncertainty, and fertility of men and women this study investigates how subjective perceptions about job stability and job prestige influence fertility intentions of both women and men living in a partnership. In addition, a mediating role of gender attitudes, defined as approval/disapproval of maternal employment, is taken into account. The results of the analyses of data from the Swiss Household Panel confirm gendered impacts of stability and prestige of jobs on fertility intentions, moderated for men by gender attitudes. Perceived job instability reduces women's intentions for a first child but motherhood sets off any employment-related effects. Contrary to expectations, job instability increases fertility intentions of men who disapprove of maternal employment. The job prestige matters only for men—its direct effect on first and subsequent child intentions is positive. However, this effect turns negative for men who do not approve of maternal employment. In searching for possible explanations, references have been made to the Liberal welfare regime promoting the family with male breadwinning, the labour market being unsupportive of reconciliation of employment and childrearing, and the gender system being at the early stage of transformation. In general, these outcomes confirm that impacts of the job instability on fertility intentions vary by gender and parity and are strongly associated with gender attitudes.

Conclusion

Because the interplay between family changes and transformation of gender roles is increasingly recognized in contemporary scholarship of the family, in this chapter we addressed both processes in Europe. We acknowledged their context dependence focusing on groups of countries by welfare regime/policy configuration types in our discussion on the evolution of family patterns and gender roles. Within this general conceptual framework we presented new evidence on implications for family dynamics generated by women's new role and changes in men's role enforced by women's emancipation. Hence, the main research outcomes discussed either from a comparative perspective or based on country-specific studies depict gendered patterns of partnership formation and transitions to parenthood as well as of the organization of family life with emphasis on involved fatherhood. As family life is increasingly influenced by labour market developments, coping strategies in family and work reconciliation under conditions of uncertainty and precariousness have been addressed as well.

Changing family patterns resulted in increasingly diverse family biographies even though originating in common trends. In addition, in most societies in Europe, transformation of gender roles in the public sphere has progressed much further than in the family. Differences in timing and intensity of gender and family changes produced differences in outcomes, especially comparing Dual-Earner regime countries with societies of the Familialistic and the Transition Post-Socialist clusters. However, within-cluster diversity cannot be neglected either. Both types of differences reflect the importance of the institutional settings, economic structures, and culture for the evolution of family patterns and gender roles alike.

As discussed, new research findings highlight the crucial role of the gender gap reversal in education for partnership formation and fertility. However, women's increasing importance as economic providers to the family is challenged by the gendered transition to parenthood. Especially fathers' entitlements to and use of leave, influenced also by workplace and job characteristics, are crucial for men's family involvement and sharing childrearing. Societal and institutional support varies across clusters, impacting family life. Similarly, patterns of housework division between women and men differ by family models based on the labour market participation of partners, and across welfare regimes.

Changes in doing family have been more affected by women's paid work engagement than by men's job characteristics. Transitions towards dual earning, in turn, may counteract negative impacts of economic uncertainty on fertility intentions, in particular on men's plans to have children. This new research evidence presented here, based predominantly on microlevel data and integrating qualitative and quantitative approaches, extends existing knowledge on new gender roles and their implications for families and societies.

Acknowledgements The research leading to these results has received funding from the European Union's Seventh Framework Programme (FP7/2007-2013) under grant agreement no. 320116 for the research project FamiliesAndSocieties. In addition, financial support for Livia Sz. Oláh via the Swedish Research Council grant to the Linnaeus Center on Social Policy and Family Dynamics in Europe, SPADE (grant number 349-2007-8701), and for Irena E. Kotowska from the Ministry of Science and High Education in Poland (grant agreement no. 2886/7.PR/2013/2) are gratefully acknowledged.

References

Allen, S. M., & Hawkins, A. J. (1999). Maternal gatekeeping. Mothers' beliefs and behaviors that inhibit greater father involvement in family work. *Journal of Marriage and the Family, 61*(1), 199–212.

Anxo, D., Mencarini, L., Paihlé, A., Solaz, A., Tanturri, M. L., & Flood, L. (2011). Gender differences in time-use over the life-course. A comparative analysis of France, Italy, Sweden and the United States. *Feminist Economist, 17*(3), 159–195.

Becker, G. S. (1991). *A Treatise on the family* (Enlarged ed.). Cambridge, MA: Harvard University Press.

Behnke, C., & Meuser, M. (2012). "Look here mate! I´m taking parental leave for a year"—involved fatherhood and images of masculinity. In M. Oechsle, U. Mueller, & S. Hess (Eds.), *Fatherhood in late modernity. cultural images, social practices, structural frames*. Opladen/Farmington Hills: Verlag Barbara Budrich.

Bengtson, V. L., Acock, A. C., Allen, K. R., Dilworth-Anderson, P., & Klein (Hg), D. M. (2005). *Sourcebook of family theory and research*. Thousand Oaks, London, New Delhi: Sage.

Berk, S. F. (1985). *The gender factory. The apportionment of work in American households*. New York: Plenum Press.

Bernhardt, E. (1993). Fertility and employment. *European Sociological Review, 9*(1), 25–42.

Bernhardt, E. (2004). Is the second demographic transition a useful concept for demography? *Vienna Yearbook of Population Research, 2004*, 25–28.

Bianchi, S. M., Milkie, M. A., Sayer, L. C., & Robinson, J. P. (2000). Is anyone doing the homework? Trends in the gender division of household labor. *Social Forces, 79*(1), 191–228.

Blossfeld, H.-P. (Ed.). (1995). *The new role of women: Family formation in modern societies*. Boulder, San Francisco, Oxford: Westview Press.

Blossfeld, H.-P., & Drobnic, S. (Eds.). (2001). *Careers of couples in contemporary societies: From male breadwinner to dual-earner families*. Oxford: Oxford University Press.

Booth, A., Crouter, A. C., & Shanahan, M. J. (Eds.) (1999). *Transitions to adulthood in a changing economy: No work, no family, no future?* Westport, CT: Praeger.

Brandt, B., & Kvande, E. (2002). Reflexive fathers. Negotiating parental leave and working life. *Gender, Work and Organization, 9*(2), 186–203.

Brewster, K. L., & Rindfuss, R. R. (2000). Fertility and women's employment in industrialized nations. *Annual Review of Sociology, 26,* 271–296.

Bruckner, H., & Mayer, K. U. (2005). De-standardization of the life course: What it might mean? And if it means anything, whether it actually took place? *Advances in Life Course Research, 9,* 27–53.

Butler, J. (1990). *Gender trouble: Feminism and the subversion of identity*. New York: Routledge.

Cerami, A., & Vanhuysse, P. (Eds.). (2009). *Post-communist welfare pathways: Theorizing social policy transformation in Central and Eastern Europe*. Basingstoke: Palgrave Macmillan.

Craig, L., & Mullan, K. (2011). How mothers and fathers share childcare: A cross-national time-use comparison. *American Sociological Review, 76*(6), 834–861.

De Hauw, Y., Piazza, F., & Van Bavel, J. (2014). *Methodological report: Measurement of education-specific mating squeeze*. FamiliesAndSocieties Working Paper 16 (2014).

De Hauw, Y., & Van Bavel, J. (2016). *The shifting gender imbalance in higher education and the timing and likelihood of union formation*. Presentation at the FamiliesAndSocieties Third Annual Consortium Meeting, Vienna, Austria, January 13–15, 2016.

Elzinga, C. H., & Liefbroer, A. C. (2007). De-standardization of family-life trajectories of young adults: A cross-national comparison using sequence analysis. *European Journal of Population, 23,* 225–250.

England, P. (2010). The gender revolution. *Uneven and Stalled. Gender & Society, 24*(2), 149–166.

Esping-Andersen, G. (1990). *The three worlds of welfare capitalism*. Cambridge: Policy Press.

Esping-Andersen, G. (2009). *The incomplete revolution: Adapting to women's new roles*. Cambridge: Policy Press.

Esping-Andersen, G., & Billari, F. C. (2015). Re-theorizing family demographics. *Population and Development Review, 41*(1), 1–31.

Esteve, A., García-Román, J., & Permanyer, I. (2012). The gender-gap reversal in education and its effect on union formation: The end of hypergamy? *Population and Development Review, 38* (3), 535–546.

Eurostat (2015). *Population and social conditions database: Demography and migration: Fertility: Fertility indicators: Total fertility rate*. http://ec.europa.eu/eurostat/data/database. Accessed September 22, 2015.

Eurostat (2016) *Population and social conditions database: Labour market: Employment and unemployment (Labour Force Surveys): LFS series—Detailed annual survey results: Activity and activity rates: Activity rates by sex, age and citizenship (%): Activity rate (20–64 years)*. http://ec.europa.eu/eurostat/data/database. Accessed February 10, 2016.

Evertsson, M., Boye, K., & Erman, J. (2015). *Fathers on call—A study on the sharing of care work among parents in Sweden. A mixed methods approach*. FamiliesAndSocieties Working Paper 27 (2015).

Fahlén, S. (2015). *Gender equality within dual-earner and dual-career couples across different policy regimes and norm systems in Europe*. FamiliesAndSocieties Working Paper 48 (2015).

Fahlén, S., & Oláh, L. Sz. (2015). *The impact of economic uncertainty on childbearing intentions in Europe*. FamiliesAndSocieties Working Paper 36 (2015).

Frejka, T., Sobotka, T., Hoem, J. M., & Toulemon, L. (Eds.). (2008). Childbearing trends and policies in Europe. *Demographic Research, Special Collection 7*, 1–1178.

Goldscheider, F. (1990). The aging of the gender revolution. What do we know and what do we need to know? *Research on Aging, 12*(4), 531–545.

Goldscheider, F. K., & Kaufman, G. (1996). Fertility and commitment: Bringing men back in. *Population and Development Review, 22*, 87–99 (Supplement: Fertility in the United States: New Patterns, New Theories).

Goldscheider, F., Bernhardt, E., & Lappegard, T. (2015). The gender revolution: A framework for understanding changing family and demographic behavior. *Population and Development Review, 41*(2), 207–239.

Goldscheider, F., Oláh, L. Sz., & Puur, A. (2010). Reconciling studies of men's gender attitudes and fertility: Response to Westoff and Higgins. *Demographic Research, 22*(1), 189–197.

Gornick, J. C., & Meyers, M. K. (2003). *Families that work: Policies for reconciling parenthood and employment*. New York: Russell Sage Foundation.

Grow, A., & Van Bavel, J. (2015). Assortative mating and the reversal of gender inequality in education in Europe: An agent-based model. *PLoS ONE, 10*(6), e0127806. https://doi.org/10.1371/journal.pone.0127806.

Haas, L., & Hwang, P. C. (2009). Is fatherhood becoming more visible at work? Trends in corporate support for fathers taking parental leave in Sweden. *Fathering, 7*(3), 303–321.

Hanappi, D., Ryser, V. -A., & Bernardi, L. (2014). *Coping strategies under uncertain, precarious employment conditions in Switzerland*. FamiliesAndSocieties Working Paper 12 (2014).

Hobson, B. (Ed.). (2002). *Making men into fathers. Men, masculinities and the social politics of fatherhood*. Cambridge, UK: Cambridge University Press.

Hobson, B. (2011). The agency gap in work-life balance: Applying Sen's capabilities framework within European contexts. *Social Politics, 18*(2), 147–167.

Hobson, B., & Fahlén, S. (2009). Competing scenarios for European fathers: Applying Sen's capabilities and agency framework to work-family balance. *The Annals of the American Academy of Political and Social Science, 624*(1), 214–233.

Hobson, B., & Oláh, L. Sz. (2006). Birthstrikes? Agency and capabilities in the reconciliation of employment and family. *Marriage and Family Review, 39*(3–4), 197–227.

Huinink, J. (2013). De-standardization or changing life course patterns? Transition to adulthood from a demographic perspective. In G. Neyer et al. (Eds.), *The Demography of Europe* (pp. 99–118). Dordrecht: Springer.

INED (2013). Developed countries database. http://www.ined.fr/en/pop_figures/developed_countries_database/. Accessed July 3, 2013.

Jurczyk, K., Lange, A., & Thiessen, B. (Eds.). (2014). *Doing family: Warum familienleben heute nicht mehr selbstverständlich ist*. Weinheim und Basel: Beltz Juventa.

Klesment, M., & Van Bavel, J. (2015). *The reversal of the gender gap in Europe and female breadwinners in Europe*. FamiliesAndSocieties Working Paper 26 (2015).

Korpi, W. (2000). Faces of inequality: Gender, class, and patterns of inequalities in different types of welfare states. *Social Politics, 7*(2), 127–191.

Korpi, W., Ferrarini, T., & Englung, S. (2013). Women's opportunities under different family policy constellations: Gender, class, and inequality tradeoffs in Western countries re-examined. *Social Politics, 20*(1), 1–40.

Lesthaeghe, R. (2010). The unfolding story of the second demographic transition. *Population and Development Review, 36*(2), 211–251.

Lewis, J. (2006). *Gender and welfare in modern Europe. Past and Present* (Suppl. 1, pp. 39–54). (The Art of Survival: Gender and History in Europe, 1450–2000).

Lewis, J. (2009). *Work–family balance, gender and policy*. Cheltenham, UK: Edward Elgar.

Liefbroer, A. C., & Corijn, M. (1999). Who, what, where and when? Specifying the impact of educational attainment and labour force participation on family formation. *European Journal of Population, 15*(1), 45–75.

Lillard, L. A., & Waite, L. J. (1993). A joint model of marital childbearing and marital disruption. *Demography, 30*(4), 653–681.

Matysiak, A. (2011). *Interdependencies between fertility and women's labour supply*. Dordrecht: Springer.

McDonald, P. (2000). Gender equity, social institutions and the future of fertility. *Journal of Population Research, 17*(1), 1–16.

McDonald, P. (2006). Low Fertility and the State: The efficacy of policy. *Population and Development Review, 32*(3), 485–510.

Mills, M., Blossfeld, H.-P., & Klijzing, E. (2005). Becoming an adult in uncertain times: A 14-country comparison of the losers of globalization. In H.-P. Blossfeld, E. Klijzing, M. Mills, & K. Kurz (Eds.), *Globalization, uncertainty and youth in society* (pp. 423–441). London: Routledge.

Morgan, D. H. J. (1999). Risk and family practices: Accounting for change and fluidity in family life. In E. B. Silva & C. Smart (Eds.), *The new family?* (pp. 13–30). London: Thousand Oaks Sage Publications.

Morgan, D. H. J. (2011). *Rethinking family practices*. Basingstoke: Palgrave Macmillan.

Moss, P. (2014). *International review of leave policies and research 2014*. http://www.leavenetwork.org/lp_and_r_reports/.

Myrskylä, M., Goldstein, J. R., & Cheng, Y.-H. A. (2013). New cohort fertility forecasts for the developed world: Rises, falls, and reversals. *Population and Development Review, 39*(1), 31–56.

Nelson, M. (2006). Single mothers "do" family. *Journal of Marriage and Family, 68,* 781–795.

Neyer, G. (2013). Welfare states, family policies, and fertility in Europe. In G. Neyer et al. (Eds.), *The demography of Europe* (pp. 29–53). Dordrecht: Springer.

Neyer, G., Lappegard T., & Vignoli, D. (2013). Gender equality and fertility: Which equality matters? *European Journal of Population, 29*(3), 245–272.

Nitsche, N., Matysiak, A., Van Bavel, J., & Vignoli, D. (2015). *Partners' educational pairings and fertility across Europe*. FamiliesAndSocieties Working Paper 38 (2015).

OECD. (2011). *Doing better for families*. Paris: OECD Publishing.

OECD. (2012). *Closing the gender gap*. Paris: OECD Publishing.

Oláh, L. Sz. (2015). *Changing families in the European Union: Trends and policy implications*. FamiliesAndSocieties Working Paper 44 (2015).

Oláh, L. Sz., & Fahlén, S. (2013). Introduction: Aspirations and uncertainties. Childbearing choices and work-life realities in Europe. In L. Sz. Oláh, & E. Fratczak (Eds.), *Childbearing, women's employment and work-life balance policies in contemporary Europe* (pp. 1–27). Basingstoke: Palgrave Macmillan.

Oláh, L. Sz., & Fratczak, E. (2013). *Childbearing, women's employment and work-life balance policies in contemporary Europe*. Basingstoke: Palgrave Macmillan.

Oppenheimer, V. K. (1994). Women's rising employment and the future of the family in industrial societies. *Population and Development Review, 20*(2), 293–342.

Oppenheimer, V. K. (1997). Women's employment and the gain to marriage: The specialization and trading model. *Annual Review of Sociology, 23,* 431–453.

Oppenheimer, V. K., Kalamijn, M., & Lim, N. (1997). Men's career development and marriage timing during a period of rising inequality. *Demography, 34,* 311–330.

Perelli-Harris, B., Sigle-Rushton, W., Kreyenfeld, M., Lappegård, T., Keizer, R., & Berghammer, C. (2010). The educational gradient of childbearing within cohabitation in Europe. *Population and Development Review, 36*(4), 775–801.

Philipov, D., & Dorbritz, J. (2003). Demographic consequences of economic transition in countries of central and eastern Europe. *Population Studies, 39*. Council of Europe Publishing.

Plantenga, J., Remery, C., Figueiredo, H., & Smith, M. (2009). Towards a European union gender equality index. *Journal of European Social Policy, 19*(1), 19–33.

Puur, A., Oláh, L. Sz., Tazi-Preve, M. I., & Dorbritz, J. (2008). Men's childbearing desires and views of the male role in Europe at the dawn of the 21st century. *Demographic Research, 19*(56), 1883–1912.

Saraceno, C. (Ed.). (2008). *Families, ageing and social policy: Intergenerational solidarity in European welfare states*. Cheltenham: Edward Elgar.

Sardon, J.-P. (1993). Women's first marriage rates in Europe: Elements for a typology. *Population: An English Selection, 5,* 120–152.

Sayer, L. C., Bianchi, S. M., & Robinson, J. P. (2004). Are parents investing less in children? Trends in mothers' and fathers' time with children. *American Journal of Sociology, 10*(1), 1–43.

Schmidt, E.-M., Rieder, I., Zartler, U., Schadler, C., & Richter, R. (2015). Parental constructions of masculinity at the transition to parenthood: The division of parental leave among Austrian couples. *International Review of Sociology, 25*(3), 373–386.

Schwartz, R. C., & Han, H. (2014). The reversal of the gender gap in education and trends in marital dissolution. *American Sociological Review, 79*(4), 605–629.

Sen, A. (1993). Capability and well-being. In M. C. Nussbaum & A. Sen (Eds.), *The quality of life* (pp. 30–53). Oxford: Oxford University Press.

Seward, R. R., Yeatts, D. E., Zottarelli, L. K., & Fletcher, R. G. (2006). Fathers taking parental leave and their involvement with children. An exploratory study. *Community, Work and Family, 9*(1), 1–9.

Skolnick, A. (1978). *The intimate environment: Exploring marriage and the family*. Boston: Little, Brown and Company.

Smart, C. (2000). Divorce and changing family practices in a post-traditional society. Moral Decline or changes to moral practices? *Family Matters, 56,* 10–19.

Smith Koslowski, A. (2011). Working fathers in Europe: Earning and caring. *European Sociological Review, 27*(2), 230–245.

Sobotka, T. (2011). Fertility in Central and Eastern Europe after 1989: Collapse and gradual recovery. *Historical Social Research, 36*(2), 246–296.

Sobotka, T., & Lutz, W. (2010). Misleading policy messages derived from the period TFR: Should we stop using it? *Comparative Population Studies, 35*(3), 637–664.

Spijker, J., & Solsona, M. (2012). *Atlas of divorce and post-divorce indicators in Europe*. Centre d'Estudis Demografics, Universitat Autonoma de Barcelona. Papers de Demografia 412. http://www.ced.uab.es/publicacions/PapersPDF/Text412.pdf.

Steel, L., Kidd, W., & Brown, A. (2012). *The family*. Basingstoke: Palgrave.

Tanturri, M. L., Donno, A., Fahlén, S., Henz, U., Paihlé, A., & Solaz, A. (2016). *D.3.10. Report on fathers' time with children, trends and determinants in France, Italy, Sweden and the UK.* FamiliesAndSocieties Deliverable report.

Thévenon, O. (2011). Family policies in OECD countries: A comparative analysis. *Population and Development Review, 37*(1), 57–87.

Thomson, E. (2004). Stepfamilies and childbearing desires in Europe. *Demographic Research, 3* (5), 117–134.

Valarino, I. (2014). *The Emergence of parental and paternity leaves in Switzerland: A Challenge to Gendered Representations and Practices of Parenthood* (Ph.D. in social sciences), University of Lausanne, Lausanne. http://serval.unil.ch/?id=serval:BIB_EC9A89C2A3A6.

Valarino, I., & Gauthier, A. (2016). Paternity leave implementation in Switzerland: A challenge to gendered representations and practices of fatherhood? *Community, Work and Family, 19*(1), 1–20.

Van Bavel, J. (2012). The reversal of gender inequality in education, union formation and fertility in Europe. *Vienna Yearbook of Population Research, 10,* 127–154.

Van de Kaa, D. J. (1987). Europe's second demographic transition. *Population Bulletin, 42*(1), 1–59.

Van de Kaa D. J. (1994). The second demographic transition revisited: Theories and expectations (1993). In G. C. N. Beets, R. L. Cliquet, G. Dooghe, & J. de Jong Gierveld (Eds.), *Population and Family in the Low Countries 1993. Late fertility and other current issues* (pp. 81–126). Amsterdam, Lisse: NIDI-CBGS Publications, Swets.

West, C., & Fenstermaker, S. (1995). Doing difference. *Gender & Society, 9*(1), 8–37.

West, C., & Zimmerman, D. H. (1987). Doing gender. *Gender & Society, 1*(2), 125–151.

Sex Differences in Health and Survival

Anna Oksuzyan, Jordi Gumà and Gabriele Doblhammer

Sex Differences in Survival

Empirical research has shown that being male is the most consistent predictor of mortality at all ages in all countries of the world (Barford et al. 2006). A female survival advantage was reported as far back as the 1750s (Glei and Horiuchi 2007). As the economic and living conditions of women in many parts of the world improved dramatically from the 1950s to the mid-1970s, the gender gap also widened rapidly in countries such as Canada, New Zealand, Australia, Japan, and most European (EU) countries, including countries in eastern Europe (Glei and Horiuchi 2007; Rigby and Dorling 2007; Oksuzyan et al. 2008). During this period, the gender gap in survival chances in the US continued to increase despite the convergence of mortality differentials across other socio-demographic characteristics, such as place of residence (urban versus rural), ethnicity (white versus non-white), and socioeconomic status (Madigan and Vance 1957). However, the

A. Oksuzyan (✉) · G. Doblhammer
Max Planck Institute for Demographic Research, Rostock, Germany
e-mail: oksuzyan@demogr.mpg.de

G. Doblhammer
e-mail: gabriele.doblhammer@uni-rostock.de

J. Gumà
Department of Political and Social Sciences, University Pompeu Fabra, Barcelona, Spain
e-mail: jordi.guma@upf.edu

G. Doblhammer
Faculty of Economics and Social Sciences, Institute of Sociology and Demography, University of Rostock, Rostock, Germany

G. Doblhammer and J. Gumà (eds.), *A Demographic Perspective on Gender, Family and Health in Europe*, https://doi.org/10.1007/978-3-319-72356-3_5

trends in sex differences in mortality in these countries were mixed in the last quarter of the 20th century. A narrowing trend was first observed in England and Wales in the early 1970s, then in other English-speaking countries in the late 1970s and the early 1980s, and slightly later in the Scandinavian countries, Austria, and the Netherlands (Trovato and Heyen 2006; Glei and Horiuchi 2007). From the 1980s to the late 1990s, the female-male differences in life expectancy narrowed in most EU countries and in the US, but expanded in certain countries, such as Greece, Hungary, and Japan (Waldron 1993; Gjonca et al. 2005). Across the developed countries, figures for 2013 indicate that the gender gap in life expectancy was largest in the Russian Federation (11.19 years) and smallest in Ireland (3.07 years) (HMD).

There are, however, fewer studies that have looked at the extent to which life expectancy at older ages differs by gender, and at how these gaps have changed over time across developed countries (Thorslund et al. 2013). The sex differences in life expectancy at age 65, when the impact of infant mortality and mortality related to reproduction (women) and high-risk behavior (men) are reduced, have been found to follow similar trends across 17 wealthy low-mortality countries, albeit with differences in timing (Thorslund et al. 2013). Until the 1950s, the gender gap in mortality in these countries was small, at around one year. But from the 1950s to the 1980s, the gap widened in most countries, to around four years. Since then, the gender gap in mortality has been narrowing in all but two countries, Japan and Spain.

Trajectories of sex differences in mortality have varied substantially across age groups and causes of death in different EU countries and over different time periods. Prior to World War II, reductions in infant mortality contributed substantially to the widening of sex differences in life expectancy (Vallin 2006). Since 1950, these differences have been mostly attributable to mortality trends at adult ages and to the causes of deaths closely related to lifestyle and health behaviors; e.g., ischemic heart disease, lung cancer, liver cirrhosis, traffic accidents, and suicide (Waldron 1993; Trovato and Heyen 2006; Glei and Horiuchi 2007; Oksuzyan et al. 2008). There is growing evidence that cigarette smoking is the factor that has played the largest role in the sex differential mortality (Preston and Glei 2011; Martikainen et al. 2014; Beltrán-Sánchez et al. 2015; Lindahl-Jacobsen et al. 2016). However, smoking alone cannot explain these trajectories, as a female advantage in life expectancy has also been observed among nonsmokers and specific populations, such as Mormons (Wingard et al. 1983; Rogers and Powell-Griner 1991; Lindahl-Jacobsen et al. 2013).

A variety of studies have provided convincing evidence that a female advantage in healthy life expectancy is less apparent [reviewed in (Oksuzyan et al. 2010a)]. Although women live longer with activity limitations at ages 15 and 50, the gender gap in healthy life expectancy is smaller than the gender gap in life expectancy in most EU countries (Van Oyen et al. 2010; Van Oyen et al. 2012). These findings suggest that women may more likely to survive despite having disabilities and chronic conditions than men.

Sex Differences in Health

Sex Differences in Physical Performance Tests

Physical performance measures have been routinely used in clinical assessments. Because handgrip strength test, gait speed test, and physical performance battery test (standing balance, gait speed, and chair rises) are quick, inexpensive, and easy to administer and are shown to be valid and reliable tools for assessing muscle strength (Mijnarends et al. 2013), they are often included in data collection instruments of population-based surveys (Innes 1999; Roberts et al. 2011).

It has been suggested that handgrip strength is a better marker of frailty than chronological age (Syddall et al. 2003), and it predicts all-cause and cause-specific mortality in community-based and patient populations (Fujita et al. 1995; Rantanen et al. 2000; Sasaki et al. 2007; Ling et al. 2010; Ortega et al. 2012; Leong et al. 2015). Moreover, handgrip strength has been found to be associated with disability at older ages (Giampaoli et al. 1999; Rantanen et al. 1999; Taekema et al. 2010), cognitive decline (Alfaro-Acha et al. 2006), and hospitalization (Cawthon et al. 2009). While there is compelling evidence that men outperform women on handgrip tests at all ages and across all continents (Bohannon et al. 2006; Dodds et al. 2014; Leong et al. 2015), the magnitude of the male advantage appears to vary across national populations, ethnicities, and age groups. It is remarkable that the grip strength of an 80-year-old Danish man is similar to that of a 45-year-old Danish woman (Frederiksen et al. 2006). The evidence that men tend to outperform women on grip strength performance seems to be inconsistent with the higher deaths rates among men at all ages. In one study that examined this apparent contradiction, the authors hypothesized that men and women differ not only in their initial grip strength levels, but also in the pace at which their grip strength declines with age. Thus, they suggested that the sex-specific associations of these parameters with lifespan may partially explain sex differences in health and mortality (Oksuzyan et al. 2010c). The results of the study indicated that men have higher initial levels of and a steeper decline in grip strength, but that the initial level was more strongly associated with lifespan than the age-related decline. These predictive effects were found to be similar in men and women.

Gender differences in other physical capability tests, such as chair rises, walking speed (or gait speed), timed get up and go (TUG), and standing balance were investigated in several cohort studies in the UK (Cooper et al. 2011; Keevil et al. 2013). Large male advantages were found for chair rising ability and standing balance, but no sex differences were observed for TUG and walking speed.

Findings on age variations in gender differences on physical performance tests have been less conclusive. Butler et al. reported that young people had similar performance levels on seven physical tests, but that older women had lower normative values than men of the same age (Butler et al. 2009). The male-female difference in grip strength was shown to increase with advancing age in the European Prospective Investigation into Cancer (EPIC)-Norfolk study, whereas a meta-analysis of eight other UK cohort studies indicated that gender differences diminished with advancing age for grip strength; did not change for TUG, chair rising ability, and standing balance; and increased for walking speed (Cooper et al. 2011; Keevil et al. 2013). These mixed patterns can be partially explained by differences in the sex-specific mortality selection in the background populations and by differences in drop-out rates due to non-response and due to the inability to perform the test across surveys (Cooper et al. 2011).

Sex Differences in Cognitive Function

The topic of gender differences in cognitive function continues to attract considerable attention from the scientific, the medical, and the political communities. Generally, the results of empirical research have suggested that men have advantages in mathematical and visuospatial abilities (Linn and Petersen 1985; Voyer et al. 1995; Halpern et al. 2016), that women have advantages in episodic memory (Halpern et al. 2016; Herlitz and Rehnman 2008) and verbal ability (Hyde and Linn 1988; Reilly 2012), and that there are no significant sex differences in category fluency (Crossley et al. 1997). Recent studies conducted in more gender-egalitarian societies have found smaller gender differences in levels of mathematical achievement (Guiso et al. 2008; Else-Quest et al. 2010; Lindberg et al. 2010). Gender differences in cognitive tasks have been found to be stable from adulthood to old age, which suggests that age-related declines in cognitive abilities have similar trajectories in men and women (Barnes et al. 2003; de Frias et al. 2006; Gerstorf et al. 2006). With respect to general intelligence, most researchers have found no or negligible sex differences in adolescent and adult populations in developed countries (Aluja-Fabregat et al. 2000; Colom et al. 2000; van der Sluis et al. 2006; Burgaleta et al. 2012).

Empirical research has consistently demonstrated that poor cognitive function is associated with increased mortality risk in older populations (Gale et al. 1996; Pavlik et al. 2003; Perna et al. 2015). In contrast, studies on predictive abilities of cognitive decline beyond current levels of cognitive function have reached competing conclusions (Maier et al. 2003; Schupf et al. 2005; Ghisletta 2008; Lavery et al. 2009). The question of whether there are sex-specific protective effects of various cognitive abilities for health and mortality also warrants further investigation.

In seeking to explain gender differences in cognitive abilities, some scholars have cited societal factors, cultural differences, and gender stereotypes; as well as biological factors, such as differences in prenatal hormonal influences and brain size and structure (Ankney 1992; Alonso-Nanclares et al. 2008; Rushton and Ankney 2009; Tapp et al. 2011; Miller and Halpern 2014). In light of evidence showing that these differences vary substantially across nations, and mirror the gender inequalities in education, employment opportunities, and career achievements in particular countries, researchers have suggested that improved standards of living and educational opportunities in populations with lower economic development levels may improve the cognitive performance levels in these populations, especially among women (Baker and Jones 1993; Else-Quest et al. 2010; Weber et al. 2014).

Sex Differences in Depression

A growing body of literature has indicated that women are more likely than men to suffer from depression, although the direction and the magnitude of these sex differences have been shown to vary across diagnostic subtypes and age (Piccinelli and Wilkinson 2000). Gender disparities have been found in the prevalence of somatic symptoms of depression, with women being more prone to experience symptoms such as appetite disturbance, sleep disorders (Roberts et al. 2000; Kockler and Heun 2002; Jaussent et al. 2011), and atypical depression (Angst et al. 2002); and men being substantially more likely than women to experience the most tragic consequence of depression: suicide (Bjerkeset et al. 2008; Brådvik et al. 2008).

A number of studies have shown that gender disparities in depression increase after early to mid-adolescence, and are especially large at reproductive ages (Nolen-Hoeksema and Girgus 1994; Hankin et al. 1998; Grigoriadis and Erlick Robinson 2007). Generally, it appears that women are more likely than men to suffer from depression though old age as well (Cairney and Wade 2002; Djernes 2006). Other studies have shown that sex differences in the prevalence of depression reverse after menopause (Bebbington et al. 1998), or become smaller at older ages (Barefoot et al. 2001; Djernes 2006; McDougall et al. 2007). These findings, which remain controversial, may be attributable to the geographic differences and the methodological challenges inherent in large-scale community-based studies of oldest-old individuals. Among these challenges are the failure to include residents of long-term care facilities, attrition due to non-response and death, and differences in the instruments used to measure depression symptomatology.

There are a number of hypotheses to explain the female preponderance in depression, including (1) artefacts, such as differential treatment-seeking and symptom-reporting behavior; (2) biological differences due to ovarian hormonal changes during puberty, postpartum periods, and menopause, and to changes in adrenal hormone levels in reaction to stressful events; (3) social factors, such as social pressure, abuse experiences during puberty and at work, role overload related to pressure to balance working full time with managing care responsibilities for children and elderly parents; and (4) psychological factors, such as having low self-esteem, low self-confidence, and high levels of neuroticism, and a greater tendency to engage in rumination (Nolen-Hoeksema and Girgus 1994; Nolen-Hoeksema 2001; Kuehner 2003; Hyde et al. 2008). Since most studies that examine the gender gap in depression focus on disentangling the effects of individual factors that contribute to this gap, there is a need for more integrative models that account for multiple pathways in the development of depression, and for the interactions of these individual factors. Understanding gender differences in depression may allow policy-makers to formulate strategies for improving women's quality of life and productivity, thereby reducing the health care costs associated with treating depression. Moreover, identifying the sources of this gender gap could help researchers better understand the origins of depression and dementia.

Sex Differences in Morbidity

The issue of sex differences in morbidity is multifaceted because the direction and the magnitude of sex differences in morbidity may vary depending on the particular disease or chronic condition under investigation, the age-related changes in the incidence rates of the disease, and the sex-specific rates of survival after the onset of the disease. It has been shown that women tend to report more symptoms and have a greater number of comorbidities that are not lethal but are disabling, whereas men have more life-threatening conditions (Macintyre et al. 1996; Case and Paxson 2005; Crimmins et al. 2011). This pattern was found in a study on opposite-sex twins that controlled for early environmental and genetic factors. Specifically, the findings indicated that men had higher rates than women of heart insufficiency, angina pectoris, and stroke; and that women had higher rates than men of cataract, knee and hip problems, and urinary tract disorders (Gold et al. 2002). There is also some evidence that the sex-specific distribution of chronic conditions is reflected at the level of biological markers of health (Oksuzyan et al. 2015). Thus, excessive morbidity in women depends to a large extent on a selected disease or illness indicator. In this chapter, we are unable to provide a comprehensive review of the patterns of sex differences for all diseases. Instead, we offer an overview of the gender gaps for the most common chronic conditions and causes of death in developed countries (Dodds et al. 2012; Go et al. 2013).

The empirical evidence has suggested that compared to men, women tend to develop cardiovascular diseases (CVD) about ten years later and to have a lower lifetime risk of CVD (Jousilahti et al. 1999; Lawlor et al. 2001; Go et al. 2013). It has also been shown that the gender gap in the incidence of coronary heart disease (CHD) and stroke diminishes with advancing age (Lerner and Kannel 1986; Petrea et al. 2009). A substantial share of the sex differences in CVD incidence can be explained by differences in the distribution among men and women of major CVD risk factors, such as smoking, HDL cholesterol levels, and hypertension; and by age-related changes in these factors (Jousilahti et al. 1999; Freedman et al. 2004; Cutler et al. 2008).

The findings regarding sex differences in survival after myocardial infarction (MI) and stroke have been less consistent. Several studies have indicated that short- and long-term post-MI (Koek et al. 2006; Milcent et al. 2007) and post-stroke mortality is higher in women than in men (Appelros et al. 2009; Lewsey et al. 2009;

Appelros et al. 2010; Andersen et al. 2011). Some studies found that the female disadvantage in post-stroke survival was limited to younger ages (Vaccarino et al. 1998, 1999, 2001; Nielsen et al. 2014), while others found that rates of post-MI and post-stroke survival did not differ significantly by gender after the baseline and clinical characteristics were taken into account (Galatius et al. 1996; Herman et al. 1997; MacIntyre et al. 2001; Di Carlo et al. 2003; Isaksson et al. 2011; Olsen et al. 2012).

Sex differences in post-stroke survival have been shown to vary across stroke types: studies have found that at younger ages ischemic and intracerebral hemorrhagic stroke deaths are less common among women than among men, but that at ages 65+ women are less likely than men to survive an ischemic stroke (Ayala et al. 2002). Compared to men, women are more likely to experience post-stroke depression and functional disabilities, to be institutionalized, and to have a poor quality of life (Di Carlo et al. 2003; Roquer et al. 2003; Appelros et al. 2009; Petrea et al. 2009).

Scholars seeking to explain these controversial findings on sex differences in post-stroke and post-MI health outcomes have speculated that these disparities could be attributable to sex-specific MI mortality prior to hospitalization; or to gender differences in the severity of the disease, in the prevalence of comorbid conditions, and in the treatment strategies used (Blomkalns et al. 2005). Strokes and MI have been found to be more severe in female than male populations (Appelros et al. 2009; Olsen et al. 2012). However, these findings have been challenged in the literature, and appear to vary depending on the measures used to define disease severity (Iezzoni et al. 1997; Barrett et al. 2007; Kardys et al. 2007; Reeves et al. 2008). Gender differences in pre-existing conditions may also contribute to survival after MI and stroke. A history of hypertension and atrial fibrillation was found to be more common among female patients who survived stroke than among their male counterparts, while a history of ischemic heart disease and diabetes was shown to be more prevalent among male than among female patients (Holroyd-Leduc et al. 2000; Di Carlo et al. 2003). In a study that compared diabetic and non-diabetic patients, the overall relative risk of dying of CHD was found to be substantially greater among women than among men (Huxley et al. 2006). This result suggests that in addition to the differences in the distribution of comorbid conditions, the relative risk associated with a comorbidity may help to explain the gender differences in the prognoses for MI and stroke. Moreover, considerably more men than women undergo invasive cardiac procedures and receive aggressive treatment (Bowling et al. 2001; Shaw et al. 2004; Blomkalns et al. 2005; Smith et al. 2009). The marked differences observed in the treatment strategies for men and women have been partially explained by differences in disease severity, comorbid conditions, symptom presentation, and patient preferences for surgical or less aggressive forms of treatment (Vaccarino et al. 2003; Anand et al. 2005). However, more research is needed to help us better understand how these factors and treatment-seeking behaviors contribute to sex differences in survival after stroke and MI.

A male preponderance in the incidence of cancer has been documented worldwide. Age-standardized incidence rates in EU countries in 2012 for all cancers (excluding non-melanoma skin cancers) was 430 and 306 per 100,000 among men and women, respectively (Ferlay et al. 2013). The Cancer Incidence in Five Continents data, which cover around 60 countries, revealed that for 32 out of 35 sites men had higher incidence rates than women, with the largest gap being for cancer of the larynx (IRR = 6.36), and the smallest gap being for other endocrine cancers (IRR = 1.19) (Edgren et al. 2012). A female disadvantage in cancer incidence was found for only a few sites: i.e., for Hodgkin's disease and for cancers of the thyroid, gallbladder, biliary tract, and anus (Edgren et al. 2012; Ferlay et al. 2013). A study for the US found that from 1975 to 2004 total cancer incidence was 37% higher among men than among women across all ages, and was 77% higher when sex-specific sites were excluded (Cook et al. 2009). Some variation in sex differences in cancer incidence across all ages was observed: for example, during the period 1975–2004, women under age 50 had higher incidence rates of all cancers and of cancers excluding sex-specific sites, whereas women over age 60 had lower incidence rates of both all cancers and cancers excluding sex-specific sites (Cook et al. 2009). When sex-specific sites and breast cancer were excluded, the total cancer rates were higher among men than among women aged 30 and older.

The age-standardized mortality rates (ASMRs) for all cancers and most cancer sites were found to be substantially higher in men than in women (Cook et al. 2011; Ferlay et al. 2013). In 2012, the ASMRs in Europe for all cancers (excluding non-melanoma skin cancers) were 223 and 129 per 100,000 among men and women, respectively. Women had higher ASMRs for cancers of the anus, the anal canal, the anorectrum, and the gallbladder, and no consistent gender patterns were observed for cancers of the peritoneum, the omentum, the mesentery, and the endocrine system. Empirical research has also shown that 5-year relative survival that cannot be explained by underlying sex differences in mortality is also higher in women than in men (Micheli et al. 1998; Albano et al. 2007). The average 5-year relative survival in Europe for eight major cancer sites (lung, melanoma, Hodgkin's disease, colorectal, breast, ovary, testis, and prostate) was found to be about 45% (44.6–45.0%) for men and 55% (54.4–54.8%) for women (Berrino et al. 2007).

These sex disparities in cancer incidence have been attributed to a range of factors, including gender differences in genetic traits, steroid hormone levels, immunocompetence, and antioxidative abilities; as well as to a range of environmental factors, such as smoking and diet, occupational exposures, and sexual practices (Cook et al. 2009; Dorak and Karpuzoglu 2012; Edgren et al. 2012). Although cancer etiology has been studied for decades, we still do not fully understand the risk factors for cancer or their mechanisms. As the known risk factors cannot fully explain the sex disparities in cancer incidence for 13 out of 35 sites, it is important that research in this area continue (Edgren et al. 2012). The reasons for and the underlying mechanisms of sex differences in survival after cancer diagnosis also remain largely unknown. While the finding that the male disadvantage in cancer-specific survival attenuates after adjusting for cancer stage and grade suggests that these factors partially account for sex disparities, the extent to which sex differences in health care utilization and comorbidities explain sex differences cancer-specific survival rates has yet to be determined (Cook et al. 2011).

Sex Differences in Self-perceived Health

For two reasons, self-perceived health is the most studied and most frequently used indicator of subjective health. First, the association between self-perceived health and mortality has been well established (McGee et al. 1999; Singh-Manoux et al. 2007). Second, it is simple and easy to include question about overall health in both health-specific surveys such as the Survey of Health, Ageing and Retirement in Europe (SHARE) and the European Health Survey, and in more general surveys such as the European Statistics on Income and Living Conditions (EU-SILC-SILC) and the European Social Survey (ESS). Because this indicator is widely used in population health studies, Jylhä proposed a conceptual model for self-perceived health designed to enhance our understanding of the different factors that may influence an individual's perception of his or her health (2009). This model is composed of three main contextual frameworks that can modify an individual's evaluation of health: differences in conceptions of health (what is good and what is poor), the reference groups chosen for comparison (external counterparts with similar socio-demographic features, and internal expectations regarding health and aging), and cultural conventions regarding the expression of opinions (positive or negative).

Multiple studies have demonstrated that at all ages, women are more likely than men to report being in poor health (Crimmins et al. 2011; Crimmins and Salto 2001; Dahlin and Härkönen 2013). Three main reasons are usually given for this gender gap: gender differences in morbidity profiles, sex differences in health reporting, and gender differences in social determinants of health. The first reason is based on the observation that women are more likely than men to have chronic conditions linked to functional capacities, whereas men are more likely than women to have chronic conditions directly linked to survival, such CVD (Case and Paxson 2005). The second reason is based on evidence that women are more knowledgeable than men about their own health status, and that men are more likely than women to avoid going to the doctor or to admit their own vulnerability (Benyamini et al. 2000; Idler 2003). The last reason is explained in more detail later in this chapter.

A number of comparative studies of EU countries found that the southern and eastern EU countries had the highest gender gaps in self-rated health (Zambon et al. 2006; Eikemo et al. 2008; Crimmins et al. 2011). One of the main explanations for these cross-country differences is rooted in levels of gender equity: the higher the degree of gender inequity in a country, the larger the gender gap in self-perceived health (Zambon et al. 2006; Eikemo et al. 2008; Crimmins et al. 2011). However, the existing evidence on this issue is inconclusive. Dahlin and Härkönen in 2013 provided no support for this hypothesis, as they found that countries in both northern and southern Europe—like Sweden and Spain—have similar gender gaps in self-perceived health (Dahlin and Härkönen 2013). The authors also showed that the odds of reporting poor health are similar for men and women after controlling for other health indicators, such as chronic conditions and indicators of functioning. After these controls were applied, the gender differences in reporting poor health not only disappeared in the majority of countries, but even reversed in some countries (Crimmins et al. 2011; Dahlin and Härkönen 2013). These findings emphasize that the abovementioned unequal health profiles of men and women are influenced by their own perceptions, and thus call for additional explanations considering gender differences in health reporting.

Sex Differences in Functional Status

Functional status can be assessed using a wide range of indicators, with the most extensively used being Activities of Daily Living (ADL) and Instrumental Activities of Daily Living (IADL). ADL are all of the activities related to an individual's capacity to take care of his or her own basic needs, such as bathing, feeding, and dressing. IADL are the activities that allow an individual to live independently in a community context, such as shopping, managing money, and using the telephone. In this chapter, we focus on age-related functional limitations as a consequence of a progressive decline over an individual's life course; i.e., on limitations resulting from the "disablement process" proposed by Verbrugge and Jette, rather than on functional limitations at younger ages, which are likely to be of a different nature (1994).

A variety of studies have provided consistent evidence that men report having fewer difficulties in performing ADL and IADL than women (Newman and Brach 1999; Murtagh and Hubert 2004; Palacios-Cena et al. 2012). However, recent empirical research suggests that a female disadvantage in functional limitations is not apparent at all ages. Analyzing individuals from the British 1946 cohort, Murray et al. found that men and women are equally likely to have limitations at age 43, but that the gender differences are greater at age 53 (2011). This finding suggests that age-related declines in functional limitations are likely to be gender-specific. Although less research has been done on sex differences in age-related declines in physical functioning, there is some evidence that the rates of decline in physical functioning are higher among men than among women (Oksuzyan et al. 2010c).

There is also some debate about a possible sex-specific bias in some of the items used to measure IADL. Especially in the older cohorts, activities like cooking or shopping are more likely to be done by women than by men. As sex differences have been found in studies that looked at both self-reported and observed disabilities (Merrill et al. 1997), it is possible that the female disadvantage in functional limitations is independent of how these limitations are measured.

There are relatively few empirical studies that have compared gender differences in the prevalence of functional limitations across countries. Cross-country comparisons of these activities are complicated by cultural differences, such as differences in typical living arrangements; differences in the availability of community services; and differences in the division of labor by gender. These factors and others could influence responses to IADL items. However, Nikula et al. showed that the differences in the dependence on IADL items (preparing meals, shopping, and doing housework) by gender, age, and occupation were similar in five EU countries (Finland, Italy, the Netherlands, Spain and Sweden); and that responses to these items are therefore comparable across different countries (2003). Existing international comparisons have shown that women tend to have more functional limitations than men of the same age, although the magnitude of these sex differences varied across countries and across the types of activities analyzed. Oksuzyan et al. found a pronounced female disadvantage in ADL in Denmark, Japan, and the United States among people aged 85 and older, even though the size of the sex difference varied across these three study populations at younger ages (2010b). Furthermore, based on three large-scale population-based surveys in the EU countries, in the UK, and in the USA, Crimmins et al. found large sex differences in IADL difficulties, but similar levels of ADL disability by gender among people aged 80 and older (2011).

Sex Differences in Health-Related Quality of Life

Health-related quality of life (HRQOL) is an indicator that is highly sensitive to differences between individuals, even in subpopulations with the same objective health profile (i.e., individuals who have been diagnosed with the same disease). This is largely because this indicator is usually derived from the compilation of information from a set of items that reflect different aspects of how an individual feels as a consequence of his/her health status (e.g.: "Does pain interfere in your daily life?" "How often do you feel calm, or full of energy?"). Different tools have been developed to measure HRQOL based on the set of items used (e.g., SF36, SF20, SF12, 15D, the Nottingham Health Profile) and the wording of questions. Since these scales are often used to monitor patient health outcomes, we provide a few examples of epidemiological studies that have assessed sex differences in HRQOL among individuals with the most prevalent diseases mentioned in the sex differences in morbidity section within this chapter: namely, CVD and cancer.

In a study of stroke survivors in Japan, HRQOL was found to be higher among men than among women because women had a higher prevalence of ADL limitations and depression (Kuroda et al. 2006). Similarly, an examination of MI survivors in Spain showed that men had higher HRQOL levels than women. This study also found that the evolution of HRQOL scores from the third to the sixth month after experiencing the attack followed a sex-specific pattern: men showed greater improvements in most dimensions of physical and social functioning, while women improved in social functioning and in only few physical dimensions (Dueñas et al. 2011). Moreover, female cancer patients (colorectal and breast cancer) have been found to have lower HRQOL levels than their male counterparts (colorectal and prostate cancer) (LeMasters et al. 2013).

The high degree of sensitivity of HRQOL to small differences enables us to use this indicator to explore health gender gaps in younger populations (i.e., children and teenagers), and thus in populations among whom health inequalities tend to be smaller than among adults. Several studies that utilized the "Kidscreen 52" questionnaire found that the gender differences in HRQOL are small among children prior to adolescence, but that adolescent girls tend to report worse levels of HRQOL than their male counterparts (Bisegger et al. 2005; Erhart et al. 2009). Most of the explanations for the emergence of these gender differences in HRQOL in adolescence refer to biological factors (e.g., that puberty is physically harder for girls), psychological factors (e.g., that girls cope with problems internally whereas boys do so externally), and social factors (e.g., that the social demands made on girls are harder to meet than those made on boys).

Explanations for Sex Differences in Health and Mortality

The most widely cited explanations for gender differences in health and survival can be classified into three general groups: biological endowments, which include hormonal and genetic factors; factors associated with lifestyle behaviors; and gender inequalities in social profiles.

Hormonal Explanations

Effects of Estrogen

A variety of studies have shown that premenopausal women have substantially lower rates of CHD, hypertensive and cerebrovascular diseases, and related mortality than men of the same age (Lerner and Kannel 1986; Appelros et al. 2009; Sandberg and Ji 2012). After menopause, sex differences in CVD become smaller, and continue to decline as men and women age. These trends suggest that estrogen plays a central role in the sex differences in CVD (Waldron 1983; Vaccarino et al. 2010). Some studies that have examined the indirect effects of female hormones have found that estrogen has positive effects on lipoprotein profiles by decreasing total cholesterol and LDL cholesterol levels and increasing HDL cholesterol levels (Knopp et al. 1994; Miller et al. 1995). The direct effects of estrogen have been mainly attributed to two estrogen receptor subtypes, ERa and ERb, which are located in vascular endothelial and myocardial cells; as well as to a recently discovered third membrane-bound estrogen receptor, the G-protein-coupled estrogen receptor (GPR30) (Babiker et al. 2002; Mendelsohn and Karas 2005; Prossnitz and Maggiolini 2009). The existing literature has provided compelling evidence that estrogen has a range of anti-inflammatory and vasoprotective effects, including improving coronary and peripheral endothelial function; reducing ischemia, reperfusion injury, and inflammatory markers; and attenuating cardiac hypertrophy (Babiker et al. 2002; Wise et al. 2005; Xing et al. 2009; Yang and Reckelhoff 2011).

Research has suggested that deficient levels of endogenous estrogen due to natural or surgical menopause are associated with elevated risks of CVD morbidity and mortality (Oliver and Boyd 1959; Bairey et al. 2003; Rivera et al. 2009). However, observational studies and randomized clinical trials that extensively examined the effects of hormone replacement therapy (HRT) on CVD risk in postmenopausal women yielded conflicting results. Some studies found that HRT reduced the risks of CVD events and mortality in postmenopausal women (Bush 1990; Stampfer and Colditz 1991; Grady et al. 1992; Wise et al. 2005); whereas two major randomized clinical trials, the Women's Health Initiative and Heart and Estrogen/Progestin Replacement Study, indicated that the overall health risks associated with HRT are greater than the health benefits of estrogen plus progestin treatment among healthy postmenopausal women with an intact uterus, as well as among women with documented CHD (Grady et al. 2002; Rossouw et al. 2002; Chlebowski et al. 2003; Heiss et al. 2008).

Effects of Testosterone

The evidence regarding the effects of endogenous testosterone on men's health has been mixed (Alexandersen et al. 1996; Vitale et al. 2009; Araujo et al. 2011; Ruige et al. 2011; Schooling 2015). Although some studies have reported negative associations between low testosterone levels and the risk of ischemic stroke and of all-cause, CVD, and cancer mortality; the question of whether these associations are causal, or whether testosterone is an important biomarker of overall male health, has yet to be fully investigated (Haring et al. 2010; Holmegard et al. 2016).

The existing findings concerning the health benefits of testosterone replacement therapy (TRT) have also been controversial (Haddad et al. 2007; Xu et al. 2013; Kelly and Jones 2014). Review studies have suggested that the most frequently observed health benefits of TRT include improvements in sexual function, mood and quality of life, muscle strength, and cognitive function; and increased bone mineral density (Nieschlag et al. 2004; Bassil et al. 2009; Fernández-Balsells et al. 2010). These studies have, however, also indicated that TRT may increase the risk of prostate and breast cancers, liver toxicity and tumors, testicular atrophy, infertility, gynecomastia, erythrocytosis, and skin diseases; may worsen benign prostatic hypertrophy; and could exacerbate sleep apnea. At present, however, there is no compelling evidence that TRT has adverse effects on prostate and CVD outcomes, and the long-term effects of TRT on the incidence of fractures and other health outcomes are under-investigated due to a lack of studies with a sufficiently long follow-up period.

Effects of Sex Hormones on the Immune System

The existing research has pointed toward a female advantage in immune protection, mainly due to the immunosuppressive effects of progesterone and testosterone and the immunoenhancing effects of estrogens (Bouman et al. 2005; Pennell et al. 2012; Giefing-Kröll et al. 2015). The incidences of many bacterial, viral, parasitic, and fungal infectious diseases (e.g., leptospirosis, brucellosis, rabies, leishmaniasis, pulmonary tuberculosis, hepatitis A, meningococcal and pneumococcal infections, and seasonal influenza) were found to be substantially higher, and some infectious diseases were shown to be more severe in men than in premenopausal women (Giefing-Kröll et al. 2015). Studies have found that autoimmune diseases are more common and that immune responses to vaccinations are often stronger in women than in men (Whitacre 2001; Giefing-Kröll et al. 2015). These findings led researchers to conclude that low levels of immunocompetence among men contributes to sex differences in mortality (Owens 2002). Although the proportion of deaths from infectious diseases in overall mortality is very small in developed countries, non-communicable diseases remain major causes of death in low-income countries (MacDonald et al. 2006). Elevated inflammatory markers were found to be associated with worse physical performance and cognition, chronic diseases, disability, and mortality (Danesh et al. 1998; Harris et al. 1999; Yaffe et al. 2003; Il'yasova et al. 2005; Schaap et al. 2009; Kaptoge et al. 2010; Singh and Newman 2011). Although substantial progress has been made in this research field, the mechanisms through which sex hormones affect both non-specific (innate) and specific (adaptive) immune responses and responses to vaccines, and the ways in which HRT can modify alterations in the immune system in humans, have not yet been fully elucidated.

Genetic Explanations

As the result of extensive mammalian evolution, in the human organism there are more than 1100 genes on the X chromosome, which are involved in various physiological processes; and fewer than 100 genes on the Y chromosome, which determine male sex (Ross et al. 2005). The presence of two copies of the X chromosome in women explains the female advantage in the risk of contracting certain X-linked diseases, such as hemophilia A, Duchenne muscular dystrophy, X-linked agammaglobulinemia; as well as the female advantage related to the modification of gene expression on the paternal or the maternal X chromosome. To equalize the expression of X gene dosage in women and men, one copy of X chromosomes is silenced (X inactivation), and this process occurs randomly with regard to the parental origin of the X chromosome (Lyon 1962; Migeon 1994). The process of random X inactivation creates so-called cellular mosaicism in women—i.e., half of a woman's cells contain active paternal X chromosome, while the other half contain active maternal X chromosome—that underlies this female biological advantage (Migeon 2007). Such a deleterious mutation of or variation in a normally functioning gene on the maternal X-chromosome will be expressed in all cells in men, but will be expressed in only half of the cells in women, as the paternal X chromosome is likely to be intact, and is likely to ameliorate the harmful effects of the gene mutation. In addition, the cellular mosaicism in women contributes to physiological diversity, which can be advantageous when encountering new immune challenges (Spolarics 2007; Morris and Harrison 2009). However, X chromosome abnormalities—e.g., extreme inactivation skewing and inactive chromosome reactivation—may also be disadvantageous for females, and may underlie the female preponderance in autoimmunity (Libert et al. 2010).

Lifestyle Explanations

Gender differences in risk-taking behaviors have been used to define, among other factors, the constructs of masculinity and femininity, with masculinity being linked to greater social acceptance of risky behaviors, and femininity being linked to higher levels of social control (De Visser and Smith 2007). These two concepts were proposed to explain why men and women behave differently based on social norms, and how these behaviors may influence health (Courtenay 2000; Lyons 2009). The greater social acceptance of men engaging in risky behaviors contributes to sex differences in health by eroding the health status of men, whereas the social control of women's behavior may protect women's health (Denton et al. 2004).

Tobacco and Alcohol Consumption

Tobacco is still known as "the single largest preventable cause of death and disease in the United States" (CDC 2012). This is the case in EU countries as well, where smoking has been described as "the most important cause of gender differences in mortality across Europe" (McCartney et al. 2011). Levels of alcohol consumption are more heterogeneous across countries (La Vecchia et al. 2014). The contribution of alcohol consumption to mortality is between 3 and 8% in EU countries (Rehm et al. 2009), and is up to 10% at working ages in the United States (Stahre et al. 2014).

There is compelling evidence that there are gender differences in both the prevalence and the levels of alcohol consumption. Across all western countries, more men than women consume tobacco and alcohol (Costanza et al. 2006; Robinson and Harris 2011), and the consumption of these substances has greater effects on health and survival among men than among women at the aggregated level (Mucha et al. 2006; Stahre et al. 2014). Men have been shown to have a greater propensity than women to engage in risky behaviors, and the link between risky behaviors and the social concept of masculinity appears to underlie the sex differences in the consumption of both alcohol and tobacco. For instance, in a qualitative study of young men in London alcohol consumption was described as a marker of masculinity (De Visser and Smith 2007). As gender-based double standards regarding alcohol consumption persist even among men and women who have similar consumption levels, there is clear evidence of a link between drinking and masculinity (De Visser and McDonnell 2012).

However, in recent generations in developed countries the gender gap in smoking (Pampel 2006) and alcohol consumption (Bloomfield et al. 2006; De Visser and McDonnell 2012) appears to have decreased, or even reversed. This gap has decreased due to both a reduction in male consumption and an increase in female consumption of both substances. The main explanations for these trends are the empowerment of women and the decline in gender inequality in western societies (Hitchman and Fong 2011). Accordingly, a number of studies have pointed to the urgent need to include women in the target populations of campaigns aimed at discouraging the consumption of these substances (Amos et al. 2011).

Diet

The effects of dietary patterns on health and survival have been extensively studied. The consumption of higher quantities of vegetables and fruits and of smaller amounts of red meat—which are typical features of the Mediterranean diet—have been shown to be strongly correlated with having better health and a longer life (Haveman-Nies et al. 2002; Knoops et al. 2004; Kourlaba and Panagiotakos 2009).

The literature that looked at the sex differences in diet has suggested that women tend to have healthier eating habits than men. Women are more likely than men at almost all ages to report eating more vegetables and fruits and fewer fatty and high-carbohydrate food products (Bere et al. 2008; Dehghan et al. 2011; Kiefer et al. 2013). One of the main explanations for why women are more likely than men to follow the dietary guidelines is that women tend to be concerned about the possible disadvantages of having an unhealthy diet, including gaining weight. Meanwhile, men tend to report that they do not care about their diet, and that they have little knowledge of what a healthy diet would be (Courtenay 2000; Gough and Conner 2006). Indeed, the gender gap in food preferences appears to be attenuated after nutrition knowledge is controlled for (Baker and Wardle 2003).

Among the social-oriented explanations for this gap are that women generally know more than men about healthy eating because they are more involved in activities like shopping or cooking (Wardle et al. 2004). Thus, women are more likely than men to be exposed to information about healthy food choices. A qualitative study showed that most men delegated the responsibility for making food choices to their female partner (Newcombe et al. 2012). But this is not the only aspect of the male approach to diet. A review of 44 UK newspaper articles on the topic of men and diet concluded that men who follow a healthy diet and express concerns about healthy eating are judged as being less masculine, whereas women are seen as being experts in healthy eating (Gough and Conner 2006). These social attitudes may partially explain why men are more reluctant than women to learn about the features of a healthy diet (Wardle et al. 2004).

Physical Activity

Epidemiological studies have provided consistent evidence regarding the relationship between physical activity and health. These studies have shown that regular activity can contribute to the prevention of certain chronic diseases (Warburton et al. 2006), the maintenance of mental well-being (Penedo and Dahn 2005), and improvements in survival among people of all ages (Löllgen et al. 2009). Current public health policies rate physical activity together with diet as the most critical issues in health promotion, especially in light of the increasing prevalence of obesity and diabetes in many high-income countries.

Gender differences in attitudes toward physical activity and sports typically appear at early ages. The number of boys enrolled in sport clubs that involve high-intensity exercise (e.g., football, basketball, bicycling) is clearly higher than the number of girls (Vilhjalmsson and Kristjansdottir 2003; Borraccino et al. 2009). This gender gap in involvement in sports translates into sex differences in the number of hours per week individuals spend doing exercise not only in childhood, but also in adulthood (Kjønniksen et al. 2009). Boys and girls also appear to have different motivations for enrolling in a youth sport club: boys tend to report engaging in physical activities for the sake of competition and in order to demonstrate their abilities (male-oriented features); while girls tend to report exercising for health reasons, for social reasons, or to improve their appearance (female-oriented features) (Vilhjalmsson and Kristjansdottir 2003).

A study that compared exercise habits in 20 countries found that young men are more likely than their female counterparts to report having high levels of physical activity (Bauman et al. 2009). However, while men are more likely than women to be active at adult ages, women are less likely than men to reduce their levels of physical activity as they age, and are thus more likely to maintain their exercise levels throughout their lives (Sjöström et al. 2006; Bauman et al. 2009).

Social Explanations

Social Determinants of Health

The factors used to define an individual's social position are commonly referred to as the social determinants of health, and are defined as follows: "The social determinants of health are the conditions in which people are born, grow, work, live, and age, and the wider set of forces and systems shaping the conditions of daily life" (WHO 2016). The social determinants of health are also related to an individual's resilience when faced with a stressful life event, such as a period of unemployment or a separation or divorce. Although sex differences in social profiles have been extensively investigated, there is little research on the implications of social profiles on the gender gap in health and mortality.

The most extensively studied social determinants of health are related to the socioeconomic status of individuals (education, income, occupation, etc.) (Raphael 2004; Marmot 2005). However, other social factors such as the family, which is described in the chapter by Hank and Steinbach in this book, may also be associated with health inequities. Evidence of such links has led researchers to propose various conceptual models for integrating a majority of these factors. The "Rainbow Model," which was proposed by Dahlgren and Whitehead, stands out from the others because of its simple but holistic approach (1991). The authors have argued that together with the demographic profile and constitutional factors (such as genetic features) of each individual, there are three levels of determinants of health: individual factors like lifestyle, which have already been introduced in this chapter; intermediate factors like social and community networks, including family and living and working conditions; and macro factors, such as the general socioeconomic, cultural, and environmental conditions into which gender inequity levels could be placed (also see Oláh, Kotowska, and Richter in this volume). In this chapter, we mainly focus on gender differences based on the social determinants of health that are of a socioeconomic nature.

Education

A large body of existing literature has emphasized the importance of education as a social determinant of health. Population-based studies have consistently shown that education is related to both health and mortality: i.e., the higher the educational status of an individual is, the better he or she is likely to perform on health measures such as self-perceived health, cancer, CVD, and other chronic diseases, and mortality (Von Dem Knesebeck et al. 2006; Albano et al. 2007; Conti et al. 2010). There are two main explanations for the association between education and health: first, better educated people are more likely than less educated people to have access to the knowledge needed to maintain a healthy lifestyle (as was previously described); and, second, education is a socioeconomic indicator that reflects people's economic capacity to gain the access to health-protective resources (e.g., better health care, higher quality food). Although the association between education and health is universal, the magnitude of this link is not homogeneous across all the countries. For instance, across EU countries social inequalities in self-perceived health and functional limitations have been shown to be relatively small in Norway, Sweden, the United Kingdom, and Austria; but relatively large in Hungary, Poland, and Portugal (Von Dem Knesebeck et al. 2006). The sources of these differences are still not completely understood.

As is the case with other measures of socioeconomic status, historical gaps between men and women have been observed in different dimensions of education, like educational attainment or even access to education at different levels, from primary school to university. In Europe, families traditionally encouraged more of their sons than of their daughters to attain high levels of education. Thus, until the 1960s men had higher rates of school and university attendance than women (European Commission 2009). Today, however, this gender gap has been closed and even reversed in western countries (Gakidou et al. 2010). A period of social development during the second half of the 20th century in Europe contributed to the spread of school access in most nations, especially for women. Currently, women exceed men with regard to access to and success at higher educational levels (van Bavel 2011). However, a study that compared gender differences in education across 37 EU countries showed that these gaps are country-specific, and that men's and women's educational attainment levels are influenced by different factors (McDaniel 2011). The study indicated that family background and country-specific fertility patterns and labor market conditions have considerable influence on the gender gaps in education. For example, men who grew up without a father present or with economic deprivation were found to be less likely than their more advantaged counterparts to complete university. In addition, a high level of general fertility in a country was shown to increase the probability of completing tertiary education for both men and women, whereby the probability was greater for women than for men if the level of fertility was low. The study also found that the labor market influences men's education more than women's education, as men were shown to be less likely to complete university in countries with more job opportunities in industry or with high unemployment rates.

The reversal of the gender gap in education has substantially influenced not just female survival rates, but child mortality rates. As women gained more knowledge about healthy lifestyles, the health of both mothers and their children from pregnancy to the first years of life improved (Cleland 2010; Gakidou et al. 2010). The outcomes of this process of female educational expansion appear to suggest that the relationships between education and health and mortality differ by gender. Recently, a study of US data showed that having a higher education is associated with improvements in survival, but not in health, in the male population; whereas the opposite pattern can be observed in the female population (Ross et al. 2012). These findings suggest that education may contribute to the reduction in the male-female health-survival paradox by acting in each of the dimensions in which men and women seem to be less favored. In the European context, a study conducted by Cacciani et al. for the city of Rome found that male mortality is more sensitive than female mortality to educational differences (Cacciani et al. 2015). However, other studies have found similar effects of education on mortality among men and women (Zajacova 2006), and variations in these effects by age (Pongiglione and Sabater 2014). An examination of 14 EU countries showed that educational inequalities in self-perceived health were relatively large among young and middle-aged men, but that education-related levels of self-perceived health tend to converge in both genders at older ages (Pongiglione and Sabater 2014).

Employment

While researchers have generally shown as much interest in investigating employment status as a proxy for an individual's socioeconomic status as they have in examining the role of education, some differences between these indictors have been identified: i.e., education is seen as a proxy for both socioeconomic status and knowledge about healthy lifestyles, whereas employment appears to be mainly related to socioeconomic status. While it is well known that employment, which is an indicator of access to a certain salary, is positively related to health, this relationship may also be a result of the selection of healthier individuals into the labor force (Smith et al. 1998; Wilkinson and Marmot 2003). Similarly, the literature has shown that within the employed sub-population, the higher a person's salary is, the better his or her health status is likely to be (Johnson 2009; Hawkins et al. 2012). It is not only the individual's own socioeconomic status that determines salary, but also parental social class influences the probability that the person will have a low or high salary (Smith 1996; Deaton 2008). Some researchers have, however, pointed out that using salary as an indicator of socioeconomic status can be problematic due to the relatively high non-response rate on this item in surveys, and the low degree of reliability of the responses (Galobardes et al. 2006).

A variety of studies have demonstrated that unemployment is related to adverse mental and physical health, unfavorable lifestyles, and increased mortality risk (McKee-Ryan et al. 2005; Cohen et al. 2007; Virtanen et al. 2008; Roelfs et al. 2011; Leist et al. 2013). Although a growing body of research has found that unemployment has differential effects on health in men and women, the results of these studies have been inconsistent. While some studies have found that the mental health of men and women is equally affected by unemployment (Hammarström and Janlert 1997; Bjarnason and Sigurdardottir 2003), other studies have shown that self-rated health is more likely to worsen among women than among men after becoming unemployed (Giatti et al. 2008; Reine et al. 2013). Contradictory results have also been found for the likelihood of using more alcohol and tobacco after becoming unemployed. While some studies have uncovered a relationship between unemployment and increased alcohol consumption and smoking in unemployed men only (Reine et al. 2013), a Swedish study found that this association was attenuated in women after controlling for having children (Janlert and Hammarstrom 1992; De Vogli and Santinello 2005; Bolton and Rodriguez 2009), and yet another study found that young women smoked more after becoming unemployed (Hammarström and Janlert 2003). An international comparison has shown that gender differences in the effects of unemployment on health differ in Ireland and Sweden. This finding suggests that the positions and the roles of men and women in the labor market and in the family are important factors explaining the negative consequences of the negative consequences of unemployment on health (Strandh et al. 2013).

Unlike education, a clear gender gap favoring men with respect to both employment and salary level continues to exist in most industrialized countries, albeit with different magnitudes (Peracchi 2001). Some observers have pointed to the uneven evolution of the gender gaps in education and labor market participation as a sign that the gender revolution is incomplete (McDonald 2000). The magnitude of the gender differences in labor market participation levels vary substantially across EU countries (Eurostat 2016). In 2014, the gap between the male and the female employment rates at ages 20–64 was 10.5% units for the whole EU-27, with Malta having the largest (25.4% units) and Finland having the smallest (1.5% units) gap. The mostly analyzed factor that explore ways to reduce this gap is the type of welfare state. Mandel and Semyonov (2006) showed that countries with a more family-oriented welfare state or with a large public service sector have relatively high female labor force participation levels, and concluded that "the impact of the state on women's employment opportunities is multidimensional and can be attributed to a series of factors, especially to the roles of the state as a legislator, as a provider of social services, and as an employer." The authors emphasized that the more women are integrated into the paid economy of a country, the higher the level of female empowerment is in the society. However, the integration of women into the labor market must be accompanied by a reduction in gender inequalities in individual wages (Weichselbaumer and Winter-Ebmer 2005; Arulampalam et al. 2007), and in the vertical segregation of the labor market to further reduce gender inequalities in both employment and salary level.

Conclusions and Future Research Directions

This review has shown that there is a growing body of research literature that has examined sex differences in health and mortality. Most existing studies on sex differences in mortality have focused on high-income countries. Meanwhile, relatively little research on this issue has been conducted in middle- and low-income countries. As more high-quality data become available, researchers will be able to investigate whether sex differences in mortality in these countries follow patterns similar to those that have been observed in high-income countries; and to examine how the magnitude of sex disparities in a given country is related to its economic development level. There is a growing need for research that summarizes recent trends in sex differences in mortality by causes of death and in specific geographic regions, such as the eastern and central EU countries, the Baltic states, Transcaucasia, and the other former Soviet republics; as well as in the most populous countries of the world, India and China.

Since health is a multidimensional concept, is not surprising that there is an increasing amount of evidence suggesting that gender differences in health vary in their directions and magnitudes. The selection of a health measure in a research study often depends on data availability. Thus, we need to gain a better understanding of how subjective and objective measures are interrelated, and how predictive these measures are of mortality at both the individual and the population levels. Solé-Auró and Crimmins showed that the best-performing countries with respect to life expectancy are not the countries that report the highest levels of health (Solé-Auró and Crimmins 2013). A similar analysis that looks at sex differences in health and in mortality may show that patterns are mixed, but it may also suggest there are some individual- and macro-level factors that affect health in women and survival in men differently.

In the epidemiological, social, and demographic studies that have so far been conducted, investigations of social disparities in health and mortality have yielded the most consistent evidence. However, less is known about the magnitude of gender differences in health and mortality across educational and socioeconomic status groups, and how changes in these gaps over the life course contribute to explanations of sex differences in mortality. Although a plethora of research has investigated the effects of marriage and reproduction on individual health and mortality risks, the number of studies that have focused on sex differences in these outcomes by childbearing status and marital status is limited.

Previous research has indicated that some migrant groups are healtheir and live longer than the host country population, the so called "healthy migrant effect" (Razum and Twardella 2002; Hedlund et al. 2008; Hill et al. 2012). It has been suggested that the health advantages of immigrants diminish at older ages and among the second generation (Sundquist and Winkleby 1999; De Maio 2010); and that these advantages vary substantially by cause of death, country of birth/origin (Stirbu et al. 2006; Wild et al. 2007; Boulogne et al. 2012), and the health measure used (Sundquist and Johansson 1997; Pudaric et al. 2003; Llacer et al. 2007; Nielsen and Krasnik 2010). While there is a large body of research on health and mortality by migration background, there is a dearth of research examining the health and the mortality of migrants through a gender lens.

It is also important that we continue an existing line of research that has been investigating the role of biological factors in explaining sex differences in health and mortality. The emotional stress associated with spousal loss has been found to negatively affect immune defenses at older ages (Khanfer et al. 2011). Considering the female advantage in immunity, it is important to investigate whether changes in immune responses due to spousal bereavement are sex-specific, and whether these differences might partially explain excess mortality and worse health outcomes after widowhood among men than among women. This issue is also an example of how biological (immune defenses) and social factors (change in marital status) may modify sex differences in health, and of how the use of multidisciplinary approaches could provide additional explanations for sex differences in health and mortality.

References

Albano, J. D., Ward, E., Jemal, A., Anderson, R., Cokkinides, V. E., Murray, T., et al. (2007). Cancer mortality in the United States by education level and race. *Journal of the National Cancer Institute, 99*(18), 1384–1394.

Alexandersen, P., Haarbo, J., et al. (1996). The relationship of natural androgens to coronary heart disease in males: A review. *Atherosclerosis, 125*(1), 1–13.

Alfaro-Acha, A., Snih, S. A., et al. (2006). Handgrip strength and cognitive decline in older Mexican Americans. *The Journals of Gerontology Series A: Biological Sciences and Medical Sciences, 61*(8), 859–865.

Alonso-Nanclares, L., Gonzalez-Soriano, J., et al. (2008). Gender differences in human cortical synaptic density. *Proceedings of the National Academy of Sciences, 105*(38), 14615–14619.

Aluja-Fabregat, A., Colom, R., et al. (2000). Sex differences in general intelligence defined as g among young adolescents. *Personality and Individual Differences, 28*(4), 813–820.

Amos, A., Greaves, L., Nichter, M., & Bloch, M. (2011). Women and tobacco: A call for including gender in tobacco control research, policy and practice. *Tobacco Control, 21,* 236–243.

Anand, S. S., Xie, C. C., et al. (2005). Differences in the management and prognosis of women and men who suffer from acute coronary syndromes. *Journal of the American College of Cardiology, 46*(10), 1845–1851.

Andersen, K. K., Andersen, Z. J., et al. (2011). Predictors of early and late case-fatality in a nationwide Danish study of 26 818 patients with first-ever ischemic stroke. *Stroke, 42*(10), 2806–2812.

Angst, J., Gamma, A., et al. (2002). Toward validation of atypical depression in the community: Results of the Zurich cohort study. *Journal of Affective Disorders, 72*(2), 125–138.

Ankney, D. C. (1992). Sex differences in relative brain size: The mismeasure of woman, too? *Intelligence, 16*(3–4), 329–336.

Appelros, P., Stegmayr, B., et al. (2009). Sex differences in stroke epidemiology: A systematic review. *Stroke, 40*(4), 1082–1090.

Appelros, P., Stegmayr, B., et al. (2010). A review on sex differences in stroke treatment and outcome. *Acta Neurologica Scandinavica, 121*(6), 359–369.

Araujo, A. B., Dixon, J. M., et al. (2011). Endogenous testosterone and mortality in men: A systematic review and meta-analysis. *The Journal of Clinical Endocrinology & Metabolism, 96*(10), 3007–3019.

Arulampalam, W., Booth, A. L., & Bryan, M. L. (2007). Is there a glass ceiling over Europe? Exploring the gender pay gap across the wage distribution. *ILR Review, 60*(2), 163–186.

Ayala, C., Croft, J. B., et al. (2002). Sex differences in US mortality rates for stroke and stroke subtypes by race/ethnicity and age, 1995–1998. *Stroke, 33*(5), 1197–1201.

Babiker, F. A., De Windt, L. J., et al. (2002). Estrogenic hormone action in the heart: Regulatory network and function. *Cardiovascular Research, 53*(3), 709–719.

Bairey, N. C. M., Johnson, B. D., et al. (2003). Hypoestrogenemia of hypothalamic origin and coronary artery disease in premenopausal women: A report from the NHLBI-sponsored WISE study. *Journal of the American College of Cardiology, 41*(3), 413–419.

Baker, D. P., & Jones, D. P. (1993). Creating gender equality: Cross-national gender stratification and mathematical performance. *Sociology of Education, 66*(2), 91–103.

Baker, A. H., & Wardle, J. (2003). Sex differences in fruit and vegetable intake in older adults. *Appetite, 40*(3), 269–275.

Barefoot, J. C., Mortensen, E. L., et al. (2001). A longitudinal study of gender differences in depressive symptoms from age 50 to 80. *Psychology and Aging, 16*(2), 342–345.

Barford, A., Dorling, D., et al. (2006). Life expectancy: Women now on top everywhere. *BMJ, 332*(7545), 808.

Barnes, L. L., Wilson, R. S., et al. (2003). Gender, cognitive decline, and risk of AD in older persons. *Neurology, 60*(11), 1777–1781.

Barrett, K. M., Brott, T. G., et al. (2007). Sex differences in stroke severity, symptoms, and Deficits after first-ever ischemic stroke. *Journal of Stroke and Cerebrovascular Diseases, 16*(1), 34–39.

Bassil, N., Alkaade, S., et al. (2009). The benefits and risks of testosterone replacement therapy: A review. *Therapeutics and Clinical Risk Management, 5,* 427–448.

Bauman, A., Bull, F., Chey, T., Craig, C. L., Ainsworth, B. E., Sallis, J. F., et al. (2009). The international prevalence study on physical activity: Results from 20 countries. *International Journal of Behavioral Nutrition and Physical Activity, 6*(1), 6–21.

Bebbington, P. E., Dunn, G., et al. (1998). The influence of age and sex on the prevalence of depressive conditions: Report from the National Survey of Psychiatric Morbidity. *Psychological Medicine, 28*(1), 9–19.

Beltrán-Sánchez, H., Finch, C. E., et al. (2015). Twentieth century surge of excess adult male mortality. *Proceedings of the National Academy of Sciences, 112*(29), 8993–8998.

Benyamini, Y., Leventhal, E. A., & Leventhal, H. (2000). Gender differences in processing information for making self-assessments of health. *Psychosomatic Medicine, 62*(3), 354–364.

Bere, E., Brug, J., & Klepp, K. I. (2008). Why do boys eat less fruit and vegetables than girls? *Public health nutrition, 11*(3), 321–325.

Berrino, F., De Angelis, R., et al. (2007). Survival for eight major cancers and all cancers combined for European adults diagnosed in 1995–99: Results of the EUROCARE-4 study. *The Lancet Oncology, 8*(9), 773–783.

Bisegger, C., Cloetta, B., von Bisegger, U., Abel, T., & Ravens-Sieberer, U. (2005). Health-related quality of life: Gender differences in childhood and adolescence. *Sozial-und Präventivmedizin, 50*(5), 281–291.

Bjarnason, T., & Sigurdardottir, T. J. (2003). Psychological distress during unemployment and beyond: Social support and material deprivation among youth in six northern European countries. *Social Science and Medicine, 56*(5), 973–985.

Bjerkeset, O., Romundstad, P., et al. (2008). Gender differences in the association of mixed anxiety and depression with suicide. *The British Journal of Psychiatry, 192*(6), 474–475.

Blomkalns, A. L., Chen, A. Y., et al. (2005). Gender disparities in the diagnosis and treatment of non-ST-segment elevation acute coronary syndromes Large-scale observations from the CRUSADE (Can rapid risk stratification of unstable angina patients suppress adverse outcomes with early implementation of the American College of Cardiology/American Heart Association Guidelines) National Quality Improvement Initiative. *Journal of the American College of Cardiology, 45*(6), 832–837.

Bloomfield, K., Gmel, G., & Wilsnack, S. (2006). Introduction to special issue 'Gender, culture and alcohol problems: a multi-national study'. *Alcohol and Alcoholism, 41*(suppl 1), i3–i7.

Bohannon, R. W., Peolsson, A., et al. (2006). Reference values for adult grip strength measured with a Jamar dynamometer: A descriptive meta-analysis. *Physiotherapy, 92*(1), 11–15.

Bolton, K. L., & Rodriguez, E. (2009). Smoking, drinking and body weight after re-employment: Does unemployment experience and compensation make a difference? *BMC Public Health, 9*(1), 77.

Borraccino, A., Lemma, P., Iannotti, R., Zambon, A., Dalmasso, P., Lazzeri, G., et al. (2009). Socio-economic effects on meeting PA guidelines: Comparisons among 32 countries. *Medicine and Science in Sports and Exercise, 41*(4), 749–756.

Boulogne, R., Jougla, E., et al. (2012). Mortality differences between the foreign-born and locally-born population in France (2004–2007). *Social Science and Medicine, 74*(8), 1213–1223.

Bouman, A., Heineman, M. J., et al. (2005). Sex hormones and the immune response in humans. *Human Reproduction Update, 11*(4), 411–423.

Bowling, A., Bond, M., et al. (2001). Equity in access to exercise tolerance testing, coronary angiography, and coronary artery bypass grafting by age, sex and clinical indications. *Heart, 85*(6), 680–686.

Brådvik, L., Mattisson, C., et al. (2008). Long-term suicide risk of depression in the Lundby cohort 1947–1997—severity and gender. *Acta Psychiatrica Scandinavica, 117*(3), 185–191.

Burgaleta, M., Head, K., et al. (2012). Sex differences in brain volume are related to specific skills, not to general intelligence. *Intelligence, 40*(1), 60–68.

Bush, T. L. (1990). The epidemiology of cardiovascular disease in postmenopausal women. *Annals of the New York Academy of Sciences, 592*(1), 263–271.

Butler, A. A., Menant, J. C., et al. (2009). Age and gender differences in seven tests of functional mobility. *Journal of NeuroEngineering and Rehabilitation, 6*(1), 1–9.

Cacciani, L., Bargagli, A. M., Cesaroni, G., Forastiere, F., Agabiti, N., & Davoli, M. (2015). Education and mortality in the Rome longitudinal study. *PLoS ONE, 10*(9), e0137576.

Cairney, J., & Wade, T. J. (2002). The influence of age on gender differences in depression further population-based evidence on the relationship between menopause and the sex difference in depression. *Social Psychiatry and Psychiatric Epidemiology, 37*(9), 401–408.

Case, A., & Paxson, C. (2005). Sex differences in morbidity and mortality. *Demography, 42*(2), 189–214.

Cawthon, P. M., Fox, K. M., et al. (2009). Do muscle mass, muscle density, strength, and physical function similarly influence risk of hospitalization in older adults? *Journal of the American Geriatrics Society, 57*(8), 1411–1419.

Centers for Disease Control and Prevention (CDC). (2012). Current cigarette smoking among adults-United States, 2011. *MMWR. Morbidity and mortality weekly report, 61*(44), 889.

Chlebowski, R. T., Hendrix, S. L., et al. (2003). Influence of estrogen plus progestin on breast cancer and mammography in healthy postmenopausal women: The women's health initiative randomized trial. *JAMA, 289*(24), 3243–3253.

Cleland, J. (2010). The benefits of educating women. *The Lancet, 376*(9745), 933–934.

Cohen, F., Kemeny, M. E., et al. (2007). Immune function declines with unemployment and recovers after stressor termination. *Psychosomatic Medicine, 69*(3), 225–234.

Colom, R., Juan-Espinosa, M., et al. (2000). Negligible sex differences in general intelligence. *Intelligence, 28*(1), 57–68.

Conti, G., Heckman, J., & Urzua, S. (2010). The education-health gradient. *The American Economic Review, 100*(2), 234–238.

Cook, M. B., Dawsey, S. M., et al. (2009). Sex disparities in cancer incidence by period and age. *Cancer Epidemiology, Biomarkers and Prevention, 18*(4), 1174–1182.

Cook, M. B., McGlynn, K. A., et al. (2011). Sex disparities in cancer mortality and survival. *Cancer Epidemiology, Biomarkers and Prevention, 20*(8), 1629–1637.

Cooper, R., Hardy, R., et al. (2011). Age and gender differences in physical capability levels from mid-life onwards: The harmonisation and meta-analysis of data from eight UK cohort studies. *PLoS ONE, 6*(11), e27899.

Costanza, M. C., Salamun, J., Lopez, A. D., & Morabia, A. (2006). Gender differentials in the evolution of cigarette smoking habits in a general European adult population from 1993–2003. *BMC Public Health, 6,* 130.

Courtenay, W. H. (2000). Constructions of masculinity and their influence on men's well-being: A theory of gender and health. *Social Science and Medicine, 50*(10), 1385–1401.

Crimmins, E. M., Kim, J. K., et al. (2011). Gender differences in health: Results from SHARE, ELSA and HRS. *The European Journal of Public Health, 21*(1), 81–91.

Crimmins, E. M., & Saito, Y. (2001). Trends in healthy life expectancy in the United States, 1970–1990: Gender, racial, and educational differences. *Social Science and Medicine, 52,* 1629–1641.

Crossley, M., D'Arcy, C., et al. (1997). Letter and category fluency in community-dwelling canadian seniors: A comparison of normal participants to those with dementia of the Alzheimer or vascular type. *Journal of Clinical and Experimental Neuropsychology, 19*(1), 52–62.

Cutler, J. A., Sorlie, P. D., et al. (2008). Trends in hypertension prevalence, awareness, treatment, and control rates in United States adults between 1988–1994 and 1999–2004. *Hypertension, 52* (5), 818–827.

Dahlgren, G., & Whitehead, M. (1991). *Policies and strategies to promote social equity in health.* Stockholm, Sweden.

Dahlin, J., & Härkönen, J. (2013). Cross-national differences in the gender gap in subjective health in Europe: Does country-level gender equality matter? *Social Science and Medicine, 98,* 24–28.

Danesh, J., Collins, R., et al. (1998). Association of fibrinogen, c-reactive protein, albumin, or leukocyte count with coronary heart disease: Meta-analyses of prospective studies. *JAMA, 279*(18), 1477–1482.

de Frias, C. M., Nilsson, L.-G., et al. (2006). Sex differences in cognition are stable over a 10-year period in adulthood and old age. *Aging, Neuropsychology, and Cognition, 13*(3–4), 574–587.

De Maio, F. (2010). Immigration as pathogenic: A systematic review of the health of immigrants to Canada. *International Journal for Equity in Health, 9*(1), 27.

De Visser, R. O., & McDonnell, E. J. (2012). 'That's OK. He's a guy': A mixed-methods study of gender double-standards for alcohol use. *Psychology and Health, 27*(5), 618–639.

De Visser, R. O., & Smith, J. A. (2007). Alcohol consumption and masculine identity among young men. *Psychology and Health, 22*(5), 595–614.

De Vogli, R., & Santinello, M. (2005). Unemployment and smoking: Does psychosocial stress matter? *Tobacco Control, 14*(6), 389–395.

Deaton, A. (2008). Income, health and wellbeing around the world: Evidence from the gallup world poll. *The Journal of Economic Perspectives: A Journal of the American Economic Association, 22*(2), 53–72.

Dehghan, M., Akhtar-Danesh, N., & Merchant, A. T. (2011). Factors associated with fruit and vegetable consumption among adults. *Journal of Human Nutrition & Dietetics, 24*(2), 128–134.

Denton, M., Prus, S., & Walters, V. (2004). Gender differences in health: A Canadian study of the psychosocial, structural and behavioural determinants of health. *Social Science and Medicine, 58*(12), 2585–2600.

Di Carlo, A., Lamassa, M., et al. (2003). Sex differences in the clinical presentation, resource use, and 3-month outcome of acute stroke in Europe: Data from a multicenter multinational hospital-based registry. *Stroke, 34*(5), 1114–1119.

Djernes, J. K. (2006). Prevalence and predictors of depression in populations of elderly: A review. *Acta Psychiatrica Scandinavica, 113*(5), 372–387.

Dodds, R., Denison, H. J., et al. (2012). Birth weight and muscle strength: A systematic review and meta-analysis. *The Journal of Nutrition, Health & Aging, 16*(7), 609–615.

Dodds, R. M., Syddall, H. E., et al. (2014). Grip strength across the life course: Normative data from twelve British studies. *PLoS ONE, 9*(12), e113637.

Dorak, M. T., & Karpuzoglu, E. (2012). Gender differences in cancer susceptibility: An inadequately addressed issue. *Frontiers in Genetics, 3,* 268.

Dueñas, M., Ramirez, C., Arana, R., & Failde, I. (2011). Gender differences and determinants of health related quality of life in coronary patients: A follow-up study. *BMC Cardiovascular Disorders, 11*(1), 11–24.

Edgren, G., Liang, L., et al. (2012). Enigmatic sex disparities in cancer incidence. *European Journal of Epidemiology, 27*(3), 187–196.

Eikemo, T. A., Huisman, M., Bambra, C., & Kunst, A. E. (2008). Health inequalities according to educational level in different welfare regimes: A comparison of 23 European countries. *Sociology of Health & Illness, 30*(8), 565–582.

Else-Quest, N. M., Hyde, J. S., et al. (2010). Cross-national patterns of gender differences in mathematics: A meta-analysis. *Psychological Bulletin, 136*(1), 103–127.

Erhart, M., Ottova, V., et al. (2009). Measuring mental health and well-being of school-children in 15 European countries using the KIDSCREEN-10 index. *International Journal of Public Health, 54*(2), 160–166.

European Commission. (2009). *Women in science*. Luxembourg: Office for Official Publications of the European Communities.

Eurostat (2016). Equality (Age and Gender): Gender Equality: Labour Market: Employment and activity by sex and age - annual data. http://ec.europa.eu/eurostat/web/equality/data/database Accessed 15 March 2016.

Ferlay, J., Steliarova-Foucher, E., et al. (2013). Cancer incidence and mortality patterns in Europe: Estimates for 40 countries in 2012. *European Journal of Cancer, 49*(6), 1374–1403.

Fernández-Balsells, M. M., Murad, M. H., et al. (2010). Adverse effects of testosterone therapy in adult men: A systematic review and meta-analysis. *The Journal of Clinical Endocrinology & Metabolism, 95*(6), 2560–2575.

Frederiksen, H., Hjelmborg, J., et al. (2006). Age trajectories of grip strength: Cross-sectional and longitudinal data among 8,342 Danes aged 46 to 102. *Annals of Epidemiology, 16*(7), 554–562.

Freedman, D. S., Otvos, J. D., et al. (2004). Sex and age differences in lipoprotein subclasses measured by nuclear magnetic resonance spectroscopy: The Framingham study. *Clinical Chemistry, 50*(7), 1189–1200.

Fujita, Y., Nakamura, Y., et al. (1995). Physical-strength tests and mortality among visitors to health-promotion centers in Japan. *Journal of Clinical Epidemiology, 48*(11), 1349–1359.

Gakidou, E., Cowling, K., Lozano, R., & Murray, C. J. (2010). Increased educational attainment and its effect on child mortality in 175 countries between 1970 and 2009: A systematic analysis. *The Lancet, 376*(9745), 959–974.

Galatius, J. S., Launbjerg, J., et al. (1996). Sex related differences in short and long term prognosis after acute myocardial infarction: 10 year follow up of 3073 patients in database of first Danish verapamil infarction trial. *BMJ, 313*(7050), 137–140.

Gale, C. R., Martyn, C. N., et al. (1996). Cognitive impairment and mortality in a cohort of elderly people. *BMJ, 312*(7031), 608–611.

Galobardes, B., Shaw, M., Lawlor, D. A., Lynch, J. W., & Smith, G. D. (2006). Indicators of socioeconomic position (part 1). *Journal of Epidemiology and Community Health, 60*(1), 7–12.

Gerstorf, D., Herlitz, A., et al. (2006). Stability of sex differences in cognition in advanced old age: The role of education and attrition. *The Journals of Gerontology Series B: Psychological Sciences and Social Sciences, 61*(4), P245–P249.

Ghisletta, P. (2008). Application of a joint multivariate longitudinal-survival analysis to examine the terminal decline hypothesis in the Swiss interdisciplinary longitudinal study on the oldest old. *Journals of Gerontology. Series B, Psychological Sciences and Social Sciences, 63*(3), P185–P192.

Giampaoli, S., Ferrucci, L., et al. (1999). Hand-grip strength predicts incident disability in non-disabled older men. *Age and Ageing, 28*(3), 283–288.

Giatti, L., Barreto, S. M., et al. (2008). Household context and self-rated health: The effect of unemployment and informal work. *Journal of Epidemiology and Community Health, 62*(12), 1079–1085.

Giefing-Kröll, C., Berger, P., et al. (2015). How sex and age affect immune responses, susceptibility to infections, and response to vaccination. *Aging Cell, 14*(3), 309–321.

Gjonca, A., Tomassini, C., et al. (2005). Sex differences in mortality, a comparison of the United Kingdom and other developed countries. *Health Statistics Quarterly, 26,* 6–16.

Glei, D. A., & Horiuchi, S. (2007). The narrowing sex differential in life expectancy in high-income populations: Effects of differences in the age pattern of mortality. *Population Studies (Cambridge), 61*(2), 141–159.

Go, A. S., Mozaffarian, D., et al. (2013). Heart disease and stroke statistics—2013 update: A report from the american heart association. *Circulation, 127*(1), e6–e245.

Gold, C. H., Malmberg, B., et al. (2002). Gender and health: A study of older unlike-sex twins. *Journals of Gerontology. Series B, Psychological Sciences and Social Sciences, 57*(3), S168–S176.

Gough, B., & Conner, M. T. (2006). Barriers to healthy eating amongst men: A qualitative analysis. *Social Science and Medicine, 62*(2), 387–395.

Grady, D., Herrington, D., et al. (2002). Cardiovascular disease outcomes during 6.8 years of hormone therapy: Heart and estrogen/progestin replacement study follow-up (hers ii). *JAMA, 288*(1), 49–57.

Grady, D., Rubin, S. M., et al. (1992). Hormone therapy to prevent disease and prolong life in postmenopausal women. *Annals of Internal Medicine, 117*(12), 1016–1037.

Grigoriadis, S., & Erlick Robinson, G. (2007). Gender issues in depression. *Annals of Clinical Psychiatry, 19*(4), 247–255.

Guiso, L., Monte, F., et al. (2008). Culture, gender, and math. *Science-New York Then Washington, 320*(5880), 1164.

Haddad, R. M., Kennedy, C. C., et al. (2007). Testosterone and cardiovascular risk in men: A systematic review and meta-analysis of randomized placebo-controlled trials. *Mayo Clinic Proceedings, 82*(1), 29–39.

Halpern, D. F., Benbow, C. P., Geary, D. C., Gur, R. C., Hyde, J. S., & Gernsbacher, M. A. (2016). The science of sex differences in science and mathematics. *Psychological Science in the Public Interest, 8*(1), 1–51.

Hammarström, A., & Janlert, U. (1997). Nervous and depressive symptoms in a longitudinal study of youth unemployment—Selection or exposure? *Journal of Adolescence, 20*(3), 293–305.

Hammarström, A., & Janlert, U. (2003). Unemployment—An important predictor for future smoking: A 14-year follow-up study of school leavers. *Scandinavian Journal of Public Health, 31,* 229–232.

Hankin, B. L., Abramson, L. Y., et al. (1998). Development of depression from preadolescence to young adulthood: Emerging gender differences in a 10-year longitudinal study. *Journal of Abnormal Psychology, 107*(1), 128–140.

Haring, R., Völzke, H., et al. (2010). Low serum testosterone levels are associated with increased risk of mortality in a population-based cohort of men aged 20–79. *European Heart Journal, 31,* 1494–1501.

Harris, T. B., Ferrucci, L., et al. (1999). Associations of elevated Interleukin-6 and C-reactive protein levels with mortality in the elderly. *The American Journal of Medicine, 106*(5), 506–512.

Haveman-Nies, A., Burema, J., Cruz, J. A. A., Osler, M., & van Staveren, W. A. (2002). Dietary quality and lifestyle factors in relation to 10-year mortality in older Europeans: The SENECA study. *American Journal of Epidemiology, 156*(10), 962–968.

Hawkins, N. M., Jhund, P. S., et al. (2012). Heart failure and socioeconomic status: Accumulating evidence of inequality. *European Journal of Heart Failure, 14*(2), 138–146.

Hedlund, E., Pehrsson, K., et al. (2008). Country of birth and survival after a first myocardial infarction in Stockholm, Sweden. *European Journal of Epidemiology, 23*(5), 341–347.

Heiss, G., Wallace, R., et al. (2008). Health risks and benefits 3 years after stopping randomized treatment with estrogen and progestin. *JAMA, 299*(9), 1036–1045.

Herlitz, A., & Rehnman, J. (2008). Sex differences in episodic memory. *Current Directions in Psychological Science, 17*(1), 52–56.

Herman, B., Greiser, E., et al. (1997). A sex difference in short-term survival after initial acute myocardial infarction. The MONICA-Bremen acute myocardial infarction register, 1985–1990. *European Heart Journal, 18*(6), 963–970.

Hill, T., Angel, J., et al. (2012). Does the "Healthy immigrant effect" extend to cognitive aging? In J. L. Angel, F. Torres-Gil, & K. Markides (Eds.), *Aging, health, and longevity in the mexican-origin population* (pp. 19–33). US: Springer.

Hitchman, S. C., & Fong, G. T. (2011). Gender empowerment and female-to-male smoking prevalence ratios. *Bulletin of the World Health Organization, 89*(3), 195–202.

HMD Human Mortality Database. University of California, Berkeley and Max Planck Institute for Demographic Research. www.mortality.org.

Holmegard, H. N., Nordestgaard, B. G., et al. (2016). Sex hormones and ischemic stroke: A prospective cohort study and meta-analyses. *The Journal of Clinical Endocrinology & Metabolism, 101*(1), 69–78.

Holroyd-Leduc, J. M., Kapral, M. K., et al. (2000). Sex differences and similarities in the management and outcome of stroke patients. *Stroke, 31*(8), 1833–1837.

Huxley, R., Barzi, F., et al. (2006). Excess risk of fatal coronary heart disease associated with diabetes in men and women: Meta-analysis of 37 prospective cohort studies. *BMJ, 332*(7533), 73–78.

Hyde, J. S., & Linn, M. C. (1988). Gender differences in verbal ability: A meta-analysis. *Psychological Bulletin, 104*(1), 53–69.

Hyde, J. S., Mezulis, A. H., et al. (2008). The ABCs of depression: Integrating affective, biological, and cognitive models to explain the emergence of the gender difference in depression. *Psychological Review, 115*(2), 291–313.

Idler, E. L. (2003). Gender differences in self-rated health, in mortality, and in the relationship between the two. *Gerontologist, 43*(3), 372–375.

Iezzoni, L. I., Ash, A. S., et al. (1997). Differences in procedure use, in-hospital mortality, and illness severity by gender for acute myocardial infarction patients: Are answers affected by data source and severity measure? *Medical Care, 35*(2), 158–171.

Il'yasova, D., Colbert, L. H., et al. (2005). Circulating levels of inflammatory markers and cancer risk in the health aging and body composition cohort. *Cancer Epidemiology, Biomarkers and Prevention, 14*(10), 2413–2418.

Innes, E. (1999). Handgrip strength testing: A review of the literature. *Australian Occupational Therapy Journal, 46*(3), 120–140.

Isaksson, R.-M., Jansson, J.-H., et al. (2011). Better long-term survival in young and middle-aged women than in men after a first myocardial infarction between 1985 and 2006. An analysis of

8630 patients in the Northern Sweden MONICA study. *BMC Cardiovascular Disorders, 11*(1), 1–8.

Janlert, U., & Hammarstrom, A. (1992). Alcohol consumption among unemployed youths: Results from a prospective study. *British Journal of Addiction, 87,* 703–714.

Jaussent, I., Dauvilliers, Y., et al. (2011). Insomnia symptoms in older adults: Associated factors and gender differences. *The American Journal of Geriatric Psychiatry, 19*(1), 88–97.

Johnson, J. V. (2009). The growing imbalance: Class, work and health in an era of increasing inequality. In P. L. Schnall, M. Dobson, & E. Rosskam (Eds.), *Unhealthy work: Causes, consequences, cures* (pp. 37–59). Amityville, NY: Baywood.

Jousilahti, P., Vartiainen, E., et al. (1999). Sex, age, cardiovascular risk factors, and coronary heart disease: A prospective follow-up study of 14 786 middle-aged men and women in Finland. *Circulation, 99*(9), 1165–1172.

Jylhä, M. (2009). What is self-rated health and why does it predict mortality? Towards a unified conceptual model. *Social Science and Medicine, 69,* 307–316.

Kaptoge, S., Di Angelantonio, E., et al. (2010). C-reactive protein concentration and risk of coronary heart disease, stroke, and mortality: An individual participant meta-analysis. *Lancet, 375*(9709), 132–140.

Kardys, I., Vliegenthart, R., et al. (2007). The female advantage in cardiovascular disease: Do vascular beds contribute equally? *American Journal of Epidemiology, 166*(4), 403–412.

Keevil, V. L., Hayat, S., et al. (2013). The physical capability of community-based men and women from a British cohort: The European prospective investigation into cancer (EPIC)-Norfolk study. *BMC Geriatrics, 13*(1), 1–11.

Kelly, D. M., & Jones, T. H. (2014). Testosterone and cardiovascular risk in men. In *Cardiovascular Issues in Endocrinology* (Vol. 43).

Khanfer, R., Lord, J. M., & Phillips, A. C. (2011). Neutrophil function and cortisol: DHEAS ratio in bereaved older adults. *Brain, Behavior, and Immunity*, *25*(6), 1182–1186.

Kiefer, I., Rathmanner, T., & Kunze, M. (2013). Eating and dieting differences in men and women. *Journal of Men's Health and Gender, 2*(2), 194–201.

Kjønniksen, L., Anderssen, Nils, & Wold, B. (2009). Organized youth sport as a predictor of physical activity in adulthood. *Scandinavian Journal of Medicine and Science in Sports, 19*(5), 646–654.

Knoops, K. T. B., de Groot, L. C. P. G. M., et al. (2004). Mediterranean diet, lifestyle factors, and 10-year mortality in elderly European men and women the HALE project. *The Journal of the American Medical Association, 292*(12), 1433–1439.

Knopp, R. H., Zhu, X., et al. (1994). Effects of estrogens on lipoprotein metabolism and cardiovascular disease in women. *Atherosclerosis, 110,* S83–S91.

Kockler, M., & Heun, R. (2002). Gender differences of depressive symptoms in depressed and nondepressed elderly persons. *International Journal of Geriatric Psychiatry, 17*(1), 65–72.

Koek, H. L., de Bruin, A., et al. (2006). Short-and long-term prognosis after acute myocardial infarction in men versus women. *The American Journal of Cardiology, 98*(8), 993–999.

Kourlaba, G., & Panagiotakos, D. B. (2009). Dietary quality indices and human health: A review. *Maturitas, 62*(1), 1–8.

Kuehner, C. (2003). Gender differences in unipolar depression: An update of epidemiological findings and possible explanations. *Acta Psychiatrica Scandinavica, 108*(3), 163–174.

Kuroda, A., Kanda, T., & Sakai, F. (2006). Gender differences in health-related quality of life among stroke patients. *Geriatrics and Gerontology International, 6*(3), 165–173.

La Vecchia, C., Bosetti, C., Bertuccio, P., Castro, C., Pelucchi, C., & Negri, E. (2014). Trends in alcohol consumption in Europe and their impact on major alcohol-related cancers. *European Journal of Cancer Prevention, 23*(4), 319–322.

Lavery, L. L., Dodge, H. H., et al. (2009). Cognitive decline and mortality in a community-based cohort: The Monongahela Valley independent elders survey. *Journal of the American Geriatrics Society, 57*(1), 94–100.

Lawlor, D. A., Ebrahim, S., et al. (2001). Sex matters: Secular and geographical trends in sex differences in coronary heart disease mortality. *BMJ, 323*(7312), 541–545.

Leist, A. K., Glymour, M. M., et al. (2013). Time away from work predicts later cognitive function: Differences by activity during leave. *Annals of Epidemiology, 23*(8), 455–462.

LeMasters, T., Madhavan, S., Sambamoorthi, U., & Kurian, S. (2013). A population-based study comparing HRQoL among breast, prostate, and colorectal cancer survivors to propensity score matched controls, by cancer type, and gender. *Psycho-Oncology, 22*(10), 2270–2282.

Leong, D. P., Teo, K. K., et al. (2015). Prognostic value of grip strength: Findings from the Prospective Urban Rural Epidemiology (PURE) study. *The Lancet, 386*(9990), 266–273.

Lerner, D. J., & Kannel, W. B. (1986). Patterns of coronary heart disease morbidity and mortality in the sexes: A 26-year follow-up of the Framingham population. *American Heart Journal, 111*(2), 383–390.

Lewsey, J. D., Gillies, M., et al. (2009). Sex differences in incidence, mortality, and survival in individuals with stroke in Scotland, 1986 to 2005. *Stroke, 40*(4), 1038–1043.

Libert, C., Dejager, L., et al. (2010). The X chromosome in immune functions: When a chromosome makes the difference. *Nature Reviews Immunology, 10*(8), 594–604.

Lindahl-Jacobsen, R., Hanson, H. A., et al. (2013). The male–female health-survival paradox and sex differences in cohort life expectancy in Utah, Denmark, and Sweden 1850–1910. *Annals of Epidemiology, 23*(4), 161–166.

Lindahl-Jacobsen, R., Rau, R., et al. (2016). Rise, stagnation, and rise of Danish women's life expectancy. *PNAS, 113,* 4015–4020.

Lindberg, S. M., Hyde, J. S., et al. (2010). New trends in gender and mathematics performance: A meta-analysis. *Psychological Bulletin, 136*(6), 1123–1135.

Ling, C. H. Y., Taekema, D., et al. (2010). Handgrip strength and mortality in the oldest old population: The Leiden 85-plus study. *Canadian Medical Association Journal, 182*(5), 429–435.

Linn, M. C., & Petersen, A. C. (1985). Emergence and characterization of sex differences in spatial ability: A meta-analysis. *Child Development, 56*(6), 1479–1498.

Llacer, A., Zunzunegui, M. V., et al. (2007). The contribution of a gender perspective to the understanding of migrants' health. *Journal of Epidemiology and Community Health, 61*(Suppl 2), ii4–10.

Löllgen, H., Böckenhoff, A., & Knapp, G. (2009). Physical activity and all-cause mortality: An updated meta-analysis with different intensity categories. *International Journal of Sports Medicine, 30*(3), 213–224.

Lyon, M. F. (1962). Sex chromatin and gene action in the mammalian X-chromosome. *American Journal of Human Genetics, 14*(2), 135–148.

Lyons, A. C. (2009). Masculinities, femininities, behaviour and health. *Social and Personality Psychology Compass, 3*(4), 394–412.

MacDonald, N. E., Halperin, B., et al. (2006). Infectious disease management: Lessons from Cuba. *The Canadian Journal of Infectious Diseases & Medical Microbiology, 17*(4), 217.

Macintyre, S., Hunt, K., et al. (1996). Gender differences in health: Are things really as simple as they seem? *Social Science and Medicine, 42*(4), 617–624.

Macintyre, K., Stewart, S., et al. (2001). Gender and survival: A population-based study of 201,114 men and women following a first acute myocardial infarction. *Journal of the American College of Cardiology, 38*(3), 729–735.

Madigan, F. C., & Vance, R. B. (1957). Differential sex mortality: A research design. *Social Forces, 35*(3), 193–199.

Maier, H., McGue, M., et al. (2003). Cognitive impairment and survival at older ages. In *Brain and longevity* (pp. 131–144). Springer.

Mandel, H., & Semyonov, M. (2006). A Welfare State Paradox: State interventions and women's employment opportunities in 22 Countries. *American Journal of Sociology, 111*(6), 1910–49.

Marmot, M. G. (2005). Social determinants of health inequalities. *The Lancet, 365,* 1099–1104.

Martikainen, P., Mäkelä, P., et al. (2014). Income differences in life expectancy: The changing contribution of harmful consumption of alcohol and smoking. *Epidemiology, 25*(2), 182–190.

McCartney, G., Mahmood, L., Leyland, A. H., Batty, G. D., & Hunt, K. (2011). Contribution of smoking-related and alcohol-related deaths to the gender gap in mortality: Evidence from 30 European countries. *Tobacco Control, 20*(2), 166–168.

McDaniel, A. (2011). *Gender differences in university completion across Europe: The influence of family background and national context*. Working paper, Institute for Social and Economic Research and Policy.

McDonald, P. (2000). Gender equity in theories of fertility transition. *Population and Development Review, 26*(3), 427–440.

McDougall, F. A., Kvaal, K., et al. (2007). Prevalence of depression in older people in England and wales: The MRC CFA study. *Psychological Medicine, 37*(12), 1787–1795.

McGee, D. L., Liao, Y., et al. (1999). Self-reported health status and mortality in a multiethnic US cohort. *American Journal of Epidemiology, 149,* 41–46.

McKee-Ryan, F. M., Song, Z., et al. (2005). Psychological and physical well-being during unemployment: A meta-analytic study. *Journal of Applied Psychology, 90*(1), 53–76.

Mendelsohn, M. E., & Karas, R. H. (2005). Molecular and cellular basis of cardiovascular gender differences. *Science, 308*(5728), 1583–1587.

Merrill, S. S., Seeman, T. E., Kasl, S. V., & Berkman, L. F. (1997). Gender differences in the comparison of self-reported disability and performance measures. *The Journals of Gerontology Series A: Biological Sciences and Medical Sciences, 52*(1), M19–M26.

Micheli, A., Mariotto, A., et al. (1998). The prognostic role of gender in survival of adult cancer patients. *European Journal of Cancer, 34*(14), 2271–2278.

Migeon, B. R. (1994). X-chromosome inactivation: Molecular mechanisms and genetic consequences. *Trends in Genetics, 10*(7), 230–235.

Migeon, B. R. (2007). Why females are mosaics, x-chromosome inactivation, and sex differences in disease. *Gender Medicine, 4*(2), 97–105.

Mijnarends, D. M., Meijers, J. M. M., et al. (2013). Validity and reliability of tools to measure muscle mass, strength, and physical performance in community-dwelling older people: A systematic review. *Journal of the American Medical Directors Association, 14*(3), 170–178.

Milcent, C., Dormont, B., et al. (2007). Gender differences in hospital mortality and use of percutaneous coronary intervention in acute myocardial infarction: Microsimulation analysis of the 1999 nationwide French hospitals database. *Circulation, 115*(7), 833–839.

Miller, D. I., & Halpern, D. F. (2014). The new science of cognitive sex differences. *Trends in Cognitive Sciences, 18*(1), 37–45.

Miller, V. T., LaRosa, J., et al. (1995). Effects of estrogen or estrogen/ progestin regimens on heart disease risk factors in postmenopausal women: The postmenopausal estrogen/progestin interventions (PEPI) trial. *JAMA, 273*(3), 199–208.

Morris, J. A., & Harrison, L. M. (2009). Hypothesis: Increased male mortality caused by infection is due to a decrease in heterozygous loci as a result of a single X chromosome. *Medical Hypotheses, 72*(3), 322–324.

Mucha, L., Stephenson, J., Morandi, N., & Dirani, R. (2006). Meta-analysis of disease risk associated with smoking, by gender and intensity of smoking. *Gender Medicine, 3*(4), 279–291.

Murtagh, K. N., & Hubert, H. B. (2004). Gender differences in physical disability among an elderly cohort. *American Journal of Public Health, 94*(8), 1406–1411.

Murray, E. T., Hardy, R., Strand, B. H., Cooper, R., Guralnik, J. M., & Kuh, D. (2011). Gender and life course occupational social class differences in trajectories of functional limitations in midlife: Findings from the 1946 British birth cohort. *The Journals of Gerontology Series A: Biological Sciences and Medical Sciences*, *66*(12), 1350–1359.

Newcombe, M. A., McCarthy, M. B., Cronin, J. M., & McCarthy, S. N. (2012). Eat like a man. A social constructionist analysis of the role of food in men's lives. *Appetite, 59*(2), 391–398.

Newman, A. B., & Brach, J. S. (1999). Gender gap in longevity and disability in older persons. *Health, 23*(2), 343–350.

Nielsen, S., Björck, L., et al. (2014). Sex-specific trends in 4-year survival in 37 276 men and women with acute myocardial infarction before the age of 55 years in Sweden, 1987–2006: A register-based cohort study. *British Medical Journal Open, 4*(5), e004598.

Nielsen, S., & Krasnik, A. (2010). Poorer self-perceived health among migrants and ethnic minorities versus the majority population in Europe: A systematic review. *International Journal of Public Health, 55*(5), 357–371.

Nieschlag, E., Behre, H. M., et al. (2004). Testosterone replacement therapy: Current trends and future directions. *Human Reproduction Update, 10*(5), 409–419.

Nikula, S., Jylhä, M., Bardage, C., Deeg, D. J., Gindin, J., Minicuci, N., et al. (2003). Are IADLs comparable across countries? Sociodemographic associates of harmonized IADL measures. *Aging Clinical and Experimental Research, 15*(6), 451–459.

Nolen-Hoeksema, S. (2001). Gender differences in depression. *Current Directions in Psychological Science, 10*(5), 173–176.

Nolen-Hoeksema, S., & Girgus, J. S. (1994). The emergence of gender differences in depression during adolescence. *Psychological Bulletin, 115*(3), 424–443.

Oksuzyan, A., Brønnum-Hansen, H., et al. (2010a). Gender gap in health expectancy. *European Journal of Ageing, 7*(4), 213–218.

Oksuzyan, A., Crimmins, E., et al. (2010b). Cross-national comparison of sex differences in health and mortality in Denmark, Japan and the US. *European Journal of Epidemiology, 25*(7), 471–480.

Oksuzyan, A., Juel, K., et al. (2008). Men: Good health and high mortality. Sex differences in health and aging. *Aging Clinical and Experimental Research, 20*(2), 91–102.

Oksuzyan, A., Maier, H., et al. (2010c). Sex differences in the level and rate of change of physical function and grip strength in the Danish 1905-cohort study. *Journal of Aging and Health, 22,* 589–610.

Oksuzyan, A., Shkolnikova, M., et al. (2015). Sex differences in biological markers of health in the study of stress, aging and health in Russia. *PLoS ONE, 10*(6), e0131691.

Oliver, M. F., & Boyd, G. S. (1959). Effect of bilateral ovariectomy on coronary-artery disease and serum-lipid levels. *The Lancet, 274*(7105), 690–694.

Olsen, T. S., Andersen, Z. J., et al. (2012). Explaining poorer stroke outcomes in women: Women surviving 3 months have more severe strokes than men despite a lower 3-month case fatality. *Gender Medicine, 9*(3), 147–153.

Ortega, F. B., Silventoinen, K., et al. (2012). Muscular strength in male adolescents and premature death: Cohort study of one million participants. *BMJ, 345,* e7279.

Owens, I. P. F. (2002). Ecology and evolution: Sex differences in mortality rate. *Science, 297*(5589), 2008–2009.

Palacios-Cena, D., Jimenez-Garcia, R., et al. (2012). Has the prevalence of disability increased over the past decade (2000–2007) in elderly people? A Spanish population-based survey. *Journal of the American Medical Directors Association, 13*(2), 136–142.

Pampel, F. C. (2006). Global patterns and determinants of sex differences in smoking. *International Journal of Comparative Sociology, 47*(6), 466–487.

Pavlik, V. N., de Moraes, S. A., et al. (2003). Relation between cognitive function and mortality in middle-aged adults: The atherosclerosis risk in communities study. *American Journal of Epidemiology, 157*(4), 327–334.

Penedo, F. J., & Dahn, J. R. (2005). Exercise and well-being: A review of mental and physical health benefits associated with physical activity. *Current opinion in psychiatry, 18*(2), 189–193.

Pennell, L. M., Galligan, C. L., et al. (2012). Sex affects immunity. *Journal of Autoimmunity, 38*(2–3), J282–J291.

Peracchi, F. (2001). Earnings inequality in international perspective. In *The causes and consequences of increasing inequality* (pp. 117–192).

Perna, L., Wahl, H.-W., et al. (2015). Cognitive impairment, all-cause and cause-specific mortality among non-demented older adults. *Age and Ageing, 44*(3), 445–451.

Petrea, R. E., Beiser, A. S., et al. (2009). Gender differences in stroke incidence and poststroke disability in the framingham heart study. *Stroke, 40*(4), 1032–1037.

Piccinelli, M., & Wilkinson, G. (2000). Gender differences in depression: Critical review. *The British Journal of Psychiatry, 177*(6), 486–492.

Pongiglione, B., & Sabater, A. (2014). The role of education at young and older ages in explaining health inequalities in Europe. *Population, Space and Place, 22,* 255–275.

Preston, S. H., & Glei, D. A., et al. (2011). Contribution of smoking to international differences in life expectancy. In *International differences in mortality at older ages: Dimensions and sources* (pp. 105–131).

Prossnitz, E. R., & Maggiolini, M. (2009). Mechanisms of estrogen signaling and gene expression via GPR30. *Molecular and Cellular Endocrinology, 308*(1–2), 32–38.

Pudaric, S., Sundquist, J., et al. (2003). Country of birth, instrumental activities of daily living, self-rated health and mortality: A Swedish population-based survey of people aged 55–74. *Social Science and Medicine, 56*(12), 2493–2503.

Rantanen, T., Guralnik, J. M., et al. (1999). Midlife hand grip strength as a predictor of old age disability. *JAMA, 281*(6), 558–560.

Rantanen, T., Harris, T., et al. (2000). Muscle strength and body mass index as long-term predictors of mortality in initially healthy men. *Journals of Gerontology. Series A, Biological Sciences and Medical Sciences, 55*(3), M168–M173.

Raphael, D. (2004). *Social determinants of health: Canadian perspectives*. Toronto: Canadian Scholars' Press.

Razum, O., & Twardella, D. (2002). Time travel with Oliver Twist. *Tropical Medicine & International Health, 7*(1), 4–10.

Reeves, M. J., Bushnell, C. D., et al. (2008). Sex differences in stroke: Epidemiology, clinical presentation, medical care, and outcomes. *The Lancet Neurology, 7*(10), 915–926.

Rehm, J., Mathers, C., Popova, S., Thavorncharoensap, M., Teerawattananon, Y., & Patra, J. (2009). Global burden of disease and injury and economic cost attributable to alcohol use and alcohol-use disorders. *The Lancet, 373*(9682), 2223–2233.

Reilly, D. (2012). Gender, culture, and sex-typed cognitive abilities. *PLoS ONE, 7*(7), e39904.

Reine, I., Novo, M., et al. (2013). Unemployment and ill health—A gender analysis: Results from a 14-year follow-up of the Northern Swedish Cohort. *Public Health, 127*(3), 214–222.

Rigby, J. E., & Dorling, D. (2007). Mortality in relation to sex in the affluent world. *Journal of Epidemiology and Community Health, 61*(2), 159–164.

Rivera, C. M., Grossardt, B. R., et al. (2009). Increased cardiovascular mortality following early bilateral oophorectomy. *Menopause (New York, NY), 16*(1), 15–23.

Roberts, H. C., Denison, H. J., et al. (2011). A review of the measurement of grip strength in clinical and epidemiological studies: Towards a standardised approach. *Age and Ageing, 40*(4), 423–429.

Roberts, R. E., Shema, S. J., et al. (2000). Sleep complaints and depression in an aging cohort: A prospective perspective. *American Journal of Psychiatry, 157*(1), 81–88.

Robinson, S., & Harris, H. (2011). *Smoking and drinking among adults, 2009*.

Roelfs, D. J., Shor, E., et al. (2011). Losing life and livelihood: A systematic review and meta-analysis of unemployment and all-cause mortality. *Social Science and Medicine, 72*(6), 840–854.

Rogers, R. G., & Powell-Griner, E. (1991). Life expectancies of cigarette smokers and nonsmokers in the United States. *Social Science and Medicine, 32*(10), 1151–1159.

Roquer, J., Campello, A. R., et al. (2003). Sex differences in first-ever acute stroke. *Stroke, 34*(7), 1581–1585.

Ross, M. T., Grafham, D. V., et al. (2005). The DNA sequence of the human X chromosome. *Nature, 434*(7031), 325–337.

Ross, C. E., Masters, R. K., & Hummer, R. A. (2012). Education and the gender gaps in health and mortality. *Demography, 49*(4), 1157–1183.

Rossouw, J. E., Anderson, G. L., et al. (2002). Risks and benefits of estrogen plus progestin in healthy postmenopausal women: Principal results from the Women's Health Initiative randomized controlled trial. *JAMA, 288*(3), 321–333.

Ruige, J. B., Mahmoud, A. M., et al. (2011). Endogenous testosterone and cardiovascular disease in healthy men: A meta-analysis. *Heart, 97*, 870–875.

Rushton, J. P., & Ankney, C. D. (2009). Whole brain size and general mental ability: A review. *International Journal of Neuroscience, 119*(5), 692–732.

Sandberg, K., & Ji, H. (2012). Sex differences in primary hypertension. *Biology of Sex Differences, 3*(1), 7.

Sasaki, H., Kasagi, F., et al. (2007). Grip strength predicts cause-specific mortality in middle-aged and elderly persons. *The American Journal of Medicine, 120*(4), 337–342.

Schaap, L. A., Pluijm, S. M. F., et al. (2009). Higher inflammatory marker levels in older persons: Associations with 5-year change in muscle mass and muscle strength. *The Journals of Gerontology Series A: Biological Sciences and Medical Sciences, 64A*(11), 1183–1189.

Schooling, C. M. (2015). Could androgens be relevant to partly explain why men have lower life expectancy than women? *Journal of Epidemiology and Community Health, 70,* 324–328.

Schupf, N., Tang, M. X., et al. (2005). Decline in cognitive and functional skills increases mortality risk in nondemented elderly. *Neurology, 65*(8), 1218–1226.

Shaw, M., Maxwell, R., et al. (2004). Gender and age inequity in the provision of coronary revascularisation in England in the 1990s: Is it getting better? *Social Science and Medicine, 59*(12), 2499–2507.

Singh, T., & Newman, A. B. (2011). Inflammatory markers in population studies of aging. *Ageing Research Reviews, 10*(3), 319–329.

Singh-Manoux, A., Gueguen, A., et al. (2007). Self-rated health and mortality: Short and long term associations in the Whitehall II Study. *Psychosomatic Medicine, 69,* 138–143.

Sjöström, M., Oja, P., Hagströmer, M., Smith, B. J., & Bauman, A. (2006). Health-enhancing physical activity across European Union countries: The Eurobarometer study. *Journal of Public Health, 14*(5), 291–300.

Smith, G. D. (1996). Income inequality and mortality: Why are they related? *BMJ. British Medical Journal, 312*(7037), 987–988.

Smith, G. D., Hart, C., Hole, D., MacKinnon, P., Gillis, C., Watt, G., et al. (1998). Education and occupational social class: Which is the more important indicator of mortality risk? *Journal of Epidemiology and Community Health, 52*(3), 153–160.

Smith, D. B., Murphy, P., et al. (2009). Gender differences in the Colorado stroke registry. *Stroke, 40*(4), 1078–1081.

Solé-Auró, A., & Crimmins, E. M. (2013). The oldest old health in Europe and the United States. *Annual Review of Gerontology and Geriatrics, 33*(1), 1–33.

Spolarics, Z. (2007). The X-files of inflammation: Cellular mosaicism of X-linked polymorphic genes and the female advantage in the host response to injury and infection. *Shock, 27*(6), 597–604.

Stahre, M. R., Roeber, J., Kanny, D., Brewer, R. D., & Zhang, X. (2014). Contribution of excessive alcohol consumption to deaths and years of potential life lost in the United States. *Preventing Chronic Disease, 11,* E109.

Stampfer, M. J., & Colditz, G. A. (1991). Estrogen replacement therapy and coronary heart disease: A quantitative assessment of the epidemiologic evidence. *Preventive Medicine, 20*(1), 47–63.

Stirbu, I., Kunst, A. E., et al. (2006). Differences in avoidable mortality between migrants and the native Dutch in the Netherlands. *BMC Public Health, 6*(1), 78.

Strandh, M., Hammarström, A., et al. (2013). Unemployment, gender and mental health: The role of the gender regime. *Sociology of Health & Illness, 35*(5), 649–665.

Sundquist, J., & Johansson, S.-E. (1997). Long-term illness among indigenous and foreign-born people in Sweden. *Social Science and Medicine, 44*(2), 189–198.

Sundquist, J., & Winkleby, M. A. (1999). Cardiovascular risk factors in Mexican American adults: A transcultural analysis of NHANES III, 1988–1994. *American Journal of Public Health, 89*(5), 723–730.

Syddall, H., Cooper, C., et al. (2003). Is grip strength a useful single marker of frailty? *Age and Ageing, 32,* 650–656.

Taekema, D. G., Gussekloo, J., et al. (2010). Handgrip strength as a predictor of functional, psychological and social health. A prospective population-based study among the oldest old. *Age and Ageing, 39*(3), 331–337.

Tapp, A. L., Maybery, M. T., et al. (2011). Evaluating the twin testosterone transfer hypothesis: A review of the empirical evidence. *Hormones and Behavior, 60*(5), 713–722.

Thorslund, M., Wastesson, J., et al. (2013). The rise and fall of women's advantage: A comparison of national trends in life expectancy at age 65 years. *European Journal of Ageing, 10,* 1–7.

Trovato, F., & Heyen, N. B. (2006). A varied pattern of change of the sex differential in survival in the G7 countries. *Journal of Biosocial Science, 38*(3), 391–401.

Vaccarino, V., Badimon, L., et al. (2010). Ischaemic heart disease in women: Are there sex differences in pathophysiology and risk factors? Position paper from the working group on coronary pathophysiology and microcirculation of the European society of cardiology. *Cardiovascular Research, 90,* 9–17.

Vaccarino, V., Horwitz, R. I., et al. (1998). Sex differences in mortality after myocardial infarction: Evidence for a sex-age interaction. *Archives of Internal Medicine, 158*(18), 2054–2062.

Vaccarino, V., Krumholz, H. M., et al. (2001). Sex differences in 2-year mortality after hospital discharge for myocardial infarction. *Annals of Internal Medicine, 134*(3), 173–181.

Vaccarino, V., Lin, Z. Q., et al. (2003). Gender differences in recovery after coronary artery bypass surgery. *Journal of the American College of Cardiology, 41*(2), 307–314.

Vaccarino, V., Parsons, L., et al. (1999). Sex-based differences in early mortality after myocardial infarction. *New England Journal of Medicine, 341*(4), 217–225.

Vallin, J. (2006). Mortality, sex, and gender. In G. Caselli, J. Vallin, & G. Wunsch (Eds.), *Demography: Analysis and synthesis* (Vol. II, pp. 177–194). Amsterdam, Boston, Heidelberg, London, New York, Oxford, Paris, San Diego, San Francisco, Singapore, Sydney, Tokyo: Elsevier.

van Bavel, J. (2011). The impact of a Mediterranean diet and healthy lifestyle on premature mortality in men and women. *The American Journal of Clinical Nutrition, 94,* 913–920.

van der Sluis, S., Posthuma, D., et al. (2006). Sex differences on the Dutch WAIS-III. *Intelligence, 34*(3), 273–289.

Van Oyen, H., Cox, B., et al. (2010). Gender gaps in life expectancy and expected years with activity limitations at age 50 in the European Union: Associations with macro-level structural indicators. *European Journal of Ageing, 7,* 229–237.

Van Oyen, H., Nusselder, W., et al. (2012). Gender differences in healthy life years within the EU: An exploration of the "health–survival" paradox. *International Journal of Public Health, 58* (1), 143–155.

Verbrugge, L. M., & Jette, A. M. (1994). The disablement process. *Social Science and Medicine, 38*(1), 1–14.

Vilhjalmsson, R., & Kristjansdottir, G. (2003). Gender differences in physical activity in older children and adolescents: The central role of organized sport. *Social Science and Medicine, 56* (2), 363–374.

Virtanen, P., Vahtera, J., et al. (2008). Employment trajectory as determinant of change in health-related lifestyle: the prospective HeSSup study. *The European Journal of Public Health, 18*(5), 504–508.

Vitale, C., Mendelsohn, M. E., et al. (2009). Gender differences in the cardiovascular effect of sex hormones. *Nature Reviews Cardiology, 6*(8), 532–542.

Von Dem Knesebeck, O., Verde, P. E., & Dragano, N. (2006). Education and health in 22 European countries. *Social Science and Medicine, 63*(5), 1344–1351.

Voyer, D., Voyer, S., et al. (1995). Magnitude of sex differences in spatial abilities: A meta-analysis and consideration of critical variables. *Psychological Bulletin, 117*(2), 250–270.

Waldron, I. (1983). Sex differences in human mortality: The role of genetic factors. *Social Science and Medicine, 17*(6), 321–333.

Waldron, I. (1993). Recent trends in sex mortality ratios for adults in developed countries. *Social Science and Medicine, 36*(4), 451–462.

Warburton, D. E., Nicol, C. W., & Bredin, S. S. (2006). Health benefits of physical activity: The evidence. *Canadian Medical Association Journal, 17*(6), 801–809.

Wardle, J., Haase, A. M., Steptoe, A., Nillapun, M., Jonwutiwes, K., & Bellisie, F. (2004). Gender differences in food choice: The contribution of health beliefs and dieting. *Annals of Behavioral Medicine, 27*(2), 107–116.

Weber, D., Skirbekk, V., et al. (2014). The changing face of cognitive gender differences in Europe. *Proceedings of the National Academy of Sciences, 111*(32), 11673–11678.

Whitacre, C. C. (2001). Sex differences in autoimmune disease. *Nature Immunology, 2*(9), 777–780.

WHO. (2016). What are social determinants of health? Retrieved June 16, 2016.

Wild, S. H., Fischbacher, C., et al. (2007). Mortality from all causes and circulatory disease by country of birth in England and Wales 2001–2003. *Journal of Public Health, 29*(2), 191–198.

Wilkinson, R. G., & Marmot, M. G. (2003). *Social determinants of health: The solid facts*.

Wingard, D. L., Suarez, L., et al. (1983). The sex differentials in mortality from all causes and ischemic heart disease. *American Journal of Epidemiology, 117*(2), 165–172.

Wise, P. M., Dubal, D. B., et al. (2005). Are estrogens protective or risk factors in brain Injury and neurodegeneration? Reevaluation after the Women's Health Initiative. *Endocrine Reviews, 26*(3), 308–312.

Weichselbaumer, D., & Winter-Ebmer, R. (2005). A meta-analysis of the international gender wage gap. *Journal of Economic Surveys*, *19*(3), 479–511.

Xing, D., Nozell, S., et al. (2009). Estrogen and mechanisms of vascular protection. *Arteriosclerosis, Thrombosis, and Vascular Biology, 29*(3), 289–295.

Xu, L., Freeman, G., et al. (2013). Testosterone therapy and cardiovascular events among men: A systematic review and meta-analysis of placebo-controlled randomized trials. *BMC Medicine, 11*(1), 1–12.

Yaffe, K., Lindquist, K., et al. (2003). Inflammatory markers and cognition in well-functioning African-American and white elders. *Neurology, 61*(1), 76–80.

Yang, X.-P., & Reckelhoff, J. F. (2011). Estrogen, hormonal replacement therapy and cardiovascular disease. *Current Opinion in Nephrology and Hypertension, 20*(2), 133–138.

Zajacova, A. (2006). Education, gender, and mortality: Does schooling have the same effect on mortality for men and women in the US?. *Social Science and Medicine*, *63*(8), 2176–2190.

Zambon, A., Boyce, W., Cois, E., Currie, C., Lemma, P., Dalmasso, P., et al. (2006). Do welfare regimes mediate the effect of socioeconomic position on health in adolescents? *International Journal of Health Services, 36*(2), 309–329.

Part II
Country Specific Chapters

Gender Differences in the Relationship Between Household Position and Health in Twelve European Countries: Are They Associated with the Value Climate?

Gabriele Doblhammer and Jordi Gumà

Introduction

John Donne's (1572–1631) words "No man is an island" form the core of this study of household arrangement and health. The household is the main social entity at the meso-level; it is where men and women decide about their involvement in employment, paid and unpaid work, and caring responsibilities. These decisions are firmly rooted in the macro-level defined by the type of welfare state, which regulates state provisions, tax regimes, transfers to family members, and the opportunity of employment and associated conditions such as flexible and family friendly working arrangements (Boje 2007). The institutional context defines the extent to which the state supports economic independence between the partners and provides formal care for children and the elderly. Decisions are also rooted in prevailing individual values and social norms, concerning family formation, work, and care, all of which influence the climate of values which governs behavior during the social life course and influences the perception and experience of decisions made, such as forming a partnership by cohabiting or marrying, or having children in or outside of marriage. Gender roles define the extent to which deviations from the gendered division of work are feasible and socially accepted (Sayer and Bianchi 2000; Cooke and Gash 2010). Although there appears to be a convergence of gender roles within the household, this process is still unfinished (McDonald 2000;

G. Doblhammer (✉)
Institute for Sociology and Demography, University of Rostock, Rostock, Germany
e-mail: gabriele.doblhammer@uni-rostock.de

J. Gumà
Department of Political and Social Sciences, University Pompeu Fabra, Barcelona, Spain
e-mail: jordi.guma@upf.edu

G. Doblhammer and J. Gumà (eds.), *A Demographic Perspective on Gender, Family and Health in Europe*, https://doi.org/10.1007/978-3-319-72356-3_6

Puur et al. 2008), and there is a lack of adaptation between the demographic behavior of partnership/family formation and the distribution of labor within the family. These macro-level factors must be taken into account when exploring the gendered association between household arrangements and individual health in different countries.

The most studied factors of health are located at the micro-level, the most prominent of which are related to social inequality in terms of education, income, and employment status (Marmot and Wilkinson 1999), life style (see e.g. von der Lippe and Rattay in this volume), and marital status (Waite 1995; Lillard and Waite 1995; Lillard and Panis 1996; Brockmann and Klein 2004; Martikainen et al. 2005). More recently the concept of marital status has expanded to include household arrangements at the meso-level which compile information about the interplay of individuals with other family members within the context of the same household (see also publications from the "Families And Societies" project). Members of a household share the same social and economic situation (Cherlin 2000; Stevenson and Wolfers 2007), and they have to negotiate their division of paid and unpaid work (Hughes and Waite 2002). Micro-level factors such as education and income, however, not only directly impact health but also shape the gender relationships in a household. In many countries women now outnumber men in terms of higher education (Vincent-Lancrin 2008), and there has been a substantial increase in female labor force participation (OECD 2012), which has reduced the differences in participation rates. Nevertheless, women still earn less than men, which is partially explained by their larger involvement in part-time work (OECD 2012). Despite their strong involvement in paid work, women are also still responsible for a disproportionately large share of household work and care, and the division of unpaid work depending on gendered norms and values in societies has changed relatively little (OECD 2012).

Health outcomes at the meso-level may be affected by the fact that in many instances micro-, meso-, and macro-level factors may counterbalance or re-inforce one another, as outlined by Oláh et al. in this volume. They give the example of women's employment, which is more likely to threaten marital stability in a country context of more traditional gender roles with particularly negative health effects for both partners. Sufficient earnings for men and high barriers of labor market entry for women would prevent women from taking up paid work, thereby losing out on the positive effects employment and increased income have on health. Having little support from the state would make employment more stressful for working parents and would reinforce the negative consequences of divorce for the economically dependent spouse.

This study tries to shed more light onto the complex relationship between household arrangements and health by concentrating on the effects of social norms. Regarding social norms, the institutionalization hypothesis originally introduced by Soons and Kalmijn (2009) proposes that in societies with a more flexible value climate, well-being is less influenced by living in a non-traditional family form. We will explore this hypothesis in the context of health, distinguishing between men

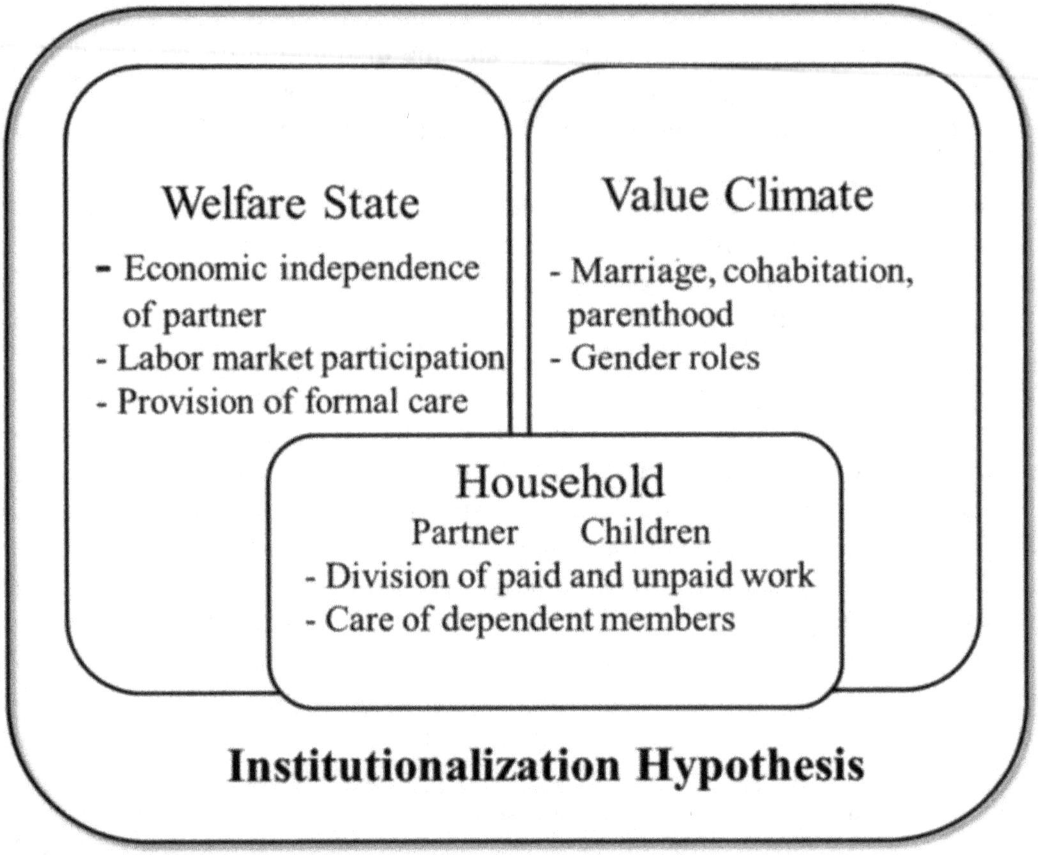

Fig. 1 Framework of the study

and women, and extend it to different family types characterized by the legal status and the presence and/or absence of a partner and of children.

This chapter is structured as follows: First, we briefly discuss health related factors at the individual level. Second, we turn to social norms and values at the macro-level, where we introduce the institutionalization hypothesis in more detail. We close this section by formulating our hypotheses in relation to health. Third, we turn to our own empirical analysis by presenting the data, the analysis strategy, and the results. Finally, we discuss to what extent the results support the institutionalization hypothesis and possible differences according to sex (Fig. 1).

Household Arrangement and Health at the Individual Level

In the European context the household arrangement among young and middle aged adults is primarily characterized by the presence or absence of a partner and/or children. There are large differences in co-residence with the parental generation, which is more widespread in Southern and Eastern Europe. We briefly discuss the health effects of partners and children below.

Partnership Effect on Health

Living with a partner is generally associated with better health (Waite 1995; Martikainen et al. 2005), which can be explained by protective factors due to individual behavior, socio-economic conditions of both partners, and social support. In addition, the selection processes into partnership might favor the healthy candidates. A detailed discussion of these explanations can be found in the overview chapter by Hank and Steinbach in this volume and is taken up in the in-depths studies of the individual countries. Whether various types of partnership, e.g. living in a consensual union or in a marriage, differ in terms oftheir health effects depends foremost on their degree of institutionalization. While marriage is more institutionalized in most countries (Nock 1995), the value climate in (post) modern societies is more open to other forms of living arrangements than in traditional ones (Soons and Kalmijn 2009). It also depends on the spread of divorce and the propensity to enter a consensual union or marriage thereafter. Whereas living with a partner enhances each partners' health status, the termination of a union typically has a short and medium term negative effect on health, due to the disappearance of the protecting factors and the erosion of mental health associated with the process of the worsening of a couple's relationship and the subsequent separation (Waldron et al. 1997; Hughes and Waite 2009). In new partnerships, the positive health levels of the first union are often not regained (Hughes and Waite 2002; Martikainen et al. 2005). Psychological distress preceding divorce as a consequence of the worsening of the relationship between both partners appears to be more prevalent among women, whereas after-divorce depression symptoms appear to be stronger and more long-lasting among men (Williams and Umberson 2004; Rotermann 2007). Again, gender roles play an important part in this, with higher levels of gender inequalities reducing women's future capacity to cope with the consequences of divorce (Gahler 2006).

Children's Effect on Health

The second main family ties within a household are children. Their effect on health differs according to the different stages related to childbirth, infancy, and adolescence, evolving from an initial worsening immediately following the birth due to the process of adaptation to the new family status, to a posterior improvement due to the effect of the increase in both the feeling of responsibility and of social control (Barnett and Hyde 2001; Bernstein 2001). For a general overview about the relationship between the number of children and early/late childbirth, see the chapter by Hank and Steinbach as well as the in-depth study of long-term fertility consequences on health by Tomassini, Di Gessa, and Egidi (both in this volume). However, beyond either pure biological effects in the case of women or variable health stages in men (from a sense of exclusion during pregnancy to improvements once they feel more involved in tasks of caring for the baby; Bartlett 2004), the health effects of children may be strongly shaped by gender roles reflecting the macro environment in terms of the welfare state and the cultural norms, the economic environment, as well as individual characteristics. For instance, children show generally a positive influence on women's health, specifically on mental health (Wang 2004; Helbig et al. 2006). Nevertheless, negative effects have also been observed in diverse countries such as Sweden or Spain in relation to an overload of childcare work (Artazcoz et al. 2001; Floderus et al. 2008).

An important dimension of change in fertility behavior is the upsurge of extramarital childbearing, in connection with new partnership patterns (for a more detailed analysis of new partnership forms, see Buber and Hanappi in this volume). Another is the increase in divorce which leads to larger numbers of single parents, particular among women, who are not engaged in new partnerships. In our own empirical study, we return to the question of whether the effect of children on the health of their parents depends on the type of partnership, i.e. whether parents raising children in consensual unions experience health advantages similar to the married, and whether this effect is modulated by the societal context in different European countries. Thus, we will explore family forms differentiating between the absence and presence of a partner, as well as the legal status of the partnership.

Values and Social Norms, and the Institutionalization Hypothesis

The complexity in studying the relationship between household arrangements and health increases when different countries are compared. The changing demographic behaviors of the Second Demographic Transition (SDT),—e.g. the rise of cohabitation instead of marriage, postponement of parenthood, higher numbers of children born out of marriage, and an increase of the acceptance of divorce (van de Kaa 1994; Lesthaege 1995)—are expanding from Northern and Western Europe to Southern and Eastern Europe with different timing (Surkyn and Lesthaeghe 2004; Liefbroer and Fokkema 2008). However, the demographic behaviors among the forerunners of the SDT do not necessarily anticipate the future pattern in the other countries due to their interplay with prevailing individual values and social norms. They all affect the evolution of the diversification of family patterns within a country as well as the acceptance of these changes (Soons and Kalmijn 2009).

Individual values play an important role when trying to understand why individuals form a certain type of union in terms of cohabitation or marriage, or extramarital childbearing. It has been shown for Europe that the value orientation of individuals is associated with certain family features (Surkyn and Lesthaeghe 2004), e.g. childless cohabitants or single individuals displayed more non-conformist[1] values than their married counterparts. Indeed, married individuals who had ever

[1]Values orientation measured by a set of different dimensions: secularization, vote to new political left, egalitarianism, unconventional civil morality and ethics, accentuation of expressive values and companionship and unconventional marital ethics.

cohabited were more non-conformist than their counterparts who had never cohabited.

In addition to individual values, social norms also influence individuals' preferences for a certain family type. Basically, these norms define how appropriate a certain behavior is, as well as possible sanctions when norms are not adhered to (Liefbroer and Merz 2009; Billari and Liefbroer 2010). These norms compile shared perceptions of social tolerance to age-specific family patterns (e.g. maximum ages at which family transitions should happen or not), how often family transitions must be experienced (e.g. how many children a couple must have), and the sequence of family trajectories (e.g. having children before or after marriage) (Hofäcker and Chaloupková 2014).

Hofäcker and Chaloupková (2014) proposed that current country differences in the degree and pace of the aforementioned family changes could be explained by the different tolerance of their population to deviations from the norms. In this sense, Soons and Kalmijn (2009) introduced the hypothesis of institutionalization. The first part of the hypothesis deals with the cohabitation gap, which states that there is a disadvantage in terms of well-being for the cohabiting compared to the married. Whereas cohabitants might profit from the presence of a partner in a similar way as the married, e.g. health selection into partnership (see Hank and Steinbach in this book), a health-promoting life-style (von der Lippe and Rattay in this book), or the pooling of resources, they might also differ from the married. It has been suggested that they are less likely to be homeowners, are less committed to their relationships, have more conflicts and a worse quality of relationships (see ref. in Soons and Kalmijn 2009).

The second part of the hypothesis states that the cohabiting gap is smaller, or even non-existent, in countries where cohabiting is more frequent. Societies were placed on a continuum from traditional to (post-) modern according to the differences in their value climate, as to how they are less or more accepting of alternative living arrangements. Investigating 30 European countries, Soons and Kalmijn (2009) found strong evidence for their hypothesis.

The Welfare State

When comparing the different countries, we follow the chapter by Olah et al. in this book and distinguish five European welfare state regimes: the *Dual-Earner* welfare state regime with extensive policy provision facilitating a work-life balance for both women and men; the *Liberal* or Market Oriented regime with limited and usually means-tested state support to families and the dominance of market-based solutions regarding welfare provision; the *General Family Support* policy configuration type or Conservative welfare regime in which men's primacy in the labor market has not really been questioned while the range of state support to families and to women aimed at combining paid work and family responsibilities varies greatly across countries; the *Familialistic* or Mediterranean welfare regime with nearly no or extremely limited policy provision to families and pronounced gender role differentiation; and the *Transition Post-Socialist* regime which is also rather heterogeneous in terms of state support to families and to women in terms of combining labor market participation and family life (Esping-Andersen 1998; Hobson and Olah 2006; Neyer 2013).

Aims and Hypotheses

The aim of this study is to assess the association between the different household arrangements and self-perceived health in individuals between 30 and 59 years of age in Europe. We compare twelve countries classified into the five welfare state regimes. Comparing different countries allows us to test whether the health differentials are related to the welfare state types that are associated with different norms and values. Men and women are analyzed separately to capture gender differences according to the norms and values applying to them. We characterize household arrangements by an individual's position within the household instead of using the household as a common context for all members. The position is defined by whether the person shares a household with a partner, children, or another person outside the family nucleus. In addition, we distinguish whether partners live in a consensual union or in a marriage.

We use self-perceived health because it reflects the integral dimension of health recommended by the World Health Organization[2] and has shown the capacity to capture differences in populations with a rather homogenous health profile in terms of objective health, such as is the case for young and middle aged adults. In addition, it has been shown that self-perceived health provides information about the evolution of an individual's health rather than only informing about the current status (Idler and Benyamini 1997; Gumà and Cámara 2014). However, self-perceived health levels differ widely between countries, reflecting not only differences in health but also culture-specific differences in answering health questions in surveys. Thus we do not explore country-differences between the health outcomes related to different household positions but rather the extent of the health gap between the most favorable household position and all others. A large number of studies have shown that the married with two or more children usually have the best health profile (see the chapters of Hank and Steinbach as well as Tomassini, Di Gessa, and Egidi in this volume), thus we use these as the reference group. We developed the following hypotheses extending the institutionalization hypothesis.

First, household position is more important for women's health than for men's due to the prevailing cultural norms and values.

Second, compared to the married living with children, all other household positions are disadvantaged.

Third, the health of individuals living in a consensual union is worse than of those who are married. However, based on the institutionalization hypothesis we

[2]Health is a state of complete physical, mental, and social well-being and not merely the absence of disease or infirmity (WHO 1946).

assume that the more common this partnership form is, the lower the disadvantage. The institutionalization hypothesis might also be true for single mothers.

Fourth, financial deprivation explains some of the disadvantage of those living alone and in particular of single mothers.

Data and Analysis

Data

We used the cross-sectional microdata of the EU statistics on income and living conditions (EU-SILC) in 2012 for twelve selected countries (Spain, Italy, Poland, Hungary, Germany, Austria, France, Netherlands, Denmark, Sweden, Norway, United Kingdom). The survey units are both the household and the individual. The household level contains information on household size, composition, and basic characteristics of household members. The individual level compiles detailed information on demographic, socioeconomic, and general health issues. We restricted our study to ages 30–59. On the one hand, age 30 permits us to distinguish between those who have already started a new family and those who will likely remain in their parents' home. For the set of countries in our study the age of leaving the parental home ranges from 19.9 for Swedish women to 30.3 for Italian men (Eurostat 2016). On the other hand, the upper age boundary avoids the possible bias retirement might have on health (Demakakos et al. 2008). In 2012, the average effective age of male retirement ranged from 59.7 in France to 66.1 in Sweden, and from 59.4 in Austria to 64.3 in Norway (OECD 2016a). We also restricted our sample to native individuals of each country, in order to avoid any possible bias due to a different sociodemographic profile of migrants, as well as heterogeneity among migrants.

Analysis Sample

The sample unit of EU-SILC is the household and we have information about the kind of ties among all its members (partner without children, father, mother, child, other). This implies that it was possible to reconstruct the household position (our variable of interest) for all the interviewees in the survey. In four countries of our analysis (Sweden, Norway, Denmark, and the Netherlands) only one reference person per household answered to the entire questionnaire, which implies that the analysis sample for these countries is considerably lower than for the others.

Table 1 describes the process of individuals included in our analysis (survey sample excluding foreign-born, and sample of individuals included in our analysis) by country and sex.

The percentage of the overall response is high for all the countries with the exception of the United Kingdom, where it is lower due to the accumulation of no information in two of the variables related to socioeconomic status (educational attainment and self-defined household capacity to make ends meet).

Table 1 Survey sample and analysis sample by country and sex

	Survey sample ages 30–59 excluding foreign-born		Analysis sample ages 30–59 excluding foreign born and missing information		Proportion of survey sample	
	Men	Women	Men	Women	Men (%)	Women (%)
Austria	2590	2861	2587	2861	99.9	100.0
Germany	5273	5995	5258	5980	99.7	99.7
Denmark[a]	1244	1372	1214	1339	97.6	97.6
Spain	6502	6875	6353	6716	97.7	97.7
France	5154	5499	5065	5419	98.3	98.5
Hungary	5718	6693	5693	6659	99.6	99.5
Italy	9272	9768	8724	9220	94.1	94.4
Netherlands[a]	2551	2948	2521	2909	98.8	98.7
Norway[a]	1575	1388	1559	1378	99.0	99.3
Poland	6783	7626	6721	7504	99.1	98.4
Sweden[a]	1333	1513	1301	1494	97.6	98.7
United Kingdom	3894	4342	2896	3296	74.4	75.9
Total	51,889	56,880	49,892	54,775	96.2	96.3

[a]The sample is based on the reference individuals who answered all the questions

Household Position

We defined household position according to three criteria: (1) the partnership situation (living or not living with a partner); (2) living with children in the household (no children, one child, two or more children) (3) the relationship with the family nucleus[3] (member of the nucleus or not). We also distinguished between cohabitation and marriage. This categorization results in the following eight household positions and two residual categories: (1) married, no children; (2) married, one child; (3) married 2+ children; (4) cohabiting, no children; (5) cohabiting, children; (6) living alone; (7) adult son/daughter living with parent(s); (8) single parent; (9) married, other; (10) not-married, other. This category of "other", married or not, includes all members of the household (relatives or not of the others) who are neither members of the nucleus nor their children (grandfather/mother, brother/sister-in-law, etc.).

[3]We consider the "family nucleus" as the adult or couple of adults who can be considered as the reference of the household (main person or persons in charge of paid and unpaid work) and who are in the age range of our study (30–59). In the case of multigenerational households, we prioritized the youngest nucleus under the assumption that they are more likely to live with school age children, who need more attention from parents.

Health

We used the question about self-perceived health "What is your state of health in general?" and combined the two answers very good and good into one category which we labelled "good health," and the three answers fair, poor, and very poor into another category labelled "poor health." In a sensitivity analysis we also explored whether assigning the middle category of fair to good health would change our results, which was not the case.

Covariates

We controlled for age by using the three age groups 30–39, 40–49, and 50–59. We used two indicators to account for individual socio-economic status: First, the highest educational attainment (defined by ISCED[4]). The original seven educational levels were aggregated into three categories: lower secondary education or lower (pre-primary education, primary education, and lower secondary education); upper secondary education (upper secondary education and post-secondary non tertiary education); and tertiary education (first stage of tertiary education (not leading directly to an advanced research qualification) and second stage of tertiary education (leading to an advanced research qualification)). Second, we used the self-defined current economic status of the individual (basic labor information on current activity status and on current job). The answers were categorized into: employed (employee working full or part-time), self-employed working full or part-time (including family workers); unemployed; fulfilling domestic tasks and care responsibilities (mainly a female situation in almost all the analyzed countries); and other economically inactive situations (in compulsory military community or service; pupil, student, further training, unpaid work experience; in retirement or in early retirement or has given up business and permanently disabled or/and unfit to work). Although this last group is the aggregation of four possible answers, the majority of individuals belong to the last two previously mentioned groups, due to the age range of analysis.

To test whether financial deprivation may account for some of the differences in health by household position, we used the information on self-defined ability to make ends meet in the household (thinking of your household's total income, is your household able to make ends meet, namely, to pay for its usual necessary expenses?). This question was posed at the household level and we categorized the answers into four categories: with difficulty (with difficulty or great difficulty); with some difficulty; fairly easily; and easily (easily and very easily). Table 2 provides information on all individual level variables.

[4]International Standard Classification of Education.

Table 2 Characteristics of the analysis sample

	Men		Women	
Age	Mean	SD	Mean	SD
	45.4	8.38	45.45	8.41
	N	%	N	%
Subjective health				
Good health	37,970	76.1	40,037	73.1
Poor health	11,922	23.9	14,738	26.9
Education				
Pre-primary and primary	2587	5.2	3093	5.6
Secondary	31,925	64.0	32,818	59.9
Post-secondary/tertiary	15,380	30.8	18,864	34.4
Self-defined current economic status				
Employee	34,076	68.3	33,710	61.5
Self-employed	7316	14.7	4057	7.4
Unemployed	4266	8.6	4586	8.4
Fulfilling domestic tasks and care responsibilities	201	0.4	7025	12.8
Other inactive person	4033	8.1	5397	9.9
Self-defined ability to make ends meet				
With difficulty	12,933	25.9	15,177	27.7
With some difficulty	13,949	28.0	15,514	28.3
Fairly easily	12,770	25.6	13,700	25.0
Easily	10,240	20.5	10,384	19.0
Total	49,892	100.0	54,775	100.0

Macro Variables

To test the institutionalization hypothesis, we used the country-specific proportion of a certain household position as noted in Table 3. To make the results comparable in our multivariate analyses we standardized the proportions over all household positions to mean zero and variance one. In a sensitivity analysis we also standardized the proportions within each household position, which did not change our results.

Analysis Strategy

The analysis strategy comprised three steps. The first step is the descriptive analysis of the household position patterns of the countries. We discuss the results on the level of the welfare state to provide the general picture, even if there are still country differences within the welfare state regions. The second step comprises the multivariate analyses, using logistic regression models of poor health, which explore the health advantage/disadvantage of a specific household position in comparison to the

Table 3 Distribution of household positions by countries and gender

Welfare state	Countries	Married, no children	Married, 1 child	Married 2 + children	Living alone	Son/ daughter	Cohabiting, no children	Cohabiting, children	Single parent	Married, other	Not married, other
Men											
Dual-earner	Denmark	15.1	18.5	20.2	27.0	0.4	7.3	6.1	2.9	1.0	1.4
	Norway	12.5	21.5	18.3	20.7	1.3	7.6	13.6	4.2	0.2	0.2
	Sweden	12.6	21.1	20.7	16.6	0.9	6.3	16.0	4.8		1.0
Liberal	United Kingdom	16.6	27.4	15.4	15.3	5.2	8.2	7.3	2.0	0.6	2.1
General family support	Austria	14.5	32.5	13.7	18.5	6.5	6.6	4.8	1.2	0.8	1.0
	France	12.8	23.4	15.4	15.9	3.5	10.2	14.8	2.2	0.4	1.2
	Germany	17.9	26.1	14.4	26.2	3.8	6.4	3.4	1.1	0.1	0.5
	Netherlands	14.0	26.5	20.5	19.7	1.3	6.9	7.2	2.3	0.4	1.2
Familialistic	Italy	8.7	37.4	15.4	13.0	16.0	2.8	3.5	1.4	0.3	1.6
	Spain	12.5	35.8	15.3	10.2	14.8	4.4	3.0	1.2	0.4	2.3
	Hungary	12.6	36.9	11.7	7.5	13.4	6.0	6.6	2.1	1.2	1.9
Transition post socialist	Poland	13.1	44.6	15.0	6.6	11.3	1.5	1.7	1.0	3.4	1.8
Women											
Dual-earner	Denmark	17.3	21.4	17.0	17.4	0.1	5.5	9.2	10.6	0.4	1.2
	Norway	14.1	21.9	16.2	13.7	0.1	5.7	15.4	12.2	0.2	0.4
	Sweden	15.4	19.8	19.6	11.8	0.3	5.9	15.9	10.4		1.0
Liberal	United Kingdom	17.5	28.4	14.4	8.8	2.0	6.3	6.9	14.3	0.6	0.8

(continued)

Table 3 (continued)

Welfare state	Countries	Married, no children	Married, 1 child	Married 2 + children	Living alone	Son/ daughter	Cohabiting, no children	Cohabiting, children	Single parent	Married, other	Not married, other
General family support	Austria	16.5	34.6	12.7	13.4	2.5	4.5	4.9	9.1	0.9	0.9
	France	15.6	23.8	14.2	11.5	2.0	6.6	14.1	10.9	0.5	0.9
	Germany	21.1	26.1	12.7	21.5	2.0	5.1	2.8	8.2	0.1	0.4
	Netherlands	15.7	29.4	17.8	12.3	0.5	4.8	8.3	9.4	0.1	1.6
Familialistic	Italy	10.7	42.1	14.9	8.5	9.2	2.6	3.0	7.2	0.4	1.5
	Spain	13.3	38.9	14.8	7.0	7.5	3.9	3.6	8.3	0.4	2.3
	Hungary	14.3	36.9	10.9	6.4	4.0	4.0	6.5	13.1	1.4	2.5
Transition post socialist	Poland	14.6	44.4	13.4	5.6	4.3	1.0	1.6	8.4	4.5	2.2

Data source SILC 2012, own calculations

position "married with children" separate for the two sexes and by individual country. All models were controlled for socio-economic characteristics and age. By entering the variable about "financial difficulties in making ends meet" we explored whether economic deprivation may be a mediator that could explain health differences between household positions. The third step consisted of a set of statistical meta-analyses which correlated the frequency of a certain household position in a country with the estimated odds ratio of poor health in comparison to the married with children. Using a relative measure such as the odds ratio rather than the level of poor health solves the problem of country-specific cultural practices and norms in answering health questions. Here we observe the relative difference in health to the married with children, which is independent from the level of health in a given country. The analyses in steps two and three use country information rather than welfare-state-specific information to take full advantage of the heterogeneity between the countries. Descriptive analyses and the multivariate regression models are performed in SPSS; the meta-regression is estimated in Stata using the command "metareg". In the meta-regression the macro variables (= frequency of the household position) is regressed on the parameter estimates of the household positions stemming from the logistic regression models estimated in step two (models without controlling for financial difficulties). The parameter estimates are weighted by their precision, i.e. the inverse of their standard deviation. Results are presented in the form of scatter plots, where the size of a data point represents its precision. The values of parameter Beta are interpreted in terms of standard deviations: e.g. a Beta of 0.05 indicates that a change of one standard deviation in the macro variable increases the parameter estimate of the logistic regression by 0.05 (say from 0.50 to 0.55, which is an increase in the odds ratio from 1.65 to 1.73). In a sensitivity analysis we ran the meta-regression using parameter estimates from the logistic regressions controlled for the effect of financial deprivation. This generally resulted in an attenuation of the correlations (results not shown).

Results

Descriptives

Household positions involving married partners

The most frequent household positions are those involving married partners (Table 3). In all welfare state regimes, the most frequent position among both women and men is "married, 1 child", which is particularly large in the Familialistic and Transition Post Socialist (TPS) countries and lowest in the Nordic Dual-Earner countries. Also for both sexes the position "married, 2+ children" comes second, and tends to be less frequent in the Familialistic and TPS countries.

Living alone and living as son/daughter with parents

For the household positions involving non-married individuals there are clear differences between the welfare state regimes. Overall, men live alone more frequently and they tend to outnumber married men without children and those with more children in the household. Again, the Familialistic and TPS countries are an exception, with low proportions living alone but a considerable number of adults of both sexes living as sons and daughters in the households of their parents. We can observe a group of countries where men living alone are more frequent than their counterparts living in their parents' home (France, Germany, and the United Kingdom); and countries where men living with their parents show higher percentages than those living alone (Spain, Italy, Poland, and Hungary). As this is cross-sectional data, we do not know whether the latter have always been living with their parents or whether they moved back.

Cohabiting and single parents

"Cohabiting, no children" is slightly more common among men than women, "cohabiting, children" appears to be equal among the two sexes. While cohabiting is rather uncommon in the Familialistic and TPS countries, is it quite frequent in the other welfare state regimes, particularly in the Nordic Dual Earner countries but also in France. In all countries, single parent mothers largely outnumber single parent fathers. With the exception of the Nordic Dual-Earner countries and France, they are more frequent than cohabiting mothers; in the Familialistic and TPS countries they are more frequent than women living alone or living as adult daughters with parents. We may hypothesize that after a partnership breaks up women tend to continue living alone with their children whereas men, depending on the welfare state regime, either live alone, go back to their parental home, or enter a cohabitation.

Multivariate Analysis

Health patterns by household position

Starting with the most common household positions, those which involve married partners, we found that married individuals with two or more children are usually the healthiest (Table 4). This holds true for all welfare state regimes and for both sexes, however, with few exceptions the effects were stronger among women. Among married women the health difference according to the number of children living in the household lacked statistical significance in the Nordic Dual-Earner countries (with the exception of the United Kingdom), was particularly pronounced in the Familialistic and TPS countries, but also present in the General Family Support regime. Among married men, differences were statistically significant only in the Familialistic and TPS countries.

Table 4 Odds ratios of poor health by household position and gender

	Dual-earner and liberal									General family support									Familialistic and transition post socialist							
	Denmark		Norway		Sweden		The UK			Austria		France		Germany		Netherlands			Italy		Spain		Hungary		Poland	
	OR	Sig	OR	Sig	OR	Sig	OR	Sig		OR	Sig	OR	Sig	OR	Sig	OR	Sig		OR	Sig	OR	Sig	OR	Sig	OR	Sig
Educational attainment (Ref: Tertiary)		**		*		a		***	Educational attainment (Ref: Tertiary)		***		***		***		***	Educational attainment (Ref: Tertiary)		***		***		***		***
Primary	–	–	4.32		3.35	a			Primary	42.66	**	1.58	**	4.42	***	4.43	***	Primary	3.23	***	2.10	***	2.06	***	2.91	***
Secondary	1.51	**	1.50	**	1.44	a	2.30	***	Secondary	2.45	***	1.52	***	1.78	***	1.87	***	Secondary	2.14	***	1.60	***	1.73	***	1.80	***
Self-defined current economic status (Ref: Employee)		***		***		***		***	Self-defined current economic status (Ref: Employee)		***		***		***		***	Self-defined current economic status (Ref: Employee)		***		***		***		***
Seld-employed	0.76		2.00	**		***	1.10		Seld-employed	1.25		1.01		0.97		0.97		Seld-employed	0.93		0.84		1.08		1.13	*
Unemployed	2.04	*	3.52	**	1.93		3.32	***	Unemployed	5.43	***	1.98	***	3.63	***	2.41	***	Unemployed	2.69	***	2.18	***	1.75	***	1.96	***
Fulfilling domestic tasks	–	–	0.00		4.11		1.25		Fulfilling domestic tasks	1.41		0.90		2.19	*	–	–	Fulfilling domestic tasks	1.53	*	1.91	**	3.33		0.00	
Other inactive	11.39	***	9.11	***	6.75	***	12.33	***	Other inactive	9.03	***	2.79	***	6.44	***	13.38	***	Other inactive	11.12	***	3.67	***	7.23	***	11.47	***
Men																										
Household position (Ref: married, 2 + children)	1.00		1.00		1.00		1.00		Household position (Ref: married, 2 + children)	1.00		1.00		1.00		1.00		Household position (Ref: married, 2 + children)	1.00		1.00		1.00		1.00	
Married no children	1.83		1.38		0.94		0.86		Married no children	1.12		1.22		1.05		1.75	a	Married no children	1.64	**	1.54	a	1.45	*	1.25	*
Married, 1 child	2.58	**	1.12		1.12		0.91		Married, 1 child	1.38	*	1.05		1.03		1.87	*	Married, 1 child	1.20	a	1.44		1.15		1.06	
Living alone	3.00	***	1.67	*	1.58	a	2.05	***	Living alone	1.42	*	1.39	a	1.52	***	1.99	***	Living alone	1.59	**	1.50	a	1.52	*	1.47	*
Son/daughter	2.39		–	–	–	–	1.21		Son/daughter	1.55	a	1.58	a	1.13		–	–	Son/daughter	1.48	a	1.76	*	1.40	a	1.36	*
Cohabiting, no children	1.58		0.98		1.11		0.92		Cohabiting, no children	0.85		1.13		0.80		2.28		Cohabiting, no children	1.11		1.75	a	1.34		1.17	
Cohabiting, children	4.22	***	1.26		0.88		1.17		Cohabiting, children	0.66		1.17		1.32		1.56		Cohabiting, children	1.17		1.15		1.17		1.32	
Single parent	0.59		1.82	a	0.85		1.32		Single parent	1.52		0.93		1.35		1.60		Single parent	1.07		1.76		1.06		1.26	

(continued)

Table 4 (continued)

	Dual-earner and liberal							
	Denmark		Norway		Sweden		The UK	
	OR	Sig	OR	Sig	OR	Sig	OR	Sig
Married, other	2.24		–	–	–	–	0.14	
Not married, other	2.67		–	–	–	–	2.91	*
Constant	0.07	***	0.07	***	0.07	***	0.05	***
Nagelkerke R square	0.25		0.17		0.09		0.28	
N	1214		1559		1301		2896	
Seld-employed	0.56		1.11			***	0.94	
Unemployed	3.10	***	3.64	**	3.31	***	2.85	***
Fulfilling domestic tasks	–	–	2.66	a	0.82		2.10	***
Other inactive	8.05	***	12.63	***	7.03	***	9.01	***
Women								
Household position (Ref: married, 2 + children)	1.00		1.00		1.00		1.00	
Married no children	1.10		1.26		1.30		1.44	*
Married, 1 child	0.99		1.40		1.29		1.78	**
Living alone	1.31	*	1.86	*	1.43		3.67	***
Son/daughter	–	–	–	–	–	–	3.19	***
Cohabiting, no children	1.19		1.21		1.34		1.68	*
Cohabiting, children	0.93		0.99		1.45		2.32	***
Single parent	1.21		2.84	***	3.16	***	2.58	***
Married, other	–	–	–	–	–	–	0.71	
Not married, other	1.92		–	–	–	–	2.97	a

	General family support							
	Austria		France		Germany		Netherlands	
	OR	Sig	OR	Sig	OR	Sig	OR	Sig
Married, other	20.46	***	0.97		1.67		–	–
Not married, other	1.91		1.89	*	0.79		1.66	
Constant	0.06	***	0.12	***	0.08	***	0.04	***
Nagelkerke R square	0.25		0.09		0.21		0.21	
N	2587		5065		5258		2521	
Seld-employed	0.76		0.84		1.10		0.92	
Unemployed	3.98	***	1.53	**	4.38	***	3.92	***
Fulfilling domestic tasks	1.33		1.23		1.28	a	2.09	***
Other inactive	5.45	***	2.52	***	7.49	***	7.10	***
Household position (Ref: married, 2 + children)	1.00		1.00		1.00		1.00	
Married no children	2.19	***	1.35	*	1.43	**	1.11	a
Married, 1 child	1.75	**	1.41	*	1.11		1.34	a
Living alone	2.46	***	1.68	***	1.76	***	3.02	***
Son/daughter	1.99		1.24		1.75	*	–	–
Cohabiting, no children	1.09		1.21		1.26		0.91	
Cohabiting, children	1.58		0.99		1.31		1.40	
Single parent	2.57	***	1.89	***	1.50	**	2.60	***
Married, other	5.43	a	5.38	**	1.52		–	–
Not married, other	2.78		3.31	*	1.38		0.78	

	Familialistic and transition post socialist							
	Italy		Spain		Hungary		Poland	
	OR	Sig	OR	Sig	OR	Sig	OR	Sig
Married, other	1.96	**	5.70	*	1.20		1.04	
Not married, other	2.62	***	1.41		0.98		1.19	
Constant	0.04	***	0.03	***	0.05	***	0.10	***
Nagelkerke R square	0.14		0.24		0.33		0.26	
N	8724		6353		5693		6721	
Seld-employed	0.77	**	1.12		0.99		1.50	**
Unemployed	2.71	***	1.84	***	2.11	***	1.60	***
Fulfilling domestic tasks	1.77	***	1.59	***	1.29	*	1.38	***
Other inactive	4.51	***	2.80	***	4.41	***	6.95	***
Household position (Ref: married, 2 + children)	1.00		1.00		1.00		1.00	
Married no children	1.74	***	1.49	***	1.89	***	1.46	*
Married, 1 child	1.35	***	1.52	***	1.59	***	1.34	**
Living alone	2.18	***	1.68	***	2.77	***	1.78	***
Son/daughter	1.64	***	2.36	***	2.59	***	1.66	***
Cohabiting, no children	2.34	a	1.95	a	1.76	***	1.42	*
Cohabiting, children	1.66	*	1.30	*	1.69	**	1.74	a
Single parent	2.22	***	2.06	***	2.46	***	1.66	***
Married, other	2.69	***	2.14	***	1.52	*	1.13	
Not married, other	1.90	***	2.25	***	2.96	***	1.90	**

(continued)

Table 4 (continued)

	Dual-earner and liberal									General family support									Familialistic and transition post socialist							
	Denmark		Norway		Sweden		The UK			Austria		France		Germany		Netherlands			Italy		Spain		Hungary		Poland	
	OR	Sig	OR	Sig	OR	Sig	OR	Sig		OR	Sig	OR	Sig	OR	Sig	OR	Sig		OR	Sig	OR	Sig	OR	Sig	OR	Sig
Age group (Ref: 30-39)		***				***		***	Age group (Ref: 30-39)		***		***		***			Age group (Ref: 30-39)		***		***		***		***
40-49	1.79	**	1.29		1.16		1.37	***	40-49	1.98	***	1.34	**	1.79	***	1.07		40-49	2.86	***	1.70	***	2.86	***	2.22	***
50–59	2.96	***	1.39		2.50	***	2.10	***	50–59	1.93	***	1.74	***	2.53	***	1.58	a	50–59	6.44	***	2.66	***	6.44	***	4.00	***
Constant	0.10	***	0.06	***	0.04	***	0.05	***	Constant	0.05	***	0.12	***	0.09	***	0.08	***	Constant	0.04	***	0.03	***	0.04	***	0.10	***
Nagelkerke R square	0.23		0.28		0.19		0.23		Nagelkerke R square	0.19		0.11		0.19		0.23		Nagelkerke R square	0.12		0.18		0.31		0.27	
N	1339		1378		1494		3296		N	2861		5419		5980		2909		N	9220		6716		6659		7504	

Data source SILC 2012, own calculations
Controlled for age; education; economic status
*** < 0.001; ** < 0.01; * < 0.05; [a] < 0.1

Compared to married individuals with children, those living alone or with their parents are generally disadvantaged in their health, independent of the welfare state regime. Effect sizes are particularly large and highly significant in the Familialistic and TPS countries, and women appear to be even more affected than men. Another highly disadvantaged group is single mothers—independent of the welfare state regime they suffer exceptional worse health than their married counterparts. For men the effect is neither consistent nor significant, probably due to small sample sizes.

In all welfare state regimes, cohabitation does not seem to involve any significant negative health effects for men. In some countries odds ratios are not even elevated. However, in the Familialistic and TPS countries cohabiting women experience a significant health disadvantage.

While the country specific results within welfare state regimes are homogenous, there are two countries that stand out. Denmark, in the group of Dual-Earner countries, shows large negative health effects for men who live with a partner and only one child (as compared to married with more children). Men in the Netherlands, a country of the general family support regime, have significantly worse health if they are married but live in households with no or only one child.

Mediator Analysis of Financial Deprivation

The health effects described above are controlled for socio-economic characteristics, however, financial deprivation might still play an important role in explaining the differences observed. Introducing the variable "difficulties in making ends meet" in the models has huge effects on the odds ratios (Table 5). A positive sign indicates that individuals occupying a certain household position are financially better off than the married with more children, which (partly) attenuates their health disadvantage. A negative sign indicates that the health disadvantage is partly due to financial deprivation. Among men positive signs tend to dominate, which indicates that the health disadvantage compared to the married with children is larger if one accounts for financial deprivation, i.e. the married with children seem to be worse off in financial terms, which affects their health. Among women, financial difficulties appear to be partly responsible for the health disadvantage of single mothers and of women living alone; as in the case of men, married women with no or one child seem to fare financially better than the married with more children, which slightly attenuates their health disadvantage.

Testing the Institutionalization Hypothesis

The institutionalization hypothesis suggests that the more frequent a certain household position is, the less it is stigmatized, thus the health disadvantage compared to the married living with two children should decrease. This implies that we are looking for a negative correlation between the odds ratio of poor health and

Table 5 Mediator effect of financial deprivation on the odds ratios of poor health by household position

	Dual-earner and liberal				General family support				Familialistic and transition post socialist			
	DK	N	SW	UK	AT	FR	GER	NE	IT	ESP	HU	PL
Men												
Married, no children	+++	+	++	+	+	+	+	++	+		+	+
Married, child	+++		+		+			+				
Living alone	+++	−	++	+				−−	+	+		+
Son/daughter	+++			+++	++	+	+		+	+		
Cohabiting, no children	+++		++	+			+	++	+		−	+
Cohabiting, children	+++	+	+				−				−	
Single parent		−−		+	++		−	−		−	−	+
Women												
Married, no children	++	+	+	++	+++	+	+	++	++	+	+	+
Married, child	+	+		+	+			+				
Living alone	−	−−−	−−	−−−	−−−	−−	−−	−−−	−	−	−−−	−
Son/daughter												
Cohabiting, no children	++			−			+	+	++		−	−
Cohabiting, children			−	−	+		−	+	−		−−	
Single parent	−−	−−−	−−−	−−−	−−−	−−−	−−	−−−	−−−	−−	−−−	−−

+ increases the odds ratio by an absolute value of 0.20–0.99; ++ increases the odds ratio by an absolute value of 1.00–1.99; +++ increases the odds ratio by an absolute value of 2.0 and more

− decreases the odds ratio by an absolute value of 0.20–0.99; −− decreases the odds ratio by an absolute value of 1.00–1.99; −−− decrease the odds ratio by an absolute value of 2.0 and more

the proportion of a certain household position in a country. Among men (Fig. 2), the correlation is indeed generally nil to negative, with the exception of men living alone. However, the negative trend is only significant for married men living without children. A change of one standard deviation in the proportion of this household position eliminates the disadvantage as compared to the married with two or more children. The result is similar for the cohabiting living without children, albeit not statistically significant. A strong positive but not significant correlation exists for men living alone, with a change of one standard deviation resulting in increasing disadvantage of 0.15, e.g. from 0.40 to 0.55, which is an increase in the odds ratio from 1.49 to 1.73.

Among women (Fig. 3), trends are mixed and not significant with two important exceptions. First, cohabiting women clearly follow the institutionalization hypothesis: the more frequent this position, the less disadvantageous it is. This trend

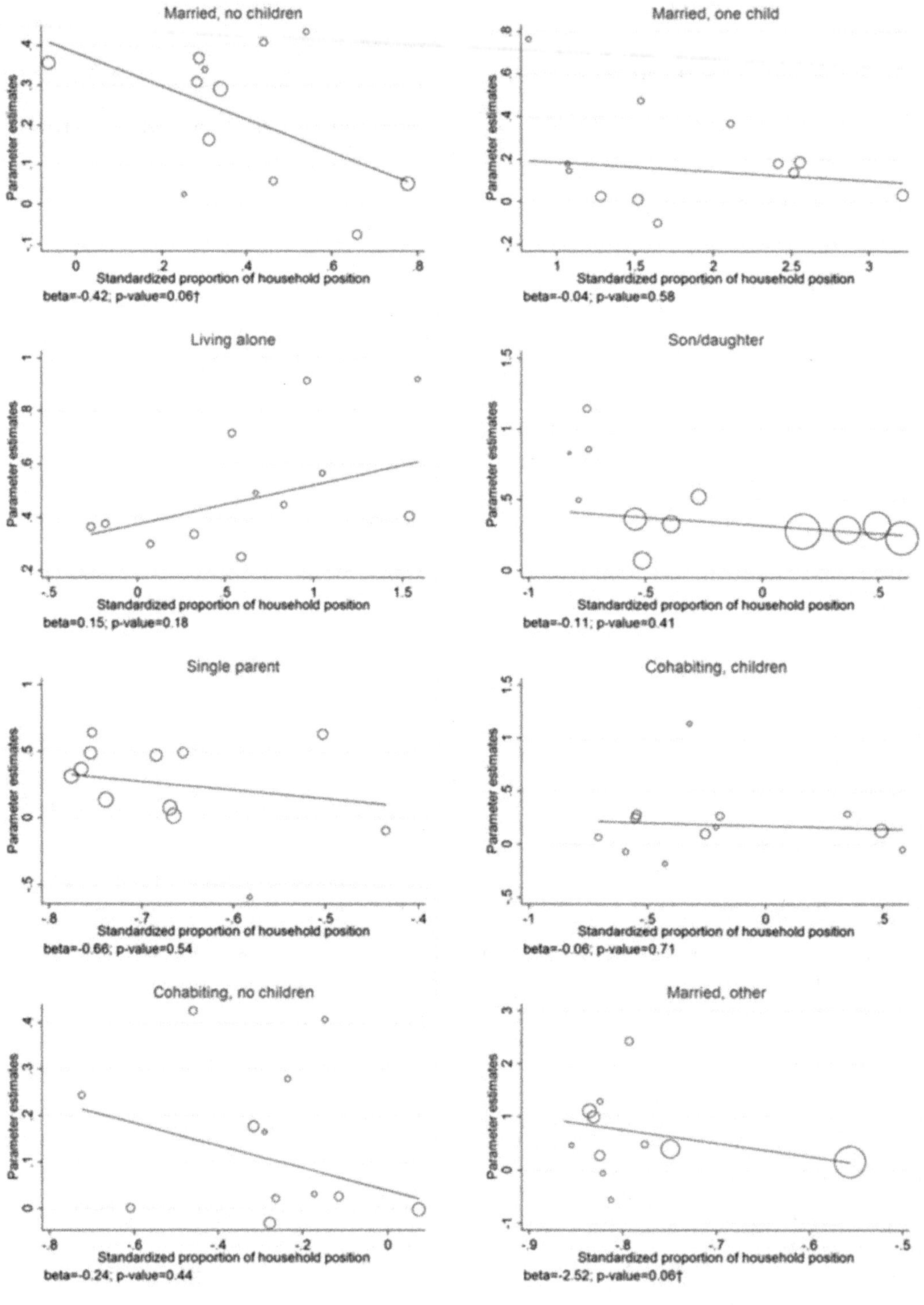

Fig. 2 Correlation between the standardized proportion of a certain household position and the parameter estimates of poor health [ln(odds ratios)] in comparison to the married with two or more children. Men. (Note: Circle size indicates the standard error of the estimate)

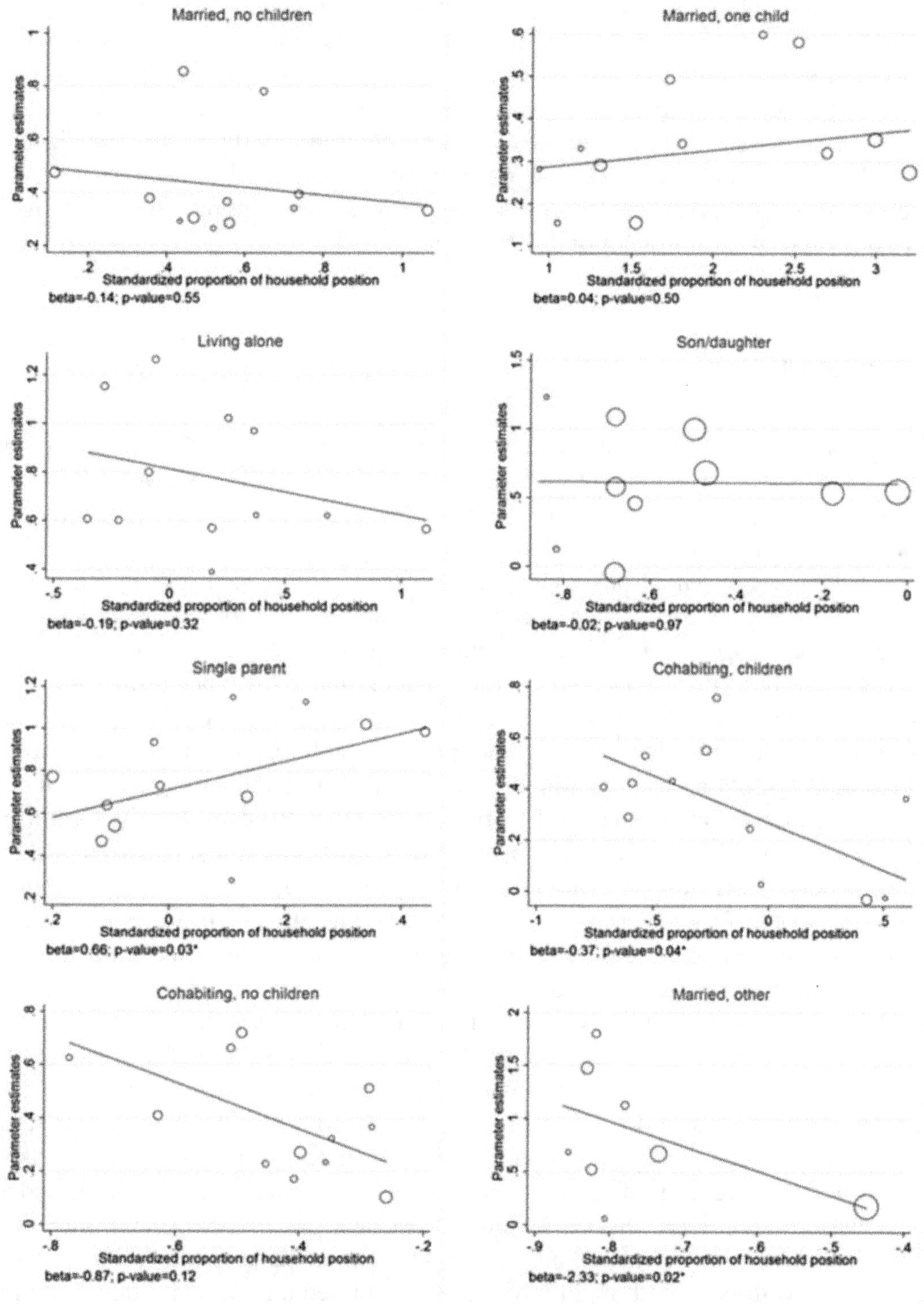

Fig. 3 Correlation between the standardized proportion of a certain household position and the parameter estimates of poor health [ln(odds ratios)] in comparison to the married with two or more children. Women. (Note: Circle size indicates the standard error of the estimate)

is particularly obvious and highly significant for cohabiting women living with children, but also exists for those living without children. A change of one standard deviation in the proportion of this position reduces the disadvantage by 0.37, i.e. reduces the odd ratio from 1.49 to 1.03. Second, women living as single parents reveal a significant positive trend, which is contrary to the institutionalization hypothesis: The more frequent the position, the more disadvantageous it is. An increase of one standard deviation increases the disadvantage by 0.66, resulting in an odds ratio of 2.89 instead of 1.49.

Discussion

The composition of the household has large repercussions for the health of an individual. This is true in addition to individual characteristics. We not only show the extent of these repercussions but also present evidence that they depend on the value climate in a society.

We defined household position by the presence of a partner and/or children as well as by being married or living in a consensual union. First, we considered the effect of the household position on health, testing the three hypotheses that the married fare best, that household position matters more for women than for men, and that some of the differentials can be explained by financial deprivation. We find large health differentials by household position and regardless of sex, married individuals with two and more children fare best, single mothers and those living alone fare worst. Differences tend to be larger and statistically highly significant among women, with the exception of the Dual-Earner countries. Our results show that financial deprivation accounts for some of the disadvantage of single mothers but not for all. This is also true for women living alone. The reverse, a better economic situation as well as the economies-of-scale advantage, may explain some of the better health of the married.

A large number of studies shows that the number of children ever born exerts a small but important effect on the health of women and partly also of men late in life, with two to three children being associated with the best health outcome (see Tomassini, Di Gessa, and Egidi, and Hank and Steinbach in this book). Our study shows that even at young and middle ages, the health of married parents is associated with the number of children in the household and that one child, and in particular no children in the household is associated with worse health outcomes. This is remarkable insofar as in our cross-sectional data those living without children or with one child might have once constituted a multi-child family during their life course. Indeed, the category living without children comprises childless persons whose worse health outcome has been repeatedly shown (see Hank and Steinbach in this volume) and parents whose children have already moved out of the household. When interpreting our results one has to be careful by taking into account the heterogeneity within the categories and the possibility of a changing effect of children on the health of their parents. For example, recent studies of happiness (Myrskylä and Margolis 2014) suggest that happiness increases prior to and in the year of having a child and decreases thereafter, with individuals who became parents at young ages having a downward happiness trajectory, while those becoming parents at older ages have a higher happiness level after the birth. The first child tends to increase happiness, the second much less, and the third may decrease happiness. This heterogeneous effect of children on happiness may also be present in terms of subjective health.

However, there are considerable differences in the association between household position and health by the welfare state regime and even by countries belonging to one regime. To further explore the country-differences we tested the institutionalization hypothesis.

The institutionalization hypothesis states that in countries where a certain partnership form is more common and thus probably more accepted, the disadvantage compared to the married is smaller. Soons and Kalmijn (2009) developed this hypothesis to study the cohabitation gap in wellbeing as compared to the married; we extended this concept to all household positions. We found strong support for the hypothesis for women living in consensual unions and for married men without children. Regarding cohabitation, both sexes face higher odds of poor health when cohabiting, and the lower the proportion living in such a partnership form, the higher the disadvantage as compared to the married living with children. The trend is even more pronounced when children are not present in the household; however, it is only statistically significant among women with children. No comparable trend exists among cohabiting men. In their study on well-being in 30 European countries, Soons and Kalmijn found that about one third of the difference of the cohabitation gap can be explained by differences in the composition between cohabiting and married people with employment, with education and religiosity playing important roles. Cohabiting people are less likely to be employed and religious and are thus less happy. A similar argument could be made for our study. We control for employment and education but not for religiosity, while it is well know that religious people have better health and live longer (e.g. Powell et al. 2003; Rew and Wong 2006). We also control for financial deprivation which, however, does not have much effect on the cohabitation gap.

Following Soons and Kalmijn (2009), the size of the cohabitation gap might be explained by the normative approval/disapproval of consensual unions, as well as the general value climate in a society ranging from traditional to (post)modern. Because the value climate is usually gendered, it is no surprise that it affects women more than men, an aspect which was not studied by the two authors.

An unexpected result is that married men living without children follow the institutionalization hypothesis but women do not. Here longitudinal data or retrospective information might help in untangling this heterogeneous group into the married childless, the married whose children have moved out, and the re-married whose children live with the former wife. Indeed, the latter is the only group where men and women differ, with re-married women usually living with the children from the previous marriage (and therefore not belonging to the group married without children). The trend might thus be an indirect indication that in societies where divorce and re-marriage is more accepted, the disadvantage to health is smaller. This, however, needs to be confirmed in future studies.

To our surprise single mothers do not follow the institutionalization hypothesis; the trend is just the opposite: The more common single mothers in a country are, the higher their health disadvantage. Some of this can be explained by financial deprivation, which is generally worse for them compared to the married, however, a sizeable effect still remains, particularly in the Scandinavian countries. One possible explanation is the distribution of unpaid work, which is more gender equal in these countries. Single mothers there may not only face financial problems but also forgo the partner as an important resource in dividing unpaid work. We will return to this below.

Another household position that does not follow the institutionalization hypothesis is living alone for men. While for women the hypothesis holds true, men face the highest disadvantage in Denmark, Sweden, and Germany, where the proportion is highest, and the lowest in the TPS and Familialistic countries, where the proportion is lowest. Financial deprivation explains much of the disadvantaged health situation in the first group of countries, little in the latter. One explanation might be that the social composition of those living alone differs between the countries. In the TPS and Familialistic countries, those facing financial difficulties might have moved back to their parental home. In these countries more than ten percent live as an adult son in the parental home; in the other countries they might stay on their own. This explanation is supported by the fact that in the Nordic countries the disadvantage is attenuated and loses significance when financial deprivation is controlled for, while there is no to little change in the Familialistic and TPS countries. Further support comes from a study by Ahn and Sánchez-Marcos (2015), who found that in Spain the proportion living alone increased during the financial crises (2009–2013) as compared to the boom years before, and that this rise was mainly driven by the full-time employed.

This study is based on cross-sectional data. Future studies on the relationship between household position and health would certainly benefit from life-course data that permit the study of both prior and current household positions. For example, in many countries cohabitation is still assumed to be a transitory phase before marriage. Marriage is perceived as a higher level of commitment and cohabitation is perceived as a testing period which is subordinated to the marriage ideal (Perelli-Harris et al. 2014). There are very different trajectories between cohabitation, marriage, and childbirth in the different European countries (Kok and Leinarte 2016) and thus far there appears to be no convergence of European life courses (Billari and Wilson 2001).

In testing the institutionalization hypothesis, we used the proportion of people living in a specific type of living arrangement as a proxy for the value climate. This hinges on the assumption that family forms are predominantly an outcome of the value structure of a society; however, there are also other determinants that influence the likelihood of family forms, such as the welfare system, the economic situation, etc. A fruitful approach for future studies might thus be to use a more direct measure of the value climate, as did Soons and Kalmijn (2009) when they explored the perceived attitude towards cohabitation in relation to well-being. Another approach might be to explore historical patterns of cohabitation, as was done by Klüsener (2016), who used these as a proxy for attitudes that are shaped by traditions of the past. In his study of extramarital births in Europe, Klüsener showed that continuity is still visible, albeit fading.

Conclusion

With the Second Demographic Transition living arrangements and household forms became more diverse, yet there seems to be no convergence to a predominantly European model. Our study shows that in Europe the household is an influential factor of health; this is particularly true for women but it is also important for men. There seem to be general patterns of advantaged and disadvantaged positions which however, are strongly modifiable. The general value climate in a society and the support by the welfare state determine to what extent certain household forms are beneficial or detrimental to health. Therefore, differences in recent evolution of family patterns across Western countries seem to influence the magnitude of the association of family with health differently, drawing a heterogeneous European map. Future country studies of living arrangement and health have to take this heterogeneity into account.

References

Ahn, N., & Sánchez-Marcos, V. (2015). Emancipation under the great recession in Spain. *Review of economics of the household.* https://doi.org/10.1007/s11150-015-9316-7.

Artazcoz, L., Borrell, C., & Benach, J. (2001). Gender inequalities in health among workers: the relation with family demands. *Journal of Epidemiology and Community Health, 55*(9), 639–647.

Barnett, R. C., & Hyde, J. S. (2001). Women, men, work, and family. *American Psychologist, 56*(10), 781–796. https://doi.org/10.1037//0003-066X.56.10.781.

Bartlett, E. E. (2004). The effects of fatherhood on the health of men. A review of the literature. *The Journal of Men's Health & Gender, 1*(2–3), 159–169. https://doi.org/10.1016/j.jmhg.2004.06.004.

Bernstein, A. B. (2001). Motherhood, health status, and health care. *Women's Health Issues, 11*(3), 173–184. https://doi.org/10.1016/S1049-3867(01)00078-0.

Billari, F. C., & Liefbroer, A. C. (2010). Towards a new pattern of transition to adulthood? *Advances in Life Course Research, 15*(2–3), 59–75. https://doi.org/10.1016/j.alcr.2010.10.003.

Billari, F. C., & Wilson, C. (2001). *Convergence towards diversity? Cohort dynamics in the transition to adulthood in contemporary Western Europe*. In Max Planck Institute for Demographic Research Rostock, Working Paper No. 2001-039.

Boje, T. P. (2007): Welfare and work. The gendered organisation of work and care in different European Countries. *European Review, 15*(03), 373. https://doi.org/10.1017/S1062798707000361.

Brockmann, H., & Klein, T. (2004). Love and death in Germany. The marital biography and its effect on mortality. *Journal of Marriage and Family, 66*(3), 567–581. https://doi.org/10.1111/j.0022-2445.2004.00038.x.

Cherlin, A. J. (2000): Toward a new home socioeconomics of union formation. In: L. J. Waite & C. Bachrach (Hg.) (Eds.), *The ties that bind. Perspectives on marriage and cohabitation* (pp. 126–144). New York: Aldine de Gruyter (Social institutions and social change).

Cooke, L. P., & Gash, V. (2010). Wives' part-time employment and marital stability in Great Britain, West Germany and the United States. *Sociology, 44*(6), 1091–1108. https://doi.org/10.1177/0038038510381605.

Demakakos, P., Nazroo, J., Breeze, E., & Marmot, M. (2008). Socioeconomic status and health. The role of subjective social status. *Social Science and Medicine, 67*(2), 330–340. https://doi.org/10.1016/j.socscimed.2008.03.038.

Esping-Andersen, G. (1998). *The three worlds of welfare capitalism*. Princeton, N.J: Princeton University Press. Online verfügbar unter http://www.loc.gov/catdir/description/prin021/89024254.html.

Eurostat (2016). Being young in Europe today. http://ec.europa.eu/eurostat/statistics-explained/index.php/Being_young_in_Europe_today_-_family_and_society. Accessed 15 March 2016.

FamilyAndSocieties. http://www.familiesandsocieties.eu/.

Floderus, B., Hagman, M., Aronsson, G., Marklund, S., & Wikman, A. (2008). Self-Reported health in mothers. The impact of age, and socioeconomic conditions. *Women and Health, 47*(2), 63–86. https://doi.org/10.1080/03630240802092308.

Gahler, M. (2006). "To divorce is to die a bit…". A longitudinal study of marital disruption and psychological distress among Swedish women and men. *The Family Journal, 14*(4), 372–382. https://doi.org/10.1177/1066480706290145.

Gumà, J., & Cámara, A. D. (2014). ¿Informa la salud autopercibida sobre las condiciones objetivas de salud? Algunas conclusiones a partir del análisis demográfico de microdatos de la Encuesta Nacional de Salud. *Revista de Estadística Española, 56*(183), 61–76.

Helbig, S., Lampert, T., Klose, M., & Jacobi, F. (2006). Is parenthood associated with mental health? Findings from an epidemiological community survey. *Social Psychiatry and Psychiatric Epidemiology, 41*(11), 889–896. https://doi.org/10.1007/s00127-006-0113-8.

Hobson, B., & Olah, L. S. (2006). Birthstrikes? Agency and capabilities in the reconciliation of employment and family. *Marriage & Family Review, 39*(3–4), 197–227. https://doi.org/10.1300/J002v39n03_01.

Hofäcker, D., & Chaloupková, J. (2014). Patterns of family life courses in Europe—between standardisation and diversity A cross-national comparison of family trajectories and life course norms in European countries. Hg. v. Federal Institute for Population Research.

Hughes, M. E., & Waite, L. J. (2002). Health in household context: Living arrangements and health in late middle age. *Journal of Health and Social Behavior, 43*(1), 1–21.

Hughes, M. E., & Waite, L. J. (2009). Marital biography and health at mid-life. *Journal of Health and Social Behavior, 50*(3), 344–358. https://doi.org/10.1177/002214650905000307.

Idler, E. L., & Benyamini, Y. (1997). Self-rated health and mortality. A review of twenty-seven community studies. *Journal of Health and Social Behavior, 38*(1), 21–37. https://doi.org/10.2307/2955359.

Klüsener, S. (2016). Spatial variation in non-marital fertility across Europe in the twentieth and twenty-first centuries. Recent trends, persistence of the past, and potential future pathways. *The History of the Family, 20*(4), 593–628. https://doi.org/10.1080/1081602X.2015.1099112.

Kok, J., & Leinarte, D. (2016). Cohabitation in Europe. A revenge of history? *The History of the Family, 20*(4), 489–514. https://doi.org/10.1080/1081602X.2015.1067240.

Lesthaege, R. (1995). The second demographic transition in Western countries: An interpretation. In: K. O. Mason & A.-M. Jensen (Hg.) (Eds.) Gender and family change in industrialized countries, (pp. 17–62). Oxford: Clarendon Press (International studies in demography).

Liefbroer, A., & Fokkema, T. (2008). Recent trends in demographic attitudes and behaviour: Is the second demographic transition moving to southern and eastern Europe? In J. Surkyn &

P. Deboosere (Hg.) (Eds.), *Demographic challenges for the 21st century: A state of the art in demography* (pp. 115–142). Brussels: VUB Press.

Liefbroer, A., & Merz, E.-M. (2009). Report on analysis of ESS data on cross-national differences in perceived norms concerning fertility-related behaviour. *REPRO deliverable, 16*(6).

Lillard, L., & Panis, C. W. A. (1996). Marital status and mortality: The role of health. *Demography, 33*(3), 313–327.

Lillard, Lee A., & Waite, Linda J. (1995). Til death do us part: Marital disruption and mortality. *American Journal of Sociology, 100*(5), 1131–1156. https://doi.org/10.1086/230634.

Marmot, M., & Wilkinson, R. G. (Eds.). (1999). *Social determinants of health*. Oxford: Oxford University Press.

Martikainen, P., Martelin, T., Nihtilä, E., Majamaa, K., & Koskinen, S. (2005). Differences in mortality by marital status in Finland from 1976 to 2000. Analyses of changes in marital-status distributions, socio-demographic and household composition, and cause of death. *Population Studies, 59*(1), 99–115. https://doi.org/10.1080/0032472052000332737.

McDonald, P. (2000). Gender equity, social institutions and the future of fertility. *Journal of Population Research, 17*(1), 1–16. https://doi.org/10.1007/BF03029445.

Myrskylä, M., & Margolis, R. (2014). Happiness. Before and after the kids. *Demography, 51*(5), 1843–1866. https://doi.org/10.1007/s13524-014-0321-x.

Neyer, G. (2013). Welfare states, family policies, and fertility in Europe. In: G. Neyer, G. Andersson, H. Kulu, L. Bernardi, & C. Bühler (Hg.) (Eds.), *The Demography of Europe* (pp. 29–53). Dordrecht: Springer.

Nock, S. L. (1995). A comparison of marriages and cohabiting relationships. *Journal of Family Issues, 16*(1), 53–76.

OECD. (2012). Closing the gender gap. Act now. Paris: OECD. Online verfügbar unter http://www.gbv.de/dms/zbw/73244778X.pdf.

OECD. (2016a). Pensions at a glance. www.oecd.org/pensions/pensionsataglance.htm. Accessed 15 March 2016.

OECD. (2016b). OECD. Stat. Full-time equivalent employment rate. Online verfügbar unter http://stats.oecd.org/index.aspx?queryid=54749.

Perelli-Harris, B., Berrington, A., Berghammer, C., Keizer, R., Lappegård, T., Mynarska, M., & et al. (2014). Towards a new understanding of cohabitation. *Demographic Research 31*, 1043–1078. https://doi.org/10.4054/DemRes.2014.31.34.

Powell, L. H., Shahabi, L., & Thoresen, C. E. (2003). Religion and spirituality. Linkages to physical health. *American Psychologist, 58*(1), 36–52. https://doi.org/10.1037/0003-066X.58.1.36.

Puur, A., Oláh, L. S., Tazi-Preve, M. I., Dorbritz, J. (2008). Men's childbearing desires and views of the male role in Europe at the dawn of the 21st century. *Demographic Research 19*, 1883–1912. https://doi.org/10.4054/DemRes.2008.19.56.

Rew, L., & Wong, Y. J. (2006). A systematic review of associations among religiosity/spirituality and adolescent health attitudes and behaviors. *Journal of Adolescent Health, 38*(4), 433–442. https://doi.org/10.1016/j.jadohealth.2005.02.004.

Rotermann, M. (2007). Marital breakdown and subsequent depression. *Health Reports, 18*(2), 33–44.

Sayer, L. C., & Bianchi, S. M. (2000). Women's economic independence and the probability of divorce. A review and reexamination. *Journal of Family Issues, 21*(7), 906–943. https://doi.org/10.1177/019251300021007005.

Soons, J. P. M., & Kalmijn, M. (2009). Is marriage more than cohabitation? Well-being differences in 30 European countries. *Journal of Marriage and Family, 71*(5), 1141–1157. https://doi.org/10.1111/j.1741-3737.2009.00660.x.

Stevenson, B., & Wolfers, J. (2007): Marriage and divorce: Changes and their driving forces. *Institute for the Study of Labor* (2602).

Surkyn, J., & Lesthaeghe, R. (2004): Value orientations and the second demographic transition (SDT) in Northern, Western and Southern Europe. An Update. *Demographic Research* (3), 45–86. https://doi.org/10.4054/DemRes.2004.S3.3.

van de Kaa, D. J. (1994). The second demographic transition revisited: Theories and expectations. In: G. Beets, H. van Den Brekel, R. L. Cliquet, G. Dooghe, & J. de Jong Gierveld (Hg.) (Eds.), Population and family in the Low Countries 1993: Late fertility and other current issues (pp. 81–126). Berwyn, Pennsylvania, Amsterdam: Swets and Zeitlinger.

Vincent-Lancrin, S. (2008): The reversal of gender inequalities in higher education. In: Demography (Vol. 1, pp. 265–298). Paris: OECD (Higher education to 2030).

Waite, L. J. (1995). Does marriage matter? *Demography, 32*(4), 483–507.

Waldron, I., Weiss, C. C., & Hughes, M. E. (1997). Marital status effects on health: are there differences between never married women and divorced and separated women? *Social Science and Medicine, 45*(9), 1387–1397.

Wang, J. L. (2004). The difference between single and married mothers in the 12-month prevalence of major depressive syndrome, associated factors and mental health service utilization. *Social Psychiatry and Psychiatric Epidemiology, 39*(1), 29–42.

Williams, K., & Umberson, D. (2004). Marital status, marital transitions, and health. A Gendered Life Course Perspective. *Journal of Health and Social Behavior, 45*(1), 81–98. https://doi.org/10.1177/002214650404500106.

World Health Organization (WHO). (1946). In minutes of the technical preparatory committee for the international health conference (pp. 03–18).

Similarity of Perceived Health Between Household Members: The "Mutual Influences" Hypothesis

Patrizia Giannantoni and Viviana Egidi

Introduction

Demographers and social epidemiologists have widely recognized that determinants of health operate on different levels (Kawachi and Subramanian 2005). Hence, a true comprehensive analysis of population health must not look only at the individual, but must also include contextual characteristics. However, only a handful of studies to date have taken the multilevel structure of health determinants properly into account and, as a consequence, findings about the impact of context on population health are sparse and inconclusive.

Existing literature has shown that, over and beyond individual characteristics, contextual factors affecting health are related to two main aspects: area of residence, i.e. *macro-level* (Stafford and McCarthy 2006; Kunst et al. 2005) and social proximity, i.e. *meso-level* (Schor et al. 1987; Cardol et al. 2005; Van Minh et al. 2010). However, a limited number of studies on population health have formally made use of a hierarchical structure accounting for both geographical and relational levels (Subramanian et al. 2003; Ferrer et al. 2005). The geographical area of residence has been studied as being potentially responsible for exposure to environmental risk factors (Martuzzi et al. 2002; Biggeri et al. 2004; Pearce and Dorling 2006), economic deprivation (Kennedy et al. 1998; Subramanian et al. 2001), social conflicts (Kawachi et al. 1999), and, in some cases, uneven health care provision (Joumard et al. 2008; Jagger et al. 2008), thus demonstrating that all of these factors have some influence on health outcomes. Less investigated is the *meso-level*, which typically refers to the network of relations binding the individual to the people close

P. Giannantoni (✉) · V. Egidi
La Sapienza University of Rome, Rome, Italy
e-mail: patrizia.giannantoni@uniroma1.it

V. Egidi
e-mail: Viviana.Egidi@uniroma1.it

G. Doblhammer and J. Gumà (eds.), *A Demographic Perspective on Gender, Family and Health in Europe*, https://doi.org/10.1007/978-3-319-72356-3_7

to him/her in everyday life (Agneessens et al. 2006; Rivellini 2006). This social/relational network influences individuals in terms of group identity, cultural background, and social support.

Among all of the relational networks, the family deserves a special place as it is the context where lifestyles and health-related behaviors (e.g. prevention, timely access to care, adherence to treatment) are generally developed and shared. Members of the same family are often found to be similar in terms of health-related lifestyles (Rice et al. 1998), help-seeking behaviors (Cardol et al. 2005), and utilization of health services (Sepheri et al. 2008). Having similar behaviors also exposes family members to similar risks (or protective factors) for health, directly deriving from those behaviors. For example, in a family where prevention is a common practice, all members share the protective effect of timely medical check-ups. Conversely, in a family where nutrition style is unbalanced in favor of consumption of fatty foods, members will be more exposed to the risk of being obese, and in turn exposed to an increased risks of cardiovascular diseases. This kind of result has been consistently illustrated in the epidemiological literature (Johnson et al. 1965; Monden 2007; Merlo et al. 2012).

Furthermore, the family is the predominant setting for the inter-exchange of resources finalized to satisfy an individual's needs and to attain wellbeing. In this perspective, the family has always played a key role in supporting its members in those specific critical periods of their lifetime when they need assistance. In short, family affects health in two main areas: the occurrence of illness and the assistance thereof. In literature, family is generally identified with the household, first because it makes it easier to define the boundaries of the concept of "family", and second because it is reasonable to assume that co-residence makes all the presented hypotheses about behaviors and assistance more intense.

Household characteristics that have been investigated in the literature as predictors of individual health include the socio-economic level of the family, housing conditions, living arrangements, and the burden of care for a cohabiting ill-health member. All of these characteristics can, to some extent, exercise influence on health as "household factors" because they operate simultaneously on all cohabiting members of the family. However, particularly when perceived health is the outcome, another hypothesis must be taken into consideration: poor health of a member can, by itself, operate as a factor influencing the perceived health status of other members. In other words, *mutual influences* of health perception can exist within a household, resulting in a high resemblance of health status for people living together, independent of (or in addition to) the effect of household covariates.

Research that has dealt with household influences on health perception (Ferrer et al. 2005; Van Minh et al. 2010) has not provided clear explanations of the mechanisms through which these influences occur. However, it is reasonable to suppose that household influences tend to be stronger in those countries where family has a strong impact on individual choices, such as Southern European Countries. Paradoxically, to the best of our knowledge, no studies of household contribution on health perception have been carried out in Italy, which is one of these familialistic countries.

Objective

The specific objectives of this study are:

- to provide an estimation of the magnitude of influence that the household has on self-perceived health, controlling for individual characteristics and the geographical context;
- to gain a better understanding of the pathways through which the household affects the perceived health of its members.

The Italian Setting

Italy is characterized by several peculiarities concerning both its territorial profile and the role of the family in an ample set of demographic and social phenomena. As a consequence, both territory and family are frequently found to have a larger influence on socio-demographic outcomes than in other countries.

Those territorial factors affecting health are closely linked to the provision of health care facilities, which have undergone profound changes in Italy in the last decades. The Italian National Health Service is currently structured on three hierarchical levels: two levels of governance (State and Regions) and one level of management (Local Health Units). It is financed through public taxation and presents centralized control together with strong federalized organization. The central governance rules the system through the national health program: it defines the priorities and guarantees homogeneity in the basic levels of assistance. At the same time, decentralization promotes regional autonomy in establishing, financing and managing health care facilities. The Region operates through the Local Health Units in transforming the economic resources in public health service for their population.

This final structure of NHS is the result of a long process of decentralization, which began in 1995 and has led Regions to contribute to their health expenses through autonomous taxation and to increase (according to resources available) the number of health services. The entire process of reform has alimented a heated debate concerning the risk of territorial health inequality. The hypothetical scenario in which health expenditures are entirely financed by Regions, without any relevant national adjustment, has further increased concerns about health equity (Egidi and Reynaud 2005).

What has been empirically observed is the existence of sharp heterogeneity between Italian Regions in both social and economic terms. Such heterogeneity is reflected also in the availability and quality of health services and it becomes apparent when viewing typical indicators of quality of care. Thirty-day mortality after a stroke, for example, varies from about 7% in Bolzano (in the North, on the Austrian border) to almost 20% in Molise (in the South). The proportion of patients receiving coronary angioplasty within 48 h ranges from 15% in Marche, Molise, and Basilicata to 50% in Valle d'Aosta (in the extreme north west part of Italy). The same indicator at the Local Health Units level reveals even more profound differences (spanning 5–60%). The waiting time for surgery after a hip fracture is 3 days in Valle d'Aosta and 7 days in Molise and Campania (South). More general indicators, commonly used as a proxy for quality in primary care, are *potentially avoidable medical admissions*, i.e. those medical conditions which are deemed fully manageable in primary care. These include conditions such as childhood asthma, for which age- and sex-adjusted hospital admissions are lowest in Toscana (0.21 per 1000 population) and highest in Sicilia (0.95) according to the data from National Outcome Programme (OECD 2014).

These variations in health provision correspond to a strong variation in health satisfaction and health outcomes. The proportion of patients who were "very satisfied" with hospital care in 2009 was about 50% in Trentino-Alto Adige and 20% in Sicilia and Puglia. This gap is reflected in the substantial flows across regional borders of patients who opt to receive health care assistance in a region other than their own.

This geography difference in health care offer is largely confirmed when we look directly at health outcomes. Differences in mortality according to Italian Regions and provinces have been extensively documented (Caselli and Egidi 1979; Divino et al. 2009), with studies consistently reporting very clear spatial trends changing over time and with minor differences according to gender. Male mortality is significantly lower in the Northern regions (especially in the eastern part of the country) and higher in the Southern regions and the Islands, with differences only slightly lower than 3 years of life expectancy at birth between the more and less favored regions. Women follow the same general trend, while showing a relative disadvantage in the northwestern part of the country. Territorial differences can be observed also for health conditions: e.g. prevalence of multiple chronic conditions, disability rates, and disability-free life expectancy have sharp geographical variations which depict the traditional North–South gradient (Fig. 1 males and Fig. 1 females).

In terms of the *familial perspective*, Italy is well-known as a characteristically familialistic country. Extensive research has documented the strong role of family ties on demographic phenomena, such as fertility, leaving the parental home, and economic conditions (Cook and Fustenberg 2002; Tomassini et al. 2003; Vignoli and Matysiak 2013). The same effects can be hypothesized as extendable to health issue.

Despite the immediacy of this hypothesis, the subject is rarely ever taken into consideration for the Italian context. In the international literature marital status and patterns of family disruption have been extensively analyzed and proven to be remarkable predictors of health; however, the family as a whole and its role on health has not yet appeared in the health demographer's agenda.

One exception is the number of emerging studies that deal with the burden of care-giving on family members (Ory et al. 2000; Bookwala and Schulz 2000; Vlachantoni 2010; Egidi et al. 2013), which present a picture of economic and health consequences of care-giving activities, in terms of wellbeing and labor

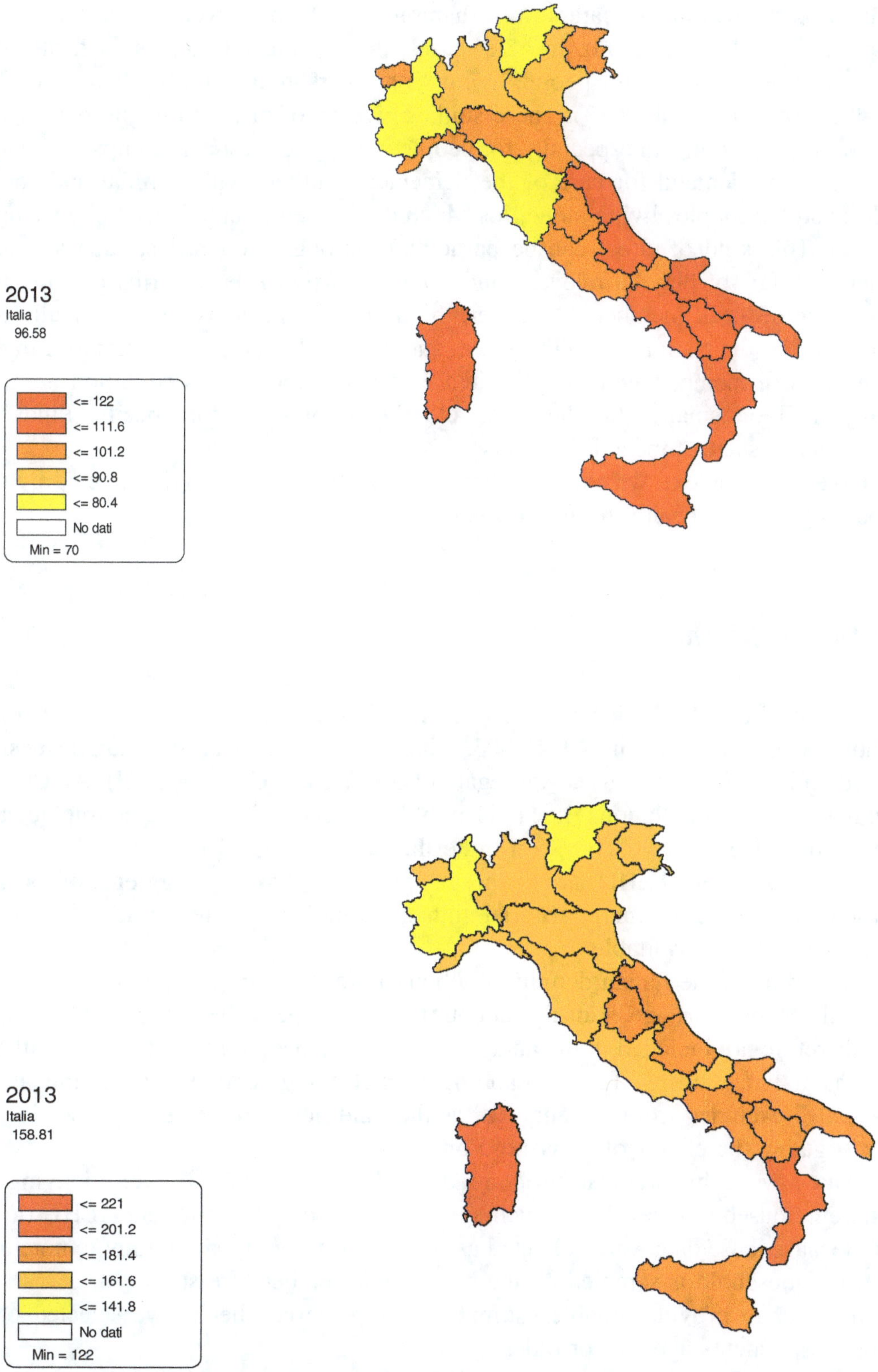

Fig. 1 A—age-standardized rate of 3 + chronic conditions per 1000 population in Italian regions for males (top) and females (bottom)—2013, ISTAT—health for all database

market participation of carers (Vlachantoni 2010) or psychological stressors (Bookwala and Shulz 2000). In other cases, they evaluated more specifically the consequences on health for people living with a person affected by dementia (Ory et al. 2000; Egidi et al. 2013). These studies give proof of a non-negligible impact on self-perceived health especially for people in the youngest age groups, up to age 64, when the demand for care of the demented conflicts with familial and social roles; and for couples living alone, for which the burden of care is faced by a single person. This kind of effect can be particularly strong in countries, such as Italy, where the family plays a relevant and often exclusive role in terms of care and assistance of an ill member. Moreover, this family-based assistance is usually not supported by the National Health System and the family is therefore left alone in the care of its ill member, with only limited external support. This condition is especially hard on smaller families, e.g. elderly couples, or for specific kinds of pathologies, such as mental disorders.

Given this context, we expected family members to be strongly affected by the emerging of poor health in one of them.

Data and Methods

Data come from the Italian Health Interview Survey carried out by the National Statistical Office (Istat) in 2004/2005. The survey used a cluster sample design based on households and uses Aggregated Local Health Units (ALHU). AHLU are aggregations of contiguous Local Health Units according to demographic and health planning criteria. They constitute the territorial level of our analysis. The reason we selected ALHU as the most appropriate territorial aggregation is that these represent the minimal territorial units granting health care facilities for which statistical data are available.

According to the Italian definition, a household is a group of people cohabiting and related by marriage, kinship, adoption, or sentiment. Institutionalized people are therefore not included in the analysis, neither are people living together with no sentimental relationship (e.g. cohabiting formal caregivers). People living alone were also excluded from the analysis, as they did not fit the research objective of investigating the effects of household on health.

Data have a hierarchical structure defined as individuals (level 1) living in different households (level 2), which are, in turns, located in different ALHU (level 3). Because these data were collected as a cluster survey, it is important to note that when a household is sampled all the household members are surveyed.

In order to provide reliable estimations of perceived health we selected only those respondents aged 18 or older.

After sample selection we had 91,391 individuals who satisfied the eligibility criteria. These resided in about 36,000 households which were, in turn, grouped into 68 ALHU. The household dimensions ranged from 2 to 8 individuals, with an average of 2.5 people per household. We selected three outcome variables to investigate perceived health: Physical Component Summary—PCS, Mental Component Summary—MCS, and poor Self-Rated Health—poor SRH. The first two measures are quantitative assessments of physical and mental health, positively oriented (the higher the score the better the health) derived from the Short Form-12 Health Survey—SF-12 included in the Italian survey. SRH is a binary variable derived from the single-item question recommended by the World Health Organization (WHO), which asks: "How is your health in general?" (De Bruin et al. 1996). Answers are distributed on a five point scale: very good, good, fair, bad, very bad. We grouped these five categories into two, creating a dummy variable (poor-SRH) of people reporting "poor" and "very poor" health conditions as opposed to those reporting "fair", "good" or "very good" conditions. This aggregation is due to the very unbalanced frequency distribution of respondents in the five categories: only a very small proportion of the population were in the two extreme categories (very good/very poor), which would have produced unreliable estimations. The choice of aggregating the category "fair" together with the positive modalities ("good" and "very good") is due to its Italian translation, which has a quite positive, rather than a neutral, connotation (Egidi and Spizzichino 2006).

We included individual and contextual (household) covariates in the analyses. As individual variables, we consider *age*, classified as <50, 50–64, 65–74, 75+; *gender*; *education* (low, i.e. primary education or lower; medium, i.e. lower secondary; and high, upper secondary education or higher); *disability* (yes/no), according to the highest limitation grade in at least one item of OECD Long-Care Disability Questionnaire; and *multichronicity* (yes/no), defined as having three or more chronic illnesses diagnosed by a medical doctor. Finally, we created a new variable from the dataset intended to capture the burden of disability of one household member on the rest of the family. It is labeled *cohabitation with disabled* and has value one when the individual cohabits with at least one disabled person.

Household covariates include: *perceived economic status* with categories good/satisfactory versus inadequate; *housing conditions,* which is based on the presence of very basic housing problems (e.g. absence of heating) and is classified as Good (no problems), Fair (1–2 problems), or Bad (more than 2 problems); *household size* with categories 2–3; 4; 5+ components; *household structure* with couple-headed families opposed to single-headed families; and *city size* with two classes based on the threshold of 50,000 inhabitants.

We adopted a multilevel approach with which we are able to disentangle the proportion of variability on different levels, i.e. the variability between individuals due to differences between individual themselves or due to household or ALHU communalities. According to the outcome characteristics, we ran linear or logistic multilevel models, with random intercepts at the household and ALHU levels. For each of the three outcomes we ran different multilevel models:

- Empty model: the model without any covariates, to evaluate the proportion of variance to be accounted for at each level, by means of the Variance Partition Coefficient (VPC).

- Model with individual covariates: to estimate the VPC controlled for compositional effects (i.e. differences due to the unequal distribution of individuals in the groups).
- Complete model: with individual and household covariates.

What remained as residual variance at the household level is the variation of perceived health between households not explained by all of those individual and household factors already included in the analysis. We should consider that the total variance is composed of the variability of individuals within the households (variance within) and the variability between households (variance between). Thus, the proportion of variance at the household level (VPC_H), as measured by the VPC, will result from:

$$VPC_H = \frac{\sigma_H}{\sigma_H + \sigma_I} * 100$$

and therefore it will be the highest, approaching 100%, when the *variance within* (σ_I) is equal to zero, i.e. when all individuals in the same household have exactly the same perceived health, and the whole variation is due to the *variation between* households (σ_H).

From this perspective one can easily understand how a high proportion of residual variance at the household level indirectly reflects a strong degree of *health homogeneity* within a household. The same formula is in fact used to calculate the Intraclass Correlation Coefficient (ICC), which is a measure of health homogeneity that expresses the correlation between two units randomly drawn from the same cluster (Snijders and Bosker 2012).

Finally, we looked at this health homogeneity as being responsible for the strong variation registered at the household level and advanced the hypothesis that *mutual influences* between household members play a major role in explaining this phenomenon. We tested this hypothesis with an analysis of health homogeneity by household structure, as we expected that the homogeneity would have been significantly different according to different typologies of households, where mutual influences have diverse magnitude.

Results

Descriptive Analyses

Whatever the measure adopted or the context of study, health is primarily affected by age. The proportion of poor-SRH ranges from 1.6% in the youngest group of people (under 50), to 27.8% in the oldest group (75 and over), and PCS and MCS scores range from 53.6 to 38.1 and from 51.0 to 45.6, on the same age interval. Looking at the range of variation of PCS and MCS, we also detect extremely large intervals between minimum and maximum values (Table 1), demonstrating the large heterogeneity in the health of the study population.

Table 1 Summary statistics for PCS by age group

Age groups	Obs	Mean	Std. dev	Min	Max
PCS					
<50	51,271	53.6	6.3	14.6	67.8
50–64	21,920	49.6	8.8	14.1	67.2
65–74	10,999	45.0	10.5	11.1	67.2
75+	7201	38.1	11.5	11.5	64.0
Total	91,391	50.4	9.3	11.1	67.8
MCS					
<50	51,271	51.0	8.7	7.5	70.4
50–64	21,920	49.4	9.6	7.6	72.0
65–74	10,999	48.2	10.3	7.5	72.3
75+	7201	45.6	11.7	11.1	71.1
Total	91,391	49.9	9.6	7.5	72.3

Multilevel Analysis

We run three nested models: the first one empty (i.e. with no covariates), the second with progressively individual covariates, and the third, which we refer to as a complete model, with individual and household covariates. We start by reporting the effects of individual and household covariates on the three health outcomes in the complete models, as illustrated in Table 2.

Objective health conditions, i.e. disability and multichronicity, have the strongest negative impact on perceived health as assessed by all three indicators. A negative effect can be detected for gender, with women having worse perceived health conditions, especially if we look at MCS, which expresses the mental/ emotional dimension of health. Education also shows a negative health gradient from the highest to the lowest school attainment. Age presents a more complex relation with perceived health, with different impacts between physical and mental dimensions: for PCS and SRH ageing is correlated with health deterioration; for MCS the worst condition is observed for people aged 50–64, whereas being older appears to be a protective factor. Not surprisingly, living together with a disabled person affects the emotional/mental dimensions of perceived health with a remarked deterioration for MCS and SRH.

Regarding household covariates, we can see that characteristics related to economic conditions (resources and housing) are those that have an impact on all three outcomes. Household size and structure impact more on MCS than PCS, with people living in larger, couple-headed households being more protected from poor mental health. Conversely, the dimension of the city is positively associated with better perceived physical health, whereas it shows no significant relationship to perceived mental health. Poor-SRH seems to be a synthesis of the other two indicators, as it is associated with all of the covariates included in the model, and in some cases (e.g. household size) with a clearer trend than the quantitative outcomes.

Table 2 Effects of household and individual covariates on PCS, MCS, and poor-SRH

	PCS		MCS		Poor-SRH	
Covariates	Coeff	p-value	Coeff	p-value	Or	p-value
Intercept	53.2	0.00	52.3	0.00	0.01	0.00
Individual variables						
Gender						
Male (ref)	0.0		0.0		1.0	
Female	–0.9	0.00	–2.0	0.00	1.2	0.00
Age in classes						
<50	2.4	0.00	0.9	0.00	0.4	0.00
50–64 *(ref)*	0.0		0.0		1.0	
65–74	–2.1	0.00	0.3	0.00	1.2	0.00
75+	–5.0	0.00	0.3	0.04	1.3	0.00
Education						
High (ref)	0.0		0.0		1.0	
Medium	–0.8	0.00	–0.1	0.08	1.4	0.00
Low	–2.1	0.00	–0.7	0.00	2.0	0.00
Disability						
no (ref)	0.0		0.0		1.0	
Yes	–12.9	0.00	–7.2	0.00	22.5	0.00
Multichronicity						
no (ref)	0.0		0.0		1.0	
Yes	–7.7	0.00	–5.2	0.00	8.6	0.00
Cohabitation with disable						
no (ref)	0.0		0.0		1.0	
Yes	0.0	0.65	–1.7	0.00	1.3	0.00
Household variables						
Household resources						
Good(ref)					1.00	
Insufficient	–0.95	0.00	–2.01	0.00	2.11	0.00
Household condition						
Good(ref)					1.00	
Fair	–0.30	0.00	–0.35	0.00	1.20	0.00
Bad	–0.55	0.00	–1.21	0.00	1.81	0.00
Household size						
2/3 comp (ref)					1.00	
4 comp	0.19	0.00	–0.09	0.00	0.75	0.00
>4 comp	0.26	0.13	1.22	0.00	0.65	0.00
Household structure						
Couple headed (ref)					1.00	
Single headed	0.05	0.49	–0.72	0.00	1.13	0.03

(continued)

Table 2 (continued)

	PCS		MCS		Poor-SRH	
Covariates	Coeff	p-value	Coeff	p-value	Or	p-value
City size						
> = 50.000 *(ref)*					1.00	
<50.000	–0.44	0.00	0.11	0.23	0.89	0.01
Likelihood ratio test	384	0.00	1016	0.00	13,500	0.00

We then looked at the proportion of variability of health perception existing on the three levels of analysis (AHLU, Households, Individuals) as measured by the Variance Partition Coefficient reported in Table 3.

On the one hand, we documented a very limited, although always significant, impact of AHLU of residence of individuals on their self-perceived health (0.3% for PCS, 0.6% for MCS, and 2.3% for poor-SRH) net from the effect of individual characteristics. Although we observed this very small influence of ALHU on health, we retained this geographical level in all subsequent analyses in order to control for the effect of territorial differences in health care facilities on health perception.

On the other hand, in the same models, the relevance of household on perceived health was quite substantive. The 14.7% of variability in PCS was a result of household differences, and MCS and poor-SRH show an even greater impact with, respectively, 32.5 and 38% of variability attributable to the household level (Table 2).

Characteristics of the household show a very weak impact on PCS (unexplained variability decreases from 14.7 to 14.3%) and only a slightly higher impact on MCS (from 32.5 to 31.5%). For poor-SRH, household covariates play a more important role (explaining an additional 5% of the variability between households). However, when all available covariates are controlled for, wide shares of SRH and MCS variability remain unexplained (34 and 32%, respectively).[1]

Seeking an explanation, we formulated the hypothesis that *mutual influences* between family members may play a major role. We hypothesized that this health homogeneity was due to mutual influences in health perception between family members, rather than exogenous factors operating on the household as a whole. It was not possible to test this hypothesis directly, therefore we designed an indirect strategy to check indirectly the robustness of the mutual influences hypothesis.

[1]The value of the SRH variability, which could be overestimated due to the small cluster sizes, is perfectly in line with the value for MCS. Although we need to be cautious in interpreting the variance of SRH between households, the resemblance of this value with the correspondent value for MCS is a cross validation for the results of the binary outcome.

Table 3 Variance partition coefficient of the household level for PCS, MCS and poor-SRH

Outcome			
Model with:	PCS	MCS	Poor-SRH
No variables	23.4	33.1	39.5
Individual variables	14.7	32.5	38.0
Individual + household variables	14.3	31.5	33.6

Our idea was that the hypothesis could be investigated indirectly by comparing the health status of individuals living in households of different sizes and structures. In fact, mutual influences should be different according to the tightness of links between household members: Where the link between members is expected to be tighter (two components, marriage-like link, mono-nucleus families) we should find also higher levels of health homogeneity.

Reciprocal Influences on Health: Evidence from the Household-Structure Analysis

We considered three main dimensions for defining the different kinds of family structures:

- household size: as it shapes the strength of the ties and determines the degree to which problems, burdens, and mutual influences are shared by the cohabiting members of the household;
- family ties: as understanding, affinity, and empathy vary greatly according to the type of familial relationship. The husband-wife relationship is expected to have a larger extent of reciprocal influence than the brother-sister relationship;
- duration of the relationships: as the emotional closeness between people is stronger according to the length of life span spent together, especially if they are a couple. Having no direct information about the relationship duration we use age as a proxy, using the age of 50 as the threshold.

In the following we verify whether the perceived health homogeneity between family members is coherent with these expectations. Health homogeneity at the household level is estimated as the Intra-class Correlation Coefficient (ICC%) at the household level. We compared specific subgroups (e.g. household composed of only two components, couples with or without children, multi-nucleus families) and we always applied the full model, in order to obtain estimations of homogeneity adjusted for territorial effects and for all individual and household observed covariates. As health measurements we use only PCS and MCS as we need robust estimation of the variability components.

Because we analyzed health resemblance only for people older than 18 years, when we analyze the household size we consider only those families where all members were older than 18. Families with children younger than 18 years are treated separately.

As expected, Fig. 2 shows that for both PCS and MCS the homogeneity is significantly higher in two-component households than in families with three or more cohabiting people. Moreover, homogeneity is higher for MCS, the indicator more sensitive to emotional influence, than for PCS.

The influence of household size on the level of homogeneity (i.e. the larger the groups the higher the probability of finding high variance) was evaluated by isolating the 2-component households and looking at the health homogeneity by family tie and duration of the relation (using age as a proxy). Our hypothesis was that homogeneity is highest for couples in a long-lasting relationship.

The hypothesis is entirely confirmed for PCS for which couples older than 50 have the highest level of homogeneity (25.1%), while their non-coupled peers have significantly lower homogeneity (11.4%) as well as young couples (14.6%) as clearly depicted in Fig. 3. People younger than 50 not in a couple were too small a group to produce reliable results.

For MCS homogeneity is not a matter of age/union duration, rather it depends on the type of relation between the two members: People in a couple have homogeneity over 36%, despite their age, while people not in a couple always have significantly lower levels of homogeneity (28.9% if younger than 50, 30% if older).

Focusing on *couples, with and without children*, our hypothesis was that the highest level of homogeneity characterizes couples without children, while it is expected to be weaker for couples with children because the ties are less tight and the network of relations wider. The duration of the link (once again approximated by the age of the individuals) should have the same effects as hypothesized before.

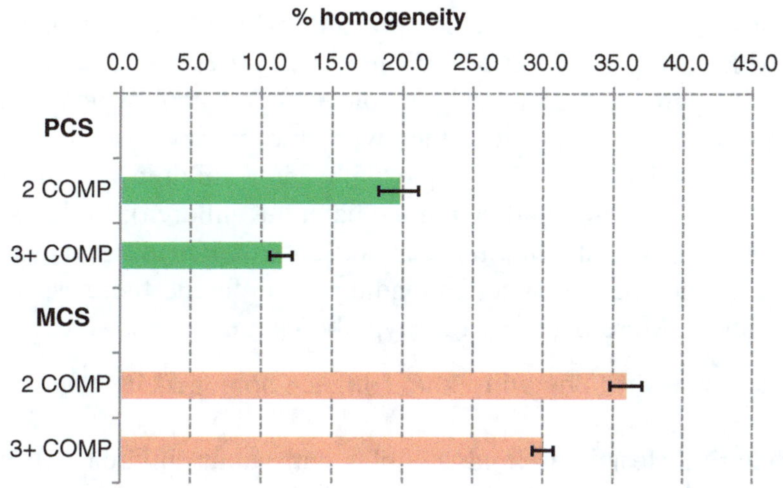

Fig. 2 Perceived health homogeneity (ICC%) between household members by household size

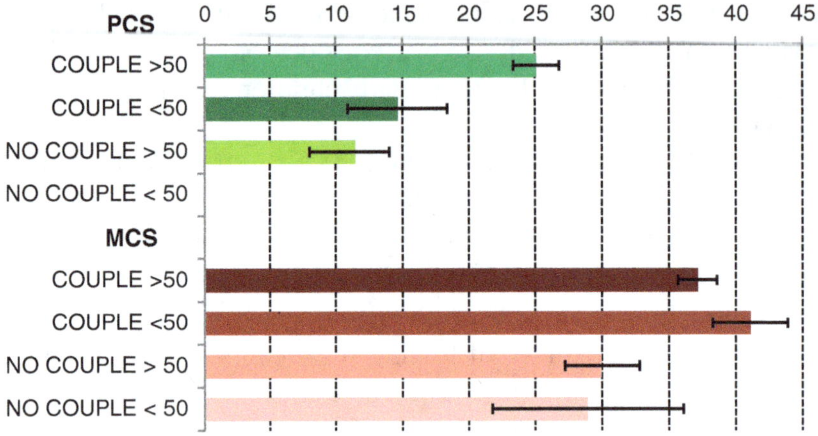

Fig. 3 Perceived health homogeneity (ICC%) between household members in two component households by typology of relation and age

In the category "couple + children", children themselves are included in the analysis of health resemblance if they are older than 18, whereas in the category "spouses in household with children" only the two partners are considered in the estimation of the homogeneity, regardless of the age of children. Our hypothesis is once again verified for PCS when we look at people over 50, while no differences are detectable for people younger than 50 (Fig. 4). This is not surprising, as in the young age group the PCS generally indicates good health and exhibits very limited variation.

For MCS, couples without children have the highest homogeneity, and this is significantly higher than that of couples with children. This result is independent of the partners' age: the homogeneity differential between *couples with and without children* is about 6–7% points both for older couples (37% vs. 30%) and for younger couples (41% vs. 35%). However, if we select only the two spouses from families with children, their level of resemblance is not statistically different than that of the level of childless couples, as the confidence intervals overlap.

Households with three or more components exhibit a wide range of different structures, which we grouped into four broad categories: (1) couple without children and with aggregated members (couple + aggregated) which consist of the main family nucleous (couple) together with one or more isolated relatives not constituing a second family; (2) couple with adult children (couple + children); (3) single parent with adult children (single parent + children); (4) households with more than one family unit (multinuclear households). Once again we expect different levels of homogeneity corresponding to different tightness of the links between members. More precisely our hypotheses are:

- mono-nuclear households will exhibit higher homogeneity than multi-nuclear ones (*hypothesis* 1);
- among multi-nuclear households couples with adult children will have higher homogeneity than couples with aggregated members (*hypothesis* 2).

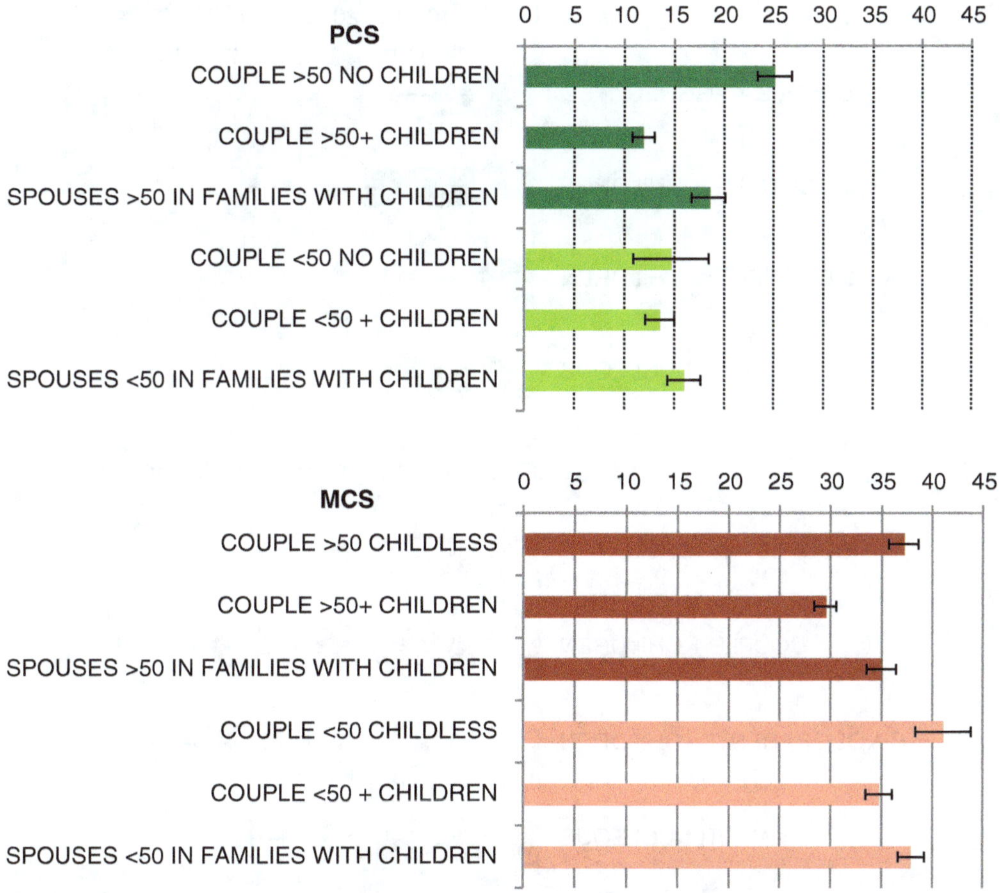

Fig. 4 Perceived health homogeneity (ICC%) between household members for couples with and without children

For single parent families with adult children two different hypotheses can be formulated:

– they may have lower homogeneity than families headed by a couple due to the absence of the two partners (*hypothesis* 3) or a mechanism of compensation could take place. In this case the link (and mutual influences) between the single-parent and the offspring could become stronger as a response to the absence of a member of the couple. If this is the case, the homogeneity in a single-parent household would not differ significantly from that of couples with children (*hypothesis* 4). Hypothesis 3 and hypothesis 4 are alternatives. However, they both appeared to be theoretically reasonable, therefore we kept both and tested empirically which one prevails.

As Fig. 5 shows, hypothesis 2 and 3 are confirmed by PCS: couples with children have a higher resemblance than couples with aggregated members and much higher similarity than one-parent households. Non-nuclear households do not

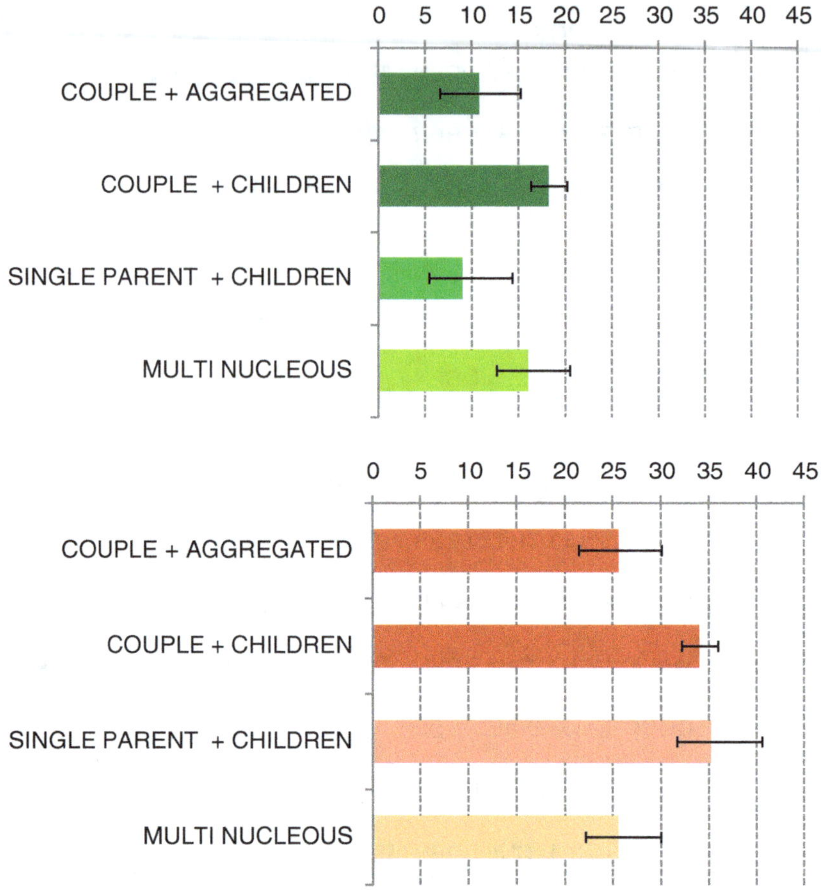

Fig. 5 Perceived health homogeneity between household members for 3 + households by structure

exhibit a level of homogeneity significantly different from the other groups according to PCS.

The picture given by MCS is entirely different: homogeneity is highest for households with adult children, despite the number of co-living parents (*hypothesis* 4). When the household comprises a couple (without children) living with relatives, the household members exhibit very different MCS, with significantly less resemblance than parents and children. People living in multinuclear households are the most heterogeneous group, confirming hypothesis 1.

Discussion

Heath is influenced not only by individual characteristics and behaviors but also by the different contexts in which the person lives. Of all of these contexts, our interest is focused on the role played by the family, which we defined as based on cohabitation. According to this definition we investigated the effects of household on health, after adjustment for available individual covariates, including age, gender, education, and objective health conditions.

In considering quantitative and qualitative perceived health outcomes, we were able to cross-validate the results, particularly those estimated for poor SRH, which could be affected by limitations related to the binary nature of the outcome. We documented an effect of household on health that ranges from 15 to 38% according to the health indicator in use.

We tried to corroborate this interpretation through an international comparison of household effects in contexts with different characteristics in terms of family role and health policy. Such a comparison is not easy, as to date only a handful of studies have looked at the issue of households influences on health, and across these studies the health outcome, the target population, and the country characteristics vary largely. Working on all-cause mortality in Sweden, Merlo et al. (2012) reported 18.6% of variability at the household level. Subramanian et al. (2003) found a very large effect of households on poor self-rated health in Chile (VPC of 47%), however they made use solely of the binary indicator (SRH). Van Minh et al. (2010) reported a share of only 15% of perceived *good* health variability among Vietnamese people over 50 which, however, is a different outcome and cannot simply be seen as the other side of the coin of our outcome (Benyamini et al. 2003; Kaplan and Baron-Epel 2003; Schüz et al. 2011). The only study concerning a developed country is based in the USA (Ferrer et al. 2005) and revealed a maximum variability share attributable to the family context of 9.9% for PCS and 15.4% for MCS, controlled for individual covariates The authors used census families, which include all persons related to the household's head by blood or marriage, disregarding the co-residence requisite. This can partially explain the lower effect of family on health with respect to our findings.

We made a further step towards a better understanding of the household effect by introducing family-covariates (i.e. a household's economic resources, size, and typology of household structure together with the size of the municipality of residence); however, we found that residual variance between households did not decrease substantially, i.e. these variables did not explain the difference in health between households. Aware of the strict dependence of variance between units at a higher level from the homogeneity of units within the groups themselves, we looked at the levels of homogeneity within households, and from this perspective we advanced the hypothesis that a major role can be played by *mutual influences* between members of the households, rather than exogenous factors. Actually, people living in the same households can have similar individual health determinants, such as nutritional choices, prevention attitude, health-seeking behavior, or health care utilization, which derive from a shared familial approach to health and care. These communalities can partially explain our results. However, there is another interpretation of mutual influences we found more stimulating and consistent with our data: the perceived health of one person can be directly affected by the perceived health of people living in the same household, especially in case of poor health. In this situation we observe mutual influences not related to similar determinants but related to the outcome itself, as happens when specific diseases or conditions affect household members asking for care from other members and altering their emotional status and subjective health (Egidi et al. 2013).

We expected these mutual influences to be of particular relevance in the Italian context, where the tightness of the links between family components and the limited support provided by the welfare state for the care of severe illnesses could emphasize the effects of "contagion" of poor health status.

It was not possible to test this hypothesis conclusively from our data; however, the analysis of homogeneity according to household structure did produce some insights in this direction. The effects of households were especially pronounced for small families and within couples.

In all, the results of homogeneity by household structure show a very clear pattern for 2-component households, while they appear more articulated when the household size increases. These results are in line with findings in social psychology, which have consistently documented a similarity in mental illness, depressive symptoms, and distress between spouses (Meyler et al. 2007; Monden 2007), and with those in sociology reporting a positive effect of partner interactions on well-being, happiness, and life satisfaction (Horwitz et al. 1998). We also documented that as the couples got older their concordance increases, which had already been noticed in studies of clinical medicine (Cheraskin et al. 1968; Johnson et al. 1965).

Furthermore, the family constellation has already been taken into consideration in relation to life satisfaction and well-being, suggesting that family structure and relations between family members are among the most important determinants of life satisfaction (Evans and Kelly 2004; Vignoli et al. 2012). Interpersonal relationships and social supports heavily shape an individual's well-being. and the most detailed investigation revealed that the effects of social support on well-being vary depending on family structure and the person providing support. We expand this framework by hypothesizing that similar mechanisms are at play when individuals rate their health. The very limited role played by the geographical context on individual perceived health was rather unexpected based on previous work illustrating a health gradient for both objective and subjective health in Italy (Costa et al. 2003; Mazzuco 2009). However, research that adopted a multilevel approach to investigate the Italian Regional and ALHU heterogeneity came to the same conclusion as we did, recognizing a proportion of variability at the ALHU level less than 3% for poor self-perceived health (Pirani and Salvini 2012).

There are also some limitations to our study, the most important of which is due to the cross-sectional nature of our data preventing us from controlling for a possible selection effect in household composition and examining the "dynamic" of mutual influences. Analyses of longitudinal data could provide valuable information about how mutual influences on health take place, particularly whether deterioration in the health perception of one member worsens the health perception of others and how long it takes for this influence to occur. These kinds of mechanisms are especially interesting when we explore health contagion from a gendered perspective. Italy, like other southern European countries, has a remarkable gender role differentiation, especially for older cohorts. Not only does this differentiation have effects on health outcomes per se, but it also determines that some typologies of activities, among which are the assistance of an ill family member, are strongly assigned to women within the families.

This asymmetry of gender roles within the family can affect the intensity and direction of the health influence between members. For example, we could expect the "contagion" of poor health to be stronger from men to women, because in the traditional family it is the woman who is requested to provide assistance and to take on the burden of her partner's disease. However, we could also expect the opposite: because the woman is used to this role of care-giver she would cope better with poor health of her partner than her partner would cope with hers.

Unfortunately, to better understand these mechanisms, longitudinal data are necessary because only if we look at temporal changes can we observe the direction of health influences; i.e. if the man or the woman worsen his/her health first and then affects the others.

Moreover, our data do not allow us to control for psychological variables, such as the personality traits of the household's members, and health related behaviors, which are often shared by family members. In conjunction with the selection effect for couples (*assortative mating*), these aspects could explain our results about health homogeneity, at least partially. However, while putting into question the primacy of the mutual influence hypothesis in explaining perceived health homogeneity inside households, these limitations do not detract from the importance played by the household context on members' health.

Conclusions

This research provides insights on the extent and the ways in which contextual factors shape subjective health. Within this general aim, we document three more specific results: (1) the geographical effect on health, examined by means of a multilevel approach, is dramatically resized compared to previous studies of the Italian case which used an ecological perspective; (2) household appears as a key-element in influencing the perceived health of individuals, with a clear gradient from physical to mental component; (3) the mechanism of the household effect on perceived health can reasonably rely on the reciprocal influences between family members.

When poor health enters into the family, even if solidarity is activated to cope with the need of the family member in poor health, cohabitation and emotional ties seem to act as a multiplier of poor health conditions, negatively altering the perceived health status of all family members. Health policies, traditionally targeted at single individuals, probably have positive effects that go far beyond the single recipient of the intervention. In fact, maintaining an individual in good health (and in good health perception) means that all of his/her family is protected from the process of health deterioration that could occur as a consequence of mutual influences on health. In this perspective, current evaluations of the benefits of social/

health interventions are consistently underestimated, as we overlook the *positive externalities* that each intervention has also on the family of the targeted recipient.

References

Agnessens, F., Waege, H., & Lievens, J. (2006). Diversity in social support by role relations: a typology. *Social Networks, 28,* 427–441.

Benyamini, Y., Leventhal, E. A., & Leventhal, H. (2003). Elderly people's rating of the importance of health-related factors to their self-assessments of health. *Social Science and Medicine, 56*, 1661–1667.

Biggeri, A., Pasetto, R., Belli, S., Bruno, C., Di Maria, G., Mastrantonio, M., et al. (2004). Mortality from chronic obstructive pulmonary disease and pleural mesothelioma in an area contaminated by natural fiber (fluoro-edenite). *Scandinavian Journal of Work Environment and Health, 30*(3), 249–252.

Bookwala, J., & Schulz, R. (2000). A comparison of primary stressors, secondary stressors, and depressive symptoms between elderly caregiving husbands and wives: the caregiver health effects study. *Psychology and Aging, 15*(4), 607–616.

Caselli, G., & Egidi, V. (1979). La geographie de la mortalite italienne: differences territoriales et milieu. *Genus, 35*(1/2), 101–153.

Cardol, M., Groenewegen, P. P., de Bakker, D. H., Spreeuwenberg, P., van Dijk, L., & van den Bosch, W. (2005). Shared help seeking behavior within families: A retrospective cohort study. *British Medical Journal, 330*(7496), 882.

Cheraskin, E., Ringsdorf, W. M., Setyaadmadja, A. T. S. H., Barrett, R. A., Sibley, G. T., & Reid, R. W. (1968). Environmental factors in blood glucose regulation. *Journal of the American Geriatrics Society, 16,* 823–825.

Cook, T. D., & Furstenberg, F. F. (2002). Explaining aspects of the transition to adulthood in Italy Sweden, Germany, and the United States: A cross-disciplinary, case synthesis approach. *The ANNALS of the American Academy of Political and Social Science, 580,* 257–287.

Costa, G., Marinacci, C., Caiazzo, A., & Spadea, T. (2003). Individual and contextual determinants of inequalities in health: The Italian case. *International Journal of Health Services, 33*(4), 635–667.

De Bruin, A., Picavet, H. S. J., & Nossikov, A. (1996). *Health interview surveys* (p. 58). European Series: Towards International Harmonization of Methods and Instruments, WHO Regional Publications.

Divino, F., Egidi, V., & Salvatore, M. A. (2009). Geographical mortality patterns in Italy: A bayesian analysis. *Demographic Research, 20*(18), 432–466.

Egidi, V., & Reynaud, C. (2005). Le politiche sanitarie nell'Italia del dopoguerra. *Popolazione e storia, 1,* 45–85.

Egidi, V., & Spizzichino, D. (2006). Perceived health and mortality: A multidimensional analysis of ECHP Italian data. *Genus, LXII*(3–4).

Egidi, V., Salvatore, M. A., Gargiulo, L., Iannucci, L., Sebastiani, G., & Tinto, A. (2013). Dementia in the elderly: Health consequences on household members. In N. Torelli, F. Pesarin, & A. Bar-Hen (Eds.), *Advances in theoretical and applied statistics*. Berlin Heidelberg: Springer-Verlag.

Evans, M. D. R., & Kelly, J. (2004). *Effects of family structure on life satisfaction: Australian evidence*. Melbourne, Vic: Melbourne Institute of Applied Economic and Social Research, University of Melbourne.

Ferrer, R. L., Palmer, R., & Burge, S. (2005). The family contribution to health status: A population-level estimate. *Annals of Family Medicine., 3*(2), 102–108.

Horwitz, A. V., McLaughlin, J., & Raskin White, H. (1998). How the negative and positive aspects of partner relationships affect the mental health of young married people. *Journal of Health and Social Behavior, 39*(2), 124–136.

Jagger. C., Gillies, C., Moscone, F., Cambois, E., Van Oyen, H., & Nusselder, W., et al.(2008). Inequalities in healthy life expectancies in EU25: A cross-national meta-regression analysis. *The Lancet, 9656*(372), 2124–2131.

Johnson, B. C., Epstein, F. H., & Kjelsberg, M. O. (1965). Distributions and familial studies of blood pressure and serum cholesterol levels in a total community—Tecumseh, Michigan. *Journal of Chronic Diseases, 18,* 147–160.

Joumard, I., André, C., Nicq, C., & Chatal, O. (2008). Health status determinants: Lifestyle, environment, health care resources and efficiency. *OECD Economics Department Working Papers, 627* (OECD Publishing).

Kaplan, G., & Baron-Epel, O. (2003). What lies behind the subjective evaluation of health status? *Social Science and Medicine, 56,* 1669–1676.

Kawachi, I., & Subramanian, S. V., (2005). Health demography. In Poston & Micklin (Eds.), *Handbook of population—handbooks of sociology and social research* (pp. 787–808). Springer.

Kawachi, I., Kennedy, B. P., & Glass, R. (1999). Social capital and self-rated health: A contextual analysis. *American Journal of Public Health, 89*(8), 1187–1193.

Kennedy, B. P., Kawachi, I., Glass, R., & Prothrow-Stith, D. (1998). Income distribution, socioeconomic status, and self-rated health in the United States: Multilevel analysis. *British Medical Journal, 317,* 917–921.

Kunst, A. E., Bos, V., Lahelma, E., Bartley, M., Lissau, I., Regidor, E., et al. (2005). Trends in socio-economic inequalities in self-assessed health in 10 European countries. *International Journal of Epidemiology, 34*(2), 295–305.

Martuzzi, M., Mitis, F., Biggeri, A., Terracini, B., & Bertollini, R. (2002). Ambiente e stato di salute nella popolazione delle aree ad alto rischio di crisi ambientale in Italia [Environment and health status of the population in areas with high risk of environmental crisis in Italy]. *Epidemiologia e Prevenzione, 26*(6), 1–53.

Mazzuco, S. (2009). Condizioni di salute nelle Regioni Italiane. In F. Ongaro & S. Salvini (Eds.), *Rapporto sulla popolazione—Salute e sopravvivenza*. Bologna: Gruppo di Coordinamento per la Demografia, Il Mulino.

Merlo, J., Viciana-Fernandez, F. J., & Ramiro-Farinas, D., Research Group of Longitudinal Database of Andalusian P. (2012). Bringing the individual back to small-area variation studies: A multilevel analysis of all-cause mortality in Andalusia, Spain. *Social Science and Medicine, 75,* 1477–1487.

Meyler, D., Stimpson, J. T., & Peek, M. C. (2007). Health concordance within couples: A systematic review. *Social Science and Medicine, 64,* 2297–2310.

Monden, C. (2007). Partners in health? Exploring resemblance in health between partners in married and cohabiting couples. *Sociology of Health & Illness, 29*(3), 391–411.

Ory, M. G., Yee, J. L., Tennestedt, S. L., & Schulz, R. (2000). The extent and impact of dementia care: Unique challenges experienced by family caregivers. In *Handbook on dementia caregiving: evidence-based interventions for family caregivers.* New York: Richard Schulz editor.

OECD. (2014). OECD reviews of health care quality: Italy 2014: Raising standard. Italy: OECD Publishing.

Pearce, J., & Dorling, D. (2006). Increasing geographical inequalities in health in New Zealand, 1980–2001. *International Journal of Epidemiology, 35*(3), 597–603.

Pirani, E., & Salvini, S. (2012). Socioeconomic inequalities and self-rated health: A multilevel study of Italian elderly. *Population Research and Policy Review, 31,* 97–117.

Rice, N., Carr-Hill, R., Dixon, P., & Sutton, M. (1998). The influence of households on drinking behaviour: A multilevel analysis. *Social Science and Medicine, 46*(8), 971–979.

Rivellini, G. (2006). *Network analysis: From theory to applications.* CLEUP, Padova (Italy): Atti della XLIII Riunione Scientifica della SIS.

Schor, E., Starfield, B., Stidley, C., & Hankin, J. (1987). Family health: Utilization and effects of family membership. *Medical Care, 25*(7), 616–626.

Schüz, B., Wurm, S., Schöllgen, I., & Tesch-Römer, C. (2011). What do people include when they self-rate their health? Differential associations according to health status in community-dwelling older adults. *Quality of Life Research, 20,* 1573–1580.

Sepehri, A., Moshiri, S., Simpson, W., & Sarma, S. (2008). Taking account of context: How important are household characteristics in explaining adult health-seeking behaviour? The case of Vietnam. *Health Policy and Planning, 23*(6), 397–407.

Snijders, T. A. B., & Bosker, R. J. (2012). *Multilevel analysis* (2nd ed.). SAGE Publications Ltd.

Stafford, M., & McCarthy, M. (2006). Neighbourhoods, housing, and health. In M. Marmot & R. G. Wilkinson (Eds.), *Social determinants of health.* Oxford University Press.

Subramanian, S. V., Kawachi, I., & Kennedy, B. P. (2001). Does the state you live in make a difference? Multilevel analysis of self-rated health in the US. *Social Science and Medicine, 53*(1), 9–19.

Subramanian, S. V., Delgado, I., Jadue, L., Vega, J., & Kawachi, I. (2003). Income inequality and health: Multilevel analysis of Chilean communities. *Journal of Epidemiology and Community Health, 57,* 844–848.

Tomassini, C., Wolf, D., & Rosina, A. (2003). Parental housing assistance and parent-child proximity in Italy. *Journal of Marriage and the Family, 65,* 700–715.

Van Minh, H., Byass, P., & Wall, S. (2010). Multilevel analysis of effects of individual characteristics and household factors on self-rated health among older adults in rural Vietnam. *Geriatrics and Gerontology International, 14,* 209–215.

Vignoli, D., & Matysiak, A. (2013). Diverse effects of women's employment on fertility: Insights from Italy and Poland. *European Journal of Population, 29,* 273–302.

Vignoli, D., Pirani, E., & Salvini, S. (2012). Family constellation and life satisfaction in Europe. In *Paper Presented at the International Society for Quality of Life Studies (ISQOLS) XI World Conference*. Venice (Italy). November 1–4.

Vlachantoni, A. (2010). The demographic characteristics and economic activity patterns of carers over 50: Evidence from the english longitudinal study of ageing. *Population Trend 2010.* Office for National Statistics (UK).

Household Position, Parenthood, and Self-reported Adult Health. Cross-Sectional and Longitudinal Evidence from the Austrian Generations and Gender Survey

Isabella Buber-Ennser and Doris Hanappi

Introduction

Family contexts have become increasingly heterogeneous in western Europe in this century, and Austria is a country of remarkable postponement of parenthood and a high prevalence of premarital cohabitation (Elzinga and Liefbroer 2007). This overall development has fueled interest among social scientists to examine the importance of family structures and the composition of a variety of societal outcomes, including health. Numerous studies have focused on well-being (captured via quality of life) (Wahrendorf and Siegrist 2010), mental health and depression (Khalaila and Litwin 2014; Ball et al. 2009), major diseases and disability as well as physical and cognitive functioning (Avendano et al. 2009; Hank et al. 2013). A central argument is that individuals' physical and mental health, and more generally their well-being, depends not only on their genetic disposition but is also influenced by social context.

From a life-course perspective, human beings share their lives with parents, siblings, partners, children, relatives, friends, neighbours, and colleagues. The relational and institutional embedding and shared events—or the lack of events—over the life course as well as personal characteristics and the needs of those involved have a large influence on an individual's health. The term "linked lives"

I. Buber-Ennser (✉)
Wittgenstein Centre (IIASA, VID/ÖAW, WU), Vienna Institute of Demography/Austrian Academy of Sciences, Vienna, Austria
e-mail: Isabella.Buber-Ennser@oeaw.ac.at

D. Hanappi
University of California, Berkeley, Berkeley, USA
e-mail: dorish@demog.berkeley.edu

D. Hanappi
Austrian Academy of Sciences (ÖAW), Vienna, Austria

G. Doblhammer and J. Gumà (eds.), *A Demographic Perspective on Gender, Family and Health in Europe*, https://doi.org/10.1007/978-3-319-72356-3_8

(Elder 1995) has become an accepted, powerful synonym for situations in which effects occurring in one life domain (e.g. the family) spill over to another domain (e.g. health, work). In a family, there are members who enter or exit a union, become parents, or who form new unions. Such transitions and family events lead to changes in the physical and mental situations of men and women, key aspects being the gendered nature of family structure and household composition and the different gender norms that govern representations and practices of appropriate family roles for men and women (see Oláh, Kotowska and Richter in this book). This indicates attitudes and norms that expect men and women to fulfill different roles in the family—as caregivers, breadwinners, or sons/daughters. Gendered practices are not necessarily perceived as unfair, instead they are mentioned in discourses on the partners' freedom of choice and preferences or their abilities to perform given tasks (Bernardi et al. 2013). In turn, these choices and preferences lead to gender-specific practices within the family context over time, which in turn produces distinct health outcomes for men and women.

In order to understand the dynamics of health in families over the life course, we adopt a longitudinal perspective. Only a few longitudinal studies to date have focused on this topic, but the launch of European panel data comprising detailed information on demographic events, partnership, socio-economic characteristics, living arrangements, and subjective well-being allows individuals to be studied over time and to examine not only the household constellation and health of women and men, but also changes over time. These data are therefore highly suitable for assessing the link between changes in family structure and household position and changes in subjective health, and to disentangle the causal relationship between the two components. Austria participates in the Generations and Gender Survey (GGS), a European longitudinal survey, the two waves of which were carried out in 2008/9 and 2012/3. This is a unique opportunity to combine micro data on demographic events, partner and socio-economic status, living arrangements, and subjective well-being which thus allows the study of changes over time. Our findings are based on the rich GGS data and examine women's and men's health in young and middle adulthood from a household and family perspective. We focus on the reproductive years of respondents in the Austrian context from a cross-sectional and a longitudinal perspective while concentrating on the household position by gender (in the cross-sectional models) and accounting for partner status and the existence of pre-union children, parity, and the arrival of a newborn child. While our primary interest is on the general relationships between individuals' family contexts and different health outcomes, we include non-standard living arrangements, especially stepfamilies and individuals living apart together.

Household Position and Adult Health

Although there are well-known universalities in the family–health nexus, it is important to place households in their particular historical social context (see also Hank and Steinbach in this book). This includes properly accounting for the growing heterogeneity of *household compositions*, which implies that considering only standard living arrangements (e.g. marriage) is no longer sufficient anymore for understanding how, for example, living with a partner within the same household or in separate households affects health (e.g. Schneider et al. 2014).

In this context, the term 'de-institutionalization' of the life course has become accepted and is now a synonym for the process by which the social and temporal organization of the life course becomes less guided by normative, legal, or organizational rules (Elzinga and Liefbroer 2007). This concept is particularly useful when studying changes in household position and the occurrence of events (union formation, separation, birth) and their effects on different life domains, such as health, as it implies that the occurrence and particularly the sequencing of events becomes less clear and that the likelihood of combining multiple roles within the family increases. Brückner and Mayer (2005) suggested that family lives are becoming more differentiated, implying an increase in the number of family-related states and an emphasis on the rise of new types of living arrangements. A second aspect in the de-standardization of family lives implies that these are becoming less similar to one another and that the domination of specific family contexts is weakening. This applies in particular to married couples living with one or two children of their own.

Marriage has largely been found to improve health in the short and long term, with numerous studies examining the association between marital status and health (for a discussion of selection issues see Hank and Steinbach in this volume). Married individuals report better self-assessed health, have lower rates of long-term illness, are less depressed, and live longer than their unmarried counterparts (Hemström 1996; Lillard and Waite 1995; Ross et al. 1990). Three explanations are given for this link between marital status with health. *First*, marriage is a *marital resource* which impacts health through better access to economic resources, social support, and regulation of health behaviours that married individuals have (Ross et al. 1990). *Second*, health selection into marriage is crucial (Goldman 1993). In a longitudinal study, Joung et al. (1998) showed that married people who reported various health complaints or chronic conditions were significantly more likely to become divorced than people without these health problems. More recently Koball et al. (2010) confirmed this health selection into marriage using data on African Americans. Similarly, a longitudinal study by Brockmann and Klein (2004) provided empirical evidence that marriage, especially a long-lasting first marriage, had positive health effects which accumulated over time and thus promoted longevity. *Third*, the marital differences in health exist primarily because the strains of marital dissolution decrease health (Booth and Amato 1991; Amato 2000). The latter perspective, however, only explains temporary health declines after a marital dissolution; it assumes similar health outcomes for the married and those long after a transition out of marriage (i.e. divorced or widowed). Previous studies of the health effects of marital status have confirmed primarily short-term effects on mental health (Booth and Amato 1991; Amato and Hohmann-Marriott 2007).

Since the 1970s, *cohabitation* has gained increasing interest as a new type of living arrangement (Beaujouan and Bhrolcháin 2011), and numerous studies have shown that its prevalence has been steadily increasing across Europe and in the US (Perelli-Harris et al. 2014; Heuveline and Timberlake 2004). Whereas premarital cohabitation delays entrance into marriage, it has not become a long-term alternative to marriage, especially when raising children (Perelli-Harris and Lyons-Amos 2015; Perelli-Harris et al. 2012). In the context of health, cohabitation is less researched than its traditional counterpart of marriage, partly because cohabitation has often been a preliminary stage to marriage and thus involves younger individuals in particular. Findings on the link between cohabitation and health are mixed. On the one hand, research finds no mental health differences between cohabiting and married or single individuals (Horwitz and White 1998), and similar results were obtained in a study comparing cohabiting and married individuals (Horwitz and White 1998; Marcussen 2005). On the other hand, in a study comparing cohabiting and married individuals using the 1998 Health and Retirement Study, Brown et al. (2005) found that cohabitors report more depressive symptoms on average than do married couples, net of economic resources, social support, and physical health. Moreover, cohabitation is associated with more risky behaviour (Horwitz and White 1998).

These differences are largely explained by whether young or older adults are examined, cross-sectional or longitudinal design are used, and by the comparison group chosen. If less emphasis is placed on marital status and more on household position, we expect that individuals living together with a partner would report better health than those not living in a couple context. A major reason for this is that living together with a partner—especially in middle adulthood—corresponds to the 'normative life course'.

There is substantial evidence linking partnership quality to health. Marital happiness and marital problems are significantly associated with physical health, and marital strain accelerates the decline in self-rated health (Miller et al. 2013; Umberson et al. 2006). Thus, we expect a positive association between partnership quality and subjective well-being.

Divorce is still a critical life event for both partners, and individual characteristics are crucial for health outcomes (Amato 2010; Holmes and Rahe 1967). Cross-sectional studies have provided evidence for the negative health effects of marital disruption (Aseltine and Kessler 1993; Ren 1997). Fewer studies have looked at the aspect of personal growth, as a psychological aspect, through divorce and separation. Perrig-Chiello and Knöpfli's longitudinal study (2015) of separation impacts on mental health finds recovery effects after divorce: They show that women reported higher depressive symptoms and perceived stress and loneliness during and after separation, whereas men were more likely to report higher levels of social isolation. At the same time, women recovered from separation within two years, whereas no similar effect was observed for men. In line with these arguments, we expect separation in Austria to harm subjective health in the short and medium term, which is expressed by lower self-assessed health after separation.

Living apart together (LAT) relationships, where partners maintain separate households and finances, are becoming more common in northern and western Europe (Davidson 2002; De Jong Gierveld 2004; Karlsson and Borell 2002; Castro-Martín et al. 2008). This type of partnership is prevalent also at older ages and is a preliminary stage of the courtship process potentially leading to cohabitation. In Europe today, unmarried cohabitation and living apart together relationships are frequently opted for on re-partnering after bereavement or divorce, even at higher ages (De Jong Gierveld 2004). Individuals in intimate non-cohabiting relationships are a heterogeneous group, including young adults, women living alone with their children after separation, and older persons. The main explanations for not sharing a household are a wish to remain independent, financial constraints, and work issues (Régnier-Loilier et al. 2009). However, studies on the link between non-cohabiting relationships and health of individuals in this living arrangement are rather scarce. We expect that having an LAT partner in young and middle adulthood to be positively associated with health as opposed to individuals reporting no intimate relationship.

Parenthood and Adult Health

A large number of family studies have focused on the association between responsibilities related to raising children and health outcomes (for an overview see Uhlenberg and Mueller 2003). In this context, scholars have also recently explored the relationship between happiness and childbearing (Baranowska and Matysiak 2011; Aassve et al. 2012; Myrskylä and Margolis 2014; Kohler et al. 2005). To explain childbearing and health, three explanations are most common: *First*, economic and rational-choice approaches to parenthood assume that individuals derive 'utility' from having children and that their decisions are based on the gains achieved by having children as compared to utility gains that are incurred from alternative allocations of resources, such as income and time, which are also required to maintain partnerships and raise children. Recent studies suggest that utility can be investigated empirically by using measures of subjective well-being (Stutzer and Frey 2010). Assuming that individuals have no misconceptions about childbearing and make conscious and informed decisions, one would expect that children would increase happiness. *Second*, Easterlin (2006) notes that significant life events, such as the birth of a child, only transitorily change an individual's well-being from a setpoint that is determined by personality traits and genetic factors. In this perspective, individuals restore their well-being to a predetermined setpoint after the birth of a child (see Kohler et al. 2005). In line with this, happiness increases in the years around the birth of a first child and then decreases to before-child levels (Myrskylä and Margolis 2014). *Third*, role-identity theory

(Stryker 1980) accounts for gender differences in social roles linked with socially constructed behavioural expectations. Fulfilling the parent role and simultaneously performing other roles as a partner, son/daughter, or employee may cause conflicting behavioural expectations leading to role overload and thus decreased well-being (Marks 1998). It is possible that having children increases demands from the family and thereby generates role overload. These demands arising from parenthood are highly gendered (Voydanoff 2005). In summary, economic and role-theoretic models expect women who take on most of the care burden to experience most of the decrease in subjective health when having children. Given the gendered division of childcare and household duties in Austria (Berghammer 2014; Buber-Ennser 2015), we anticipate negative health outcomes for mothers of two or more children. There is, however, sufficient variation in health outcomes depending on the age of the youngest child in the home (Hanappi 2012), the positive health effect of having school children (Mason and Kuhltau 1989), and the overall number of children in a household. Especially the birth of the first child has a positive effect on the subjective well-being of mothers (Baranowska and Matysiak 2011; Myrskylä and Margolis 2014). Accordingly, we expect a positive effect of the birth of a child on health.

Lone parents are an increasingly important group in contemporary Western populations. Numerous studies have shown that lone parents have a poorer health status than the general population (Franz and Lensche 2003; Benzeval 1998; Witvliet et al. 2014; Van de Velde et al. 2014). Although health differences mirror variations in socioeconomic circumstances, lone mothers in particular have significantly poorer health than couple mothers, even after controlling for a wide range of demographic and socioeconomic circumstances. The absence of an intimate relationship, the stress and stigma associated with being a lone parent, and health selection might be alternative explanations for health differences between lone and couple parents (Benzeval 1998; Vingilis et al. 1998). We anticipate lone mothers will have worse self-perceived health compared to mothers co-residing with a partner.

A last group of interest are *stepfamilies*—a group that has higher rates of separation and divorce, with childbearing extending over several partnerships (Beaujouan and Solaz 2013; Beaujouan 2011; Bumpass et al. 1995; Thomson et al. 2002, 2012). Stepfamilies have become an important object of study (Thomson 1997, 2004; Vikat et al. 1999; Thomson 2014; Thomson et al. 2014). In the late 1970s, Furstenberg (1979) already observed that this process of "recycling the family" had replaced the nuclear family with distinct implications for kinship systems. Due to changes in traditional family structures, the term stepfamilies, formerly restricted to marriages, has been extended and now includes cohabiting unions with at least one child from a previous union (Bumpass et al. 1995). Recently, the terms 'multi-partner fertility' and 'complex families' have been used to describe adults having children with more than one person (Meyer et al. 2005; Evenhouse and Reilly 2012; Thomson 2014). Studies on stepfamilies in demography have focused mainly on childbearing and dissolution. Another vein of research examines children's health, behaviour, support, and school achievement in such families (Bronte-Tinkew et al. 2009; Guzzo 2009; Osborne and McLanahan 2007). Empirical evidence from the US shows that children and adolescents in single-parent or stepfather families reported significantly poorer physical and mental health than persons living with both biological parents (Heard et al. 2008; Dawson 1991). The health of parents in complex families has rarely been investigated, and insights from the well-being of (mainly) mothers and fathers in stepfamilies largely stem from the US and also reveal negative effects for adults. Mothers with children by more than one father report lower support and are more prone to depressive symptoms than mothers with children by only one partner (Harknett and Knab 2007; Turney and Carlson 2011). Parental health in stepfamilies still constitutes an area open for research in the European context. The potential negative effect of the well-being of individuals in multipartnered families is expected to correlate with economic, psychological, and social deprivation. Social selection may comprise part of the link between well-being and multi-partnered families; health disadvantages and stepfamilies may be "reciprocally related and part of broader processes of social disadvantage" (Turney and Carlson 2011, p. 570). If people of a lower socio-economic status and well-being are more likely to enter into multi-partnered families (see. e.g. Treviño and Gumà (2013) for disadvantaged divorced individuals entering remarriage in Spain), we might easily associate such a multi-partnered context with lower well-being.

Data and Methods

The current study is based on the first two waves of the Austrian Generations and Gender Survey (GGS). The first wave took place in 2008/9 and included 5001 respondents aged 18–44, the second wave was carried out four years later in 2012/13. In total 78% of wave 1 respondents were interviewed again in wave 2, corresponding to a relatively low panel dropout of 22% (Buber-Ennser 2014). Overall, the Austrian GGS panel data can be used without (significant) concern about selectivity (Buber-Ennser 2014) and are a valuable source for studying living arrangements and health as well as their dynamics over a period of four years.

The main variables used in our study include two crucial dimensions, living arrangements and health. Individuals' health is measured based on self-perceived health status, from the question "How is your health in general?" Possible answers were (1) very good, (2) good, (3) fair, (4) bad, and (5) very bad. This is a powerful measure of health, as studies have consistently found that it is an independent predictor of mortality (Idler and Benyamini 1997). Nevertheless, recent findings indicate that the predictive capacity of self-perceived health on mortality decreases for old and late old ages (Woo and Zajacova 2015). For the descriptive results we keep part of the detailed levels and give means. For multivariate analyses these are categorized into a binary health variable "(very) good" and "fair or worse". For the sake of simplicity, we denote those with fair, bad, or very bad health as being in poor health, and those with good or very good health as being in good health.

We focus on the individual's position within the household according to (1) partnership situation (living or not with a partner), (2) living with children, and (3) the relationship within the family nucleus (member or not of the nucleus). As the age of the target population is 18–44, this differentiation is important for this period encompassing the transition to adulthood. The position in the household is a more appropriate way to capture the advantages and disadvantages a person faces in a particular household composition. The distinction between being an adult son or daughter or being the mother or father in a household allows the role of (mainly) the recipient and provider of resources to be taken into account. Additionally, the differentiation between childless couples, couples with one child, and those with two or more children assesses the responsibilities associated with childrearing within couples. Lone mothers and lone fathers, constituting a key group in family studies, are associated with a higher risk of poverty and a variety of health problems (Curtis and Pennock 2006; Curtis 2001; Benzeval 1998). We distinguish between (1) living alone, (2) adult son/daughter, (3) living with a partner and no children in the household, (4) living with a partner and one child, (5) living with a partner and two or more children, (6) single parent, and (7) other. The latter group includes various arrangements of shared living. As non-cohabiting relationships are not captured when focusing on household, an indicator equalling one for living apart together relationships was incorporated into the model in order to include this type of partnership.[1]

Available detailed information on children allows for a distinction to be made between families where parents have shared child(ren) only and stepfamilies, where at least one partner has a pre-union child, either living or not living in the household. In the remainder of the chapter, stepfamilies, patchwork families, and complex families are used synonymously. Several indicators for the existence of stepfamily context were considered, namely (1) a binary variable distinguishing whether respondents' children with a previous partner are living in the household (to avoid collinearity with single parents, this variable takes the value of one only if the respondent is living with a partner), (2) a binary variable indicating if pre-union children of the partner (i.e. respondents' stepchildren) are living in the household, (3) a binary variable indicating if the respondent has pre-union children not living in the household, and (4) a binary variable indicating if the partner has pre-union children not living in the household (i.e. respondents' stepchildren). These indicators were first analysed separately and then combined with a further dichotomous variable capturing patchwork families. The latter variable took value one if the respondent or his/her partner had pre-union children either living in or outside the household.

Various socio-demographic variables crucial for individuals' health status are included in the analyses, such as age, educational attainment, and economic situation (Ross and Wu 1995). We chose education as our measure of socioeconomic status. National-specific levels are classified into four categories according to the international standard classification of education (ISCED): levels 0–2 (lower secondary

[1]In Austria, among persons aged 18–44 in LAT relationships, the wish for independence and not being ready to live together were by far the reasons cited most often for not cohabiting.

school or lower), 3 (upper secondary school), 4 (post-secondary non-tertiary education) and 5–6 (tertiary education). These categories represent milestones in the educational process, important in determining health and commonly used in health research (Galobardes et al. 2006). The individuals' financial situation[2] is captured via the question: "Thinking about your household's total monthly income, is your household able to make ends meet (1) with great difficulty, (2) with difficulty, (3) with some difficulty, (4) fairly easily, (5) easily, or (6) very easily." This self-rated economic status is a valuable general indicator for financial capacity (Litwin and Sapir 2009). Quality of partnership measured via "How satisfied are you with your relationship with your partner/spouse?", ranging from 0 (not satisfied) to 10 (very satisfied) is another important aspect. A dichotomous variable distinguishing between satisfied (8–10) and not satisfied (0–7) was included in the analyses.[3]

In a first step, the household position and the health status at wave 1 are analysed from a cross-sectional perspective (see Section "Cross-Sectional Perspective: Health at Wave 1"). Descriptive statistics give an overview on what household forms Austrians aged 18–44 years live in and how they evaluate their health. Mean self-perceived health and share of persons in poor health by household position and sex provide insights into differences across groups. In multivariate analyses, self-perceived health at wave 1 is regressed on the study variables. The dependent variable, self-perceived health, was dichotomized into good versus poor health. Analyses are carried out for women and men separately in order to detect possible differences in the association between the sexes. We focus on household position and control for important background variables such as age, education, financial situation, and quality of partnership. Moreover, indicators for stepfamily context and LAT are included in the models.

In a second step (see Section "Longitudinal Perspective: Changes Over Time"), we adopt a longitudinal perspective in order to analyse changes in household position and in health over a period of four years. Descriptive results provide insights into the dynamics over time regarding health and household position. In a multivariate framework, logistic regressions depict how health at wave 2 is associated with household position and health in wave 1 and further socio-demographic characteristics. Crucial events such as the birth of a child or a change in partnership are taken into consideration. In the regression model, the independent variable is health at wave 2, measured—in line with the cross-sectional model—as a dichotomous variable (0 for good versus 1 for poor health). Binary logistic regression analyses with poor health at wave 2 as a dependent variable were calculated. Household position, health at wave 1 and further socio-economic determinants (both at wave 1 and wave 2) are explanatory variables, following an approach by Khalaila and Litwin (2014). By controlling for health at wave 1, we are able to capture

[2]As mentioned earlier, one individual per household was interviewed, thus data are independent in terms of households.

[3]A different grouping with 'satisfied' for 7–10 and 'not satisfied' for 0–6 leads to similar results in multivariate analyses.

changes in health over time. As results for household position are similar for women and men, we run joint regressions for both sexes, controlling for sex.

Stepwise models for cross-sectional and longitudinal approaches allow insights in the mediating effects of various explanatory variables. Positive coefficients in the regression models indicate a higher risk of reporting bad health.

Results

Cross-Sectional Perspective: Health at Wave 1

In the overall sample, four in ten people were living as a couple with one or more children, one in four were (still) living in the parental home, 15% were living alone and roughly the same number were living with a partner and no children (Table 1). Four percent were single parents and the remaining 3% reported other shared living arrangements (flat-sharing with relatives was more common than with non-relatives, like students).

A differentiation by age and gender depicts the transition to adulthood, including leaving the parental home to live alone or with a partner, and the family formation process (Table 2). Whereas below age 20 the majority was living in the parental home, this proportion decreased to one-half and two-thirds for women and men in the early twenties, and 16% and one-third, respectively, in the late twenties. From age 20 onwards, about 10–25% lived with a partner and without children. From age 25 onwards, roughly 20% shared the household with the partner and a child, and households with couples and two and more children were most frequent in the thirties and forties. Women experienced major demographic events, such as leaving the parental home, having a first, and eventually a second child, earlier than men did. Children were mainly raised in a couple context: in the age group 30–44 years, 10–13% of women were single mothers and only a minority of men were single fathers.

In young and middle adulthood, 57% perceive their health as very good, 34% as good, 8% as fair, 1% as bad, and 0.2% as very bad (Table 1). Therefore, nine in ten people in this age group reported good health, the remaining 10% reported poor health. Poor health was more frequently stated by women (12%) than by men (7%) (Table 1). Even at this age, we find statistically significant differences in health among women and men[4] (Fig. 2).

When calculating means of self-rated health measured on a five-point scale (with 1 representing very good and 5 very bad health), the variation across household position and gender becomes evident. Men and women aged 18–44 living with their parents evaluated their health best, single mothers and mothers of two and more children living with a partner worst. Although for various household arrangements differences between men and women exist, these were statistically significant only

[4]Confidence intervals are [6.2%; 8.4%] for men and [10.7%; 13.0%] for women.

Table 1 Household position and self-perceived health of Austrian population aged 15–44

	Percentages (weighted)			Totals (N unweighted)		
	Men (%)	Women (%)	Total (%)	Men	Women	Total
Household position						
Living alone	17	12	15	305	339	644
Son/daughter	29	19	24	489	397	886
Living with partner no children	12	14	13	334	446	829
Living with partner and child	13	15	14	272	437	679
Living with partner and children	26	29	28	534	1045	1560
Single parent	0	8	4	10	264	274
Other	3	2	3	56	73	129
Total	100	100	100	2000	3001	5001
Self-perceived health						
Very good	57.9	55.3	56.6	1165	1664	2829
Good	34.8	32.9	33.8	694	990	1684
Fair	6.3	10.0	8.1	124	295	419
Bad	0.8	1.7	1.2	14	45	59
Very bad	0.2	0.2	0.2	3	7	10
Total	100	100	100	2000	3001	5001

Source Austrian GGS 2008/9, wave 1

for men and women living with a partner and children, while for the other groups the confidence intervals overlap (Fig. 1). An alternative way of depicting differences in health is to state the share of persons in poor health (Fig. 2). Differences by gender and household position become even more evident: 10% among men as opposed to 15% among women living with a partner and children reported poor health. The highest share of poor health was reported by single mothers (18%). Moreover, gender differences for those living alone and living with a partner and no children were large, although not statistically significant, as the confidence intervals overlap (Fig. 2).

Turning to the stepfamily context, mean self-perceived health was significantly worse in patchwork families (Table 3): In households where at least one partner had pre-union children either living or not living in the household, adults evaluated their own health worse than adults not living in complex families (mean self-rated health 1.67 and 1.53, respectively; the share of people in poor health was 14 and 9%, respectively; confidence intervals do not overlap, see Table 3). Specification by various types of patchwork families reveals that this was especially the case for those where stepchildren were not living in the household but with the other parent.

Table 2 Household positions of Austrian population aged 18–44 by age and gender

		Living alone (%)	Son/ daughter (%)	Living with partner no children (%)	Living with partner and child (%)	Living with partner and children (%)	Single parent (%)	Other (%)	Total (%)
All	Total	15	24	13	14	28	4	3	100
Women	18–19	5	88	2	1	0	2	2	100
	20–24	13	47	18	9	3	4	7	100
	25–29	18	16	25	19	15	4	3	100
	30–34	12	6	16	18	36	10	2	100
	35–39	11	4	8	18	47	11	1	100
	40–44	12	2	11	15	46	13	0	100
	Total	12	19	14	15	29	8	2	100
Men	18–19	4	90	1	0	0	1	4	100
	20–24	14	65	11	4	1	0	5	100
	25–29	21	34	19	12	9	0	5	100
	30–34	22	17	15	19	25	0	2	100
	35–39	21	10	9	18	41	0	1	100
	40–44	15	7	10	14	51	2	2	100
	Total	17	29	12	13	26	0	3	100

Source Austrian GGS 2008/9, wave 1

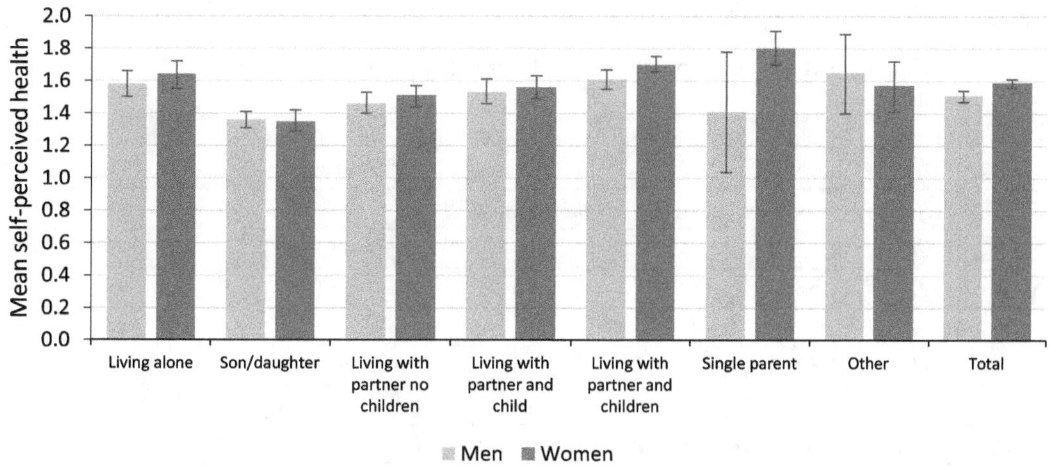

Fig. 1 Mean self-perceived health by position in household and gender. *Source* Austrian GGS 2008/9, wave 1

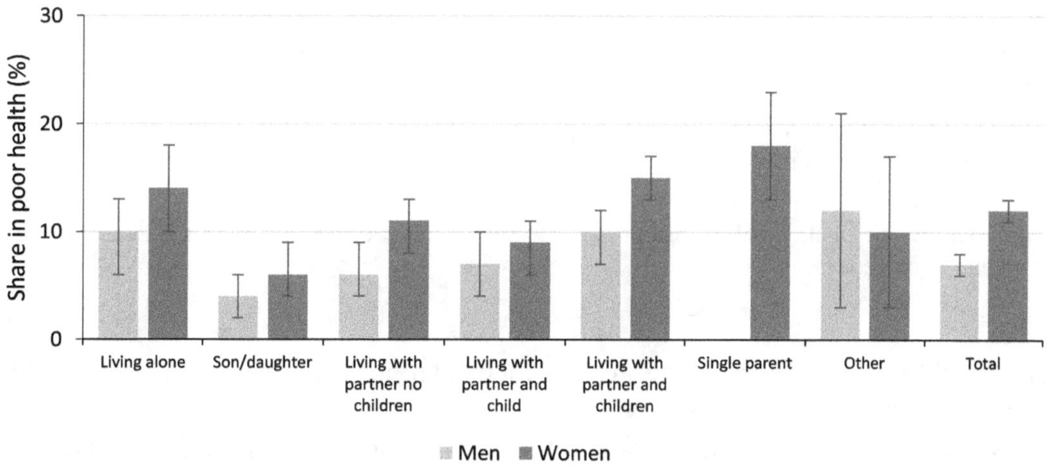

Fig. 2 Share of people in poor health by position in household and gender. *Source* Austrian GGS 2008/9, wave 1

A further differentiation by gender shows significant health differences for patchwork families for both women and men.[5]

We explored an interaction of health with education, as divorce rates are higher and available resources to handle complex family situations are fewer among less educated persons. It turned out that people with low and medium education living in stepfamilies evaluated their own health as poor (16%) substantially more often, compared to their peers not in complex families (10%). Moreover, highly educated

[5]Mean self-perceived health for women in patchwork families: 1.69 [1.60; 1.78]; for women not in patchwork families: 1.57 [1.55; 1.60]; for men in patchwork families: 1.65 [1.54; 1.76]; for men not in patchwork families: 1.49 [1.46; 1.52].

Table 3 Self-perceived health in stepfamily context

	Self-perceived health (5-point scale)		Poor self-perceived health (binary)		N
	Mean	95% Confidence interval	Mean (%)	95% Confidence interval	
Children with previous partner living in the household					
No	1.54	[1.52; 1.56]	9	[8%; 10%]	4847
Yes	1.69	[1.55; 1.82]	15	[9%; 20%]	154
Stepchildren living in the household					
No	1.54	[1.52; 1.56]	9	[9%; 10%]	4920
Yes	1.68	[1.51; 1.86]	16	[8%; 24%]	81
Children with previous partner not living in the household					
No	1.54	[1.52; 1.56]	10	[9%; 10%]	4884
Yes	1.58	[1.44; 1.72]	11	[5%; 17%]	117
Stepchildren not living in the household					
No	1.54	[1.52; 1.56]	9	[9%; 10%]	4780
Yes	1.75	[1.64; 1.85]	15	[10%; 20%]	221
Patchwork family					
No	1.53	[1.51; 1.55]	9	[8%; 10%]	4501
Yes	1.67	[1.60; 1.74]	14	[11%; 17%]	500

Source Austrian GGS 2008/9, wave 1

Note Due to the small number, results are not shown for women and men separately but are available upon request

people did not vary in the perception of their own health whether they were living in patchwork families or not (Fig. 3).

Next, multivariate models examine the association between household position and health. In a stepwise procedure, age, educational level, stepfamily context, economic constraints (e.g. having to make ends meet), existence of LAT relationship, and partnership quality were included. Individuals living with a partner and one child in the household are the reference group. In a basic model including only household position, women living alone, women living with a partner and two or more children, and single mothers statistically significantly reported poor health more often, whereas men living in the parental home did so less often (Table 4, Models 1). As expected, age and education are strongly associated with self-perceived health (Table 4, Models 2): Poor health was more often reported with increasing age. Results for education are less straightforward. With upper secondary school as the reference group, the association between women's health and education is evident; i.e. health outcomes are poor especially for those with low levels of education. In contrast, more highly educated men report poor health significantly less often. In other words, education and health are positively associated across gender, although less educated women report significantly lower health compared to their more highly educated peers, but it is the men with higher education who report more positive health outcomes. When controlling for age, the

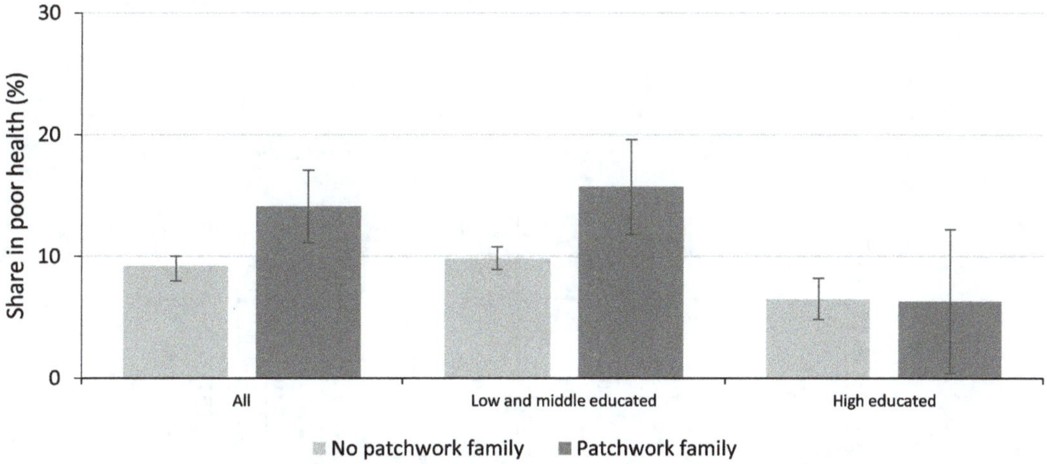

Fig. 3 Share of people in poor health by patchwork family status and education. *Source* Austrian GGS 2008/9, wave 1

estimated coefficient for women living in the parental home becomes positive and statistically significant. This indicates that the originally good self-perceived health of adult women living as daughters in the parental home is due to their young age. The same holds true for women and men living in shared households with relatives or non-relatives, but not parents, children, or partners. On the opposite side, the significant negative coefficient for sons becomes non-significant, showing again that the good health of men living in the parental home is mainly due to age and educational differences.

Furthermore, we find that women living in patchwork families more often reported poor health than those who are not (Table 4, Models 3). For men, the estimated coefficient is also positive, but lacks statistical significance. When introducing LAT partnership, the estimated coefficient is negative both for women and men, but statistically significant only for men (Table 4, Models 4). This indicates that men who have a romantic relationship, but who do not live together with that person, report good health. Moreover, people having an LAT partnership report positively on their health. We also find that economic constraints are important: the easier young and middle-aged adults can make ends meet, the better their health (Table 4, Models 5). In Model 5 we included the variable "making ends meet" to account for financial constraints. This operation reduces the size and significance of the status "being a single mother", showing that part of their less favourable health is due to financial constraints. Moreover, the smaller and less significant coefficient for education in Model 5 compared to Model 4 shows that educational level correlates with one's financial situation. Similarly, the coefficient for patchwork families becomes smaller in size and statistical significance, indicating correlations between stepfamily context and economic constraints. Finally, we only consider individuals with a partner (either cohabiting or LAT) and find that men and women who are less satisfied with their partnership more often report poor health (Table 4, Models 6).

Table 4 Binary logistic regression with poor self-perceived health as dependent variable

	Women						Men					
	Model 1	Model 2	Model 3	Model 4	Model 5	Model 6	Model 1	Model 2	Model 3	Model 4	Model 5	Model 6
Household position												
Living alone	0.56*	0.71**	0.79**	0.88***	0.73**	–	0.30	0.43	0.44	0.70*	0.54	–
Son/daughter	−0.26	0.50+	0.58+	0.68*	0.77*	–	−0.57+	0.02	0.05	0.33	0.51	–
Living with partner no children	0.33	0.55*	0.55*	0.55*	0.58*	0.58*	−0.22	−0.07	-0.07	−0.07	0.14	0.15
Living with partner and child	0	0	0	0	0	0	0	0	0	0	0	0
Living with partner and children	0.58**	0.30	0.33	0.33	0.29	0.32	0.27	0.08	0.10	0.11	0.07	0.10
Single parent	0.89***	0.63*	0.72**	0.80**	0.40	–	–	–	–	–	–	–
Other	0.20	0.90*	0.97*	1.04*	0.97*	2.45*	0.64	0.84+	0.84+	1.03*	1.15*	1.26*
Age in years		0.07***	0.07***	0.07***	0.08***	0.07***		0.07***	0.06***	0.06***	0.07***	0.06***
Education												
ISCED 1 + 2		0.74***	0.76***	0.76***	0.61***	0.51***		0.33	0.32	0.23	0.02	−0.19
ISCED 3		0	0	0	0	0		0	0	0	0	0
ISCED 4		−0.37+	−0.34+	−0.34+	−0.25	−0.22		−1.32**	−1.31**	−1.32**	−1.06*	−1.04*
ISCED 5 + 6		−0.20	−0.19	−0.18	−0.03	−0.02		−1.09***	−1.09***	−1.08***	−0.83**	−0.85*
Patchwork family												
No			0	0	0	0			0	0	0	0
Yes			0.41*	0.41*	0.33+	0.28			0.32	0.33	0.24	0.20
Has LAT relationship[a]												
No				0	0					0	0	
Yes				−0.23	−0.21					−0.90*	−0.87*	

(continued)

Table 4 (continued)

	Women						Men					
	Model 1	Model 2	Model 3	Model 4	Model 5	Model 6	Model 1	Model 2	Model 3	Model 4	Model 5	Model 6
Making ends meet					−0.36***	−0.33***					−0.45***	−0.45***
Satisfaction with partnership												
Satisfied						0						0
Not satisfied						0.43**						1.38***
Constant	−2.44***	−5.02***	−5.08***	−5.08***	−3.74***	−3.63***	−2.59***	−4.71***	−4.71***	−4.70***	−3.15***	−2.99***
R^2	0.0147	0.0622	0.0645	0.0651	0.0923	0.0742	0.0152	0.0636	0.0651	0.0723	0.1060	0.1047
N	3001	3001	3001	3001	2997	1929	1990	1990	1990	1990	1990	1145

Remark Models 6 only include individuals with a partner (either cohabiting or LAT)
Source Austrian GGS 2008/9, wave 1
[a]If not living in a couple
Significance levels: $+p < 0.10$; $*p < 0.05$; $**p < 0.01$; $***p < 0.001$

Our multivariate models show that health outcomes are related to different living arrangements for women and men. Women living with a partner and one or more children in the household reported better health than their peers in other household positions. Those women living with a partner and two or more children evaluated their health in a similar way as those cohabiting with one child and a partner. This is in contrast to women living alone, in the parental household, with a partner but no children, single mothers, as well as women in shared households who reported bad health significantly more often than women living with a partner and one child. Among men, those living alone and in shared households reported poor health more often. Apart from significant associations with age, education, financial constraints, and partnership quality for both sexes, patchwork context further determines the subjective health of young and middle aged women negatively, whereas LAT relationships are associated with better health among men. The fact that the coefficient for single mothers changes in the stepwise setup of the model when including LAT and making ends meet indicates a complex interaction of these dimensions and mediating effects. In summary, our results show that socio-economic factors and health characteristics generate household contexts that mediate the way household structure and self-rated health in young and middle adulthood plays out.

Longitudinal Perspective: Changes Over Time

In this section, we focus on the longitudinal sample. As mentioned earlier, panel attrition in the Austrian GGS was comparably low (22%). Of the 5001 wave 1 respondents interviewed in 2008/9, a total of 3908 individuals participated in wave 2 four years later (2012/13). About eight in ten reported good health at both interviews, for roughly one in ten health had deteriorated from good to poor, whereas for 4% health improved from poor to good. A small, but not negligible group (5%) declared poor health at both interview time points (Table 5). Against the argument that health outcomes vary by gender in late adulthood and old age, our data show apparent gender differences even in early and middle adulthood: Whereas 85% of men reported good health in both waves, this proportion is significantly smaller among women (80%). In other words, two in ten women reported fair or bad health at least once when interviewed four years apart. As expected, changes in health vary substantially by age: Whereas below age 20, nine in ten reported good health at both waves, this was the case for roughly seven in ten in their early forties (Table 5). The longitudinal approach supports our cross-sectional evidence (Fig. 3) that poor health in complex families mainly involves low educated persons, whereas their highly educated peers do not report worse health (Table 5).

Differentiating among seven different household types would have made the interpretation of changes in household position very complex (49 possible combinations). We thus distinguished first between those who had no change and those who had one change in the household position between waves: Roughly two thirds

Table 5 Change in health between wave 1 and wave 2 by gender, age, and stepfamily context

	Good → good (%)	Poor → good (%)	Good → poor (%)	Poor → poor (%)	Total (%)
Gender					
Men	85	3	8	4	100
Women	80	5	9	6	100
Total	83	4	8	5	100
Age					
18–19	91	3	5	1	100
20–24	90	3	4	2	100
25–29	88	4	6	2	100
30–34	84	4	8	4	100
35–39	79	4	11	6	100
40–44	73	7	11	9	100
Patchwork in wave 1 and low or middle level of education					
No	83	4	8	5	100
Yes	75	6	10	9	100
Patchwork in wave 1 and high level of education					
No	86	5	8	2	100
Yes	84	5	7	4	100

Source Austrian GGS 2008/9 and 2012/13, wave 1 and wave 2

did not change their household position and about one third did over the four-year period. Part of these changes were from “childless couple” to “couple with child (ren)” or from “couple with one child” to “couple with two and more children”. In addition, in some households an adult child left the parental home. We find that 12% had changes due (mainly) to the arrival of a newborn, whereas 24% had a change in the household position due to other reasons, including the formation of a new partnership, moving together with a partner, separation, and divorce (Fig. 4). Changes in household position were frequent for those initially living in the parental home and living alone—and therein more often among women than men. Also shared living arrangements with friends, students, or relatives (e.g. siblings) turned out to be more transitory living arrangements. The observation that changes in the household position differed over the life course is reflected in the mean age across groups: People without change in household position had mean age of 34 years, those reporting a change were either substantially younger, 28 years on average, or substantially older (42 years) if experiencing empty nest (Table 6). People who had a newborn between the two waves were about 30 years at wave 1.

The majority of the respondents reported good health at both interviews, and this was more often the case if a change in the household position took place (86%, compared to 81% of those remaining in the same household position). The share of people who recently transitioned to parenthood and who were in good health at both

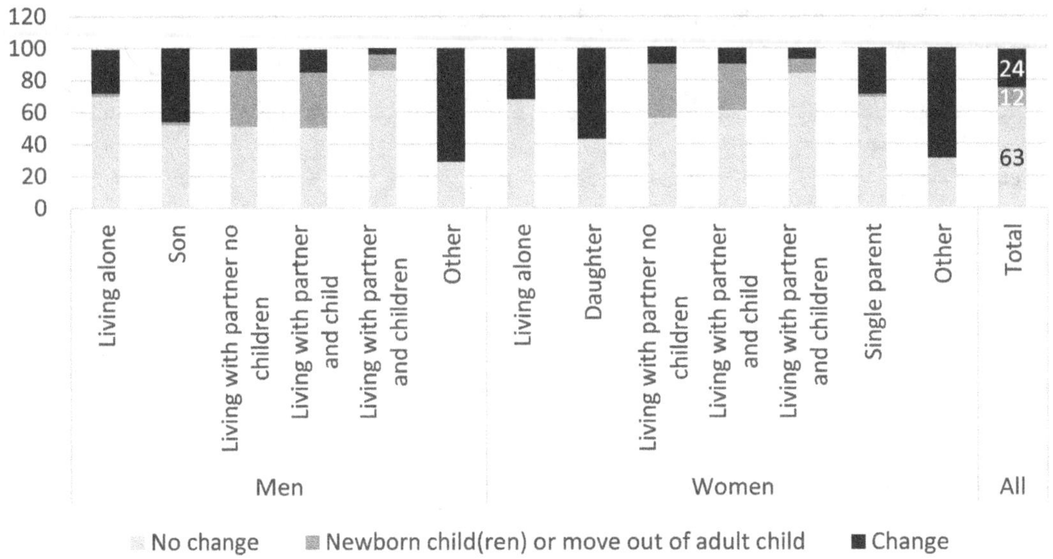

Fig. 4 Change in the household position. *Source* Austrian GGS 2008/9 and 2012/13, wave 1 and wave 2. Remark 1: Single fathers are omitted due to the small number remaining in wave 2. Remark 2: In the group "Newborn child(ren) or move out of adult child", the majority (92%) comprises 92% arrival of a newborn, a minority (8%) move out of adult child(ren)

Table 6 Change in the household position and change in health between wave 1 and wave 2

	No change	Change	Newborn child (ren)	Adult child(ren) moved out	Total
Good → good	81%	86%	89%	60%	83%
Poor → good	5%	4%	2%	8%	4%
Good → poor	9%	7%	7%	8%	8%
Poor → poor	6%	3%	2%	23%	5%
Total	100%	100%	100%	100%	100%
Mean age at wave 1	34	28	30	42	32
N	2507	849	513	39	3908

Source Austrian GGS 2008/9 and 2012/13, wave 1 and wave 2

waves even amounted to 89% (Table 6). The small group of respondents where an adult child had left the parental home between waves had worst self-perceived health, as only six out of ten reported good health both times. As mean age substantially varies within groups, with changes in household position and transition to parenthood being more frequent in young adulthood, age is an important determinant for changes in health over time.

Change in Health If No Change in the Household Position

Changes in the partnership do not necessarily change a person's household position, but can still affect individual health outcomes: 6% of respondents were living as a couple but with different partners at both waves, 5% reported an LAT partner in wave 1, but not so in wave 2, and 9% had no LAT partner at wave 1 but did so at wave 2. The remaining persons either had the same partner (64%) or no partner (16%) in both waves. This distinction was taken into account.

Model 1 that regresses effects of household position on health in wave 2 suggests that persons living continuously alone and especially single parents reported poor health at wave 2 more often, whereas living in the parental home was associated with better health (Table 7, Model 1). As only a few single fathers remained in the longitudinal sample, the single parents are mainly single mothers. Model 2 introduces health at wave 1, which is crucial for health reported four years later: The estimated coefficient is large in size and highly statistically significant, showing that persons who reported bad health at wave 1, also did so substantially more often at wave 2 (Table 7, Model 2). Next, parents in stepfamily context at wave 1 reported poor health at wave 2 more often, even after controlling for health at baseline (Table 7, Model 3).

In Models 4 and 5 we included the socio-demographic variables of sex, age, and education. Women and men did not significantly differ in self-perceived health at wave 2, once the initial health status at wave 1 was controlled for, whereas age and education have further explanatory power (Table 7, Models 4 and 5). Having no partner at all in both waves, breaking up a LAT partnership and a partner change (either cohabiting or non-cohabiting) are also associated with bad health (Table 7, Model 6). Not only the financial situation at wave 2, but also economic constraints at wave 1 (still) are related with poor health at wave 2 (Table 7, Model 7). As in the cross-sectional model, current partnership quality is related with current self-perceived health (Table 7, Model 8). In the final model, poor health at wave 1, age, education, economic constraints at both observations, having no partner (not even a non-co-residing one) at both interview times, breaking up with a partner as well as partnership quality at wave 2 are all associated with bad health at wave 2. We might conclude that from a longitudinal perspective the association with age, education, economic constraints, and having no partner even got stronger. Once these determinants are taken into account, the only household position significantly associated with health is living in the parental home, whereas stepfamily context no longer has explanatory power. The stepwise model specification shows that especially educational differences and economic constraints associated with certain household positions and with stepfamilies are mediating factors for poor health.

In young and middle adulthood, a substantial number of people experienced first or repeated parenthood over a period of four years, whereas some early parents witnessed empty nests as their adult children moved out. People who became parents evaluated their health best: Nine in ten were in good health at both waves (Table 6). Parents whose children moved out reported poor health more often compared with the parents of newborn children (Table 6). In multivariate analyses,

Table 7 Binary logistic regression analyses with poor health at wave 2 as dependent variable (for respondents without change in the household position between wave 1 and wave 2)

	Model 1	Model 2	Model 3	Model 4	Model 5	Model 6	Model 7	Model 8
Household position in wave 1								
Living alone	0.49*	0.31	0.35	0.46+	0.50+	−0.51	−0.61	−0.65
Son/daughter	−0.69*	−0.72*	−0.65*	−0.11	−0.16	−1.18*	−1.02*	−1.06*
Living with partner no children	0.14	0.07	0.06	0.16	0.20	0.17	0.26	0.27
Living with partner and child	0	0	0	0	0	0	0	0
Living with partner and children	0.24	0.15	0.18	0.13	0.12	0.13	0.07	0.08
Single parent	0.92***	0.63*	0.70*	0.62*	0.60*	−0.37	−0.69	−0.71
Other	−0.59	−0.44	−0.39	−0.01	0.00	−1.15	−1.23	−1.26
Poor health in wave 1								
No		0	0	0	0	0	0	0
Yes		2.30***	2.29***	2.18***	2.15***	2.14***	1.96***	1.96***
Patchwork family in wave 1								
No			0	0	0	0	0	0
Yes			0.39*	0.36+	0.33+	0.33+	0.28	0.28
Sex								
Male				0	0	0	0	0
Female				0.11	0.09	0.12	0.18	0.16
Age in years				0.04***	0.05***	0.05***	0.05***	0.05***
Education								
ISCED 1 + 2					0.33+	0.32+	0.16	0.16
ISCED 3					0	0	0	0
ISCED 4					−0.20	−0.21	−0.14	−0.15
ISCED 5 + 6					−0.52**	−0.51**	−0.37+	−0.38*

(continued)

Table 7 (continued)

	Model 1	Model 2	Model 3	Model 4	Model 5	Model 6	Model 7	Model 8
Partner at wave 1 and wave 2								
Different partner at w2						0.75*	0.73+	0.75*
Same partner at w1 and w2						0	0	0
LAT → No LAT						1.11*	0.89+	0.97+
No LAT at w1 and w2						1.38**	1.32**	1.39**
No LAT → LAT						0.57	0.56	0.55
Making ends meet at wave 1							−0.15*	−0.14*
Making ends meet at wave 2							−0.22***	−0.22***
Satisfied with partnership in wave 2								
Satisfied								0
Not satisfied								0.47+
Constant	−1.93***	−2.28***	−2.35***	−4.14***	−4.12***	−4.14***	−2.84***	−2.86***
R^2	0.0196	0.1413	0.1432	0.1520	0.1595	0.1670	0.1838	0.1854
N	2507	2507	2507	2507	2507	2507	2505	2505

Source Austrian GGS 2008/9 and 2012/13, wave 1 and wave 2
Significance levels: $+p < 0.10$; $*p < 0.05$; $**p < 0.01$; $***p < 0.001$

health at wave 1 was the main explanatory factor for health at wave 2. Moreover, low education was associated with poor health, further indicating increasing educational differences over time (results available on request). Stepwise multivariate models showed that health at wave 1 and age were the main mediating factor for poor health of parents experiencing an empty nest.

Change in Health If Household Position Changes

We now turn to the analyses of changes in health if changes in the household position occurred. This dynamic group encompasses rather young adults, with a mean age of 28 at wave 1. As changes across the detailed household positions become too complex, we distinguish between living as a couple and not living as a couple: One in two people moved together with a partner in a joint household (Table 8). About one in four separated (were living with a partner at wave 1, but not at wave 2), and another one in four changed within the non-couple-context, including living in the parental home, in a single household or in a shared household with non-relatives. Moving together with a partner and changing non-couple-living arrangement was more common among younger adults (mean age 27 and 25 years), persons involved in separations were significantly older (34 years) (Table 8).

In multivariate analyses, people moving together with a partner are the reference group. In the basic model, separation is associated with poor health at wave 2 (Table 9, Model 1). As expected, self-perceived health at wave 1 is important (Table 9, Model 2). Patchwork family at wave 1 and gender have no explanatory power, whereas age is an important determinant for health at wave 2 (Table 9, Models 3–5). Although the estimated coefficients for education fail statistical significance, they do point in the expected direction, with better health among higher educated (Table 9, Model 6). With the inclusion of age, the estimated coefficient for "couple → no couple" decreases in size and statistical significance (from 0.83** to 0.51+). With the further inclusion of education, it becomes insignificant (0.46). First bivariate analyses mentioned above showed substantial differences in mean ages across groups, and multivariate regressions confirmed that age is an important mediator for the relation between household dynamics and health. As adults were

Table 8 Distribution and mean age by couple context

	Mean age	
Couple → couple	4%	35
No couple → couple	51%	27
Couple → no couple	22%	34
No couple → no couple	23%	25
Total	100%	28

Source Austrian GGS 2008/9 and 2012/13, wave 1 and wave 2; N = 849 respondents with a change in household position between wave 1 and wave 2

Table 9 Binary logistic regression analyses with poor health at wave 2 as dependent variable (for respondents with change in the household position between wave 1 and wave 2)

	m1	m2	m3	m4	m5	m6	m7	m8	m9	m10	N
Couple at wave 1 and wave 2											
Couple → couple	0.89+	0.74	0.87	0.89+	0.56	0.53	0.47	0.53	0.59	0.88	35
No couple → couple	0	0	0	0	0	0	0	0			436
Couple → no couple	0.99***	0.76**	0.83**	0.83**	0.51+	0.46	0.22	0.16	−0.05	−0.19	183
No couple → no couple	0.36	0.27	0.26	0.28	0.38	0.34	0.27	0.23	0.09	0.29	195
Poor health in wave 1											
No		0	0	0	0	0	0	0	0	0	754
Yes		2.01***	2.06***	2.05***	2.02***	1.94***	2.01***	2.03***	2.02***	2.52***	95
Patchwork family in wave 1											
No			0	0	0	0	0	0	0	0	755
Yes			−0.34	−0.32	−0.47	−0.46	−0.61	−0.61	−0.56	−0.88	94
Sex											
Male				0	0	0	0	0	0	0	359
Female				0.26	0.24	0.26	0.25	0.17	0.13	0.70+	490
Age in years					0.06***	0.06***	0.05**	0.04*	0.05*	0.05*	
Education											
ISCED 1 + 2						0.33	0.39	0.38	0.20	0.58	103
ISCED 3						0	0	0			470
ISCED 4						−0.69	−0.59	−0.60	−0.45	−0.76	138
ISCED 5 + 6						−0.21	−0.05	−0.04	0.09	−0.12	138
Number of children in wave 1											
Childless							0	0	0	0	610
1 child							0.59	0.77+	0.63	0.70	122

(continued)

Table 9 (continued)

	m1	m2	m3	m4	m5	m6	m7	m8	m9	m10	N
2 children							0.29	0.45	0.22	−0.18	81
3+ children							0.47	0.62	0.37	0.25	36
Arrival of newborn after wave 1											
No newborn							0	0	0	0	691
1 newborn							−0.85*	−0.88*	−0.99*	−0.77	139
2 newborn							0.30	0.32	0.19	0.14	19
Patchwork family in wave 2											
No patchwork								0	0	0	770
Patchwork								−0.48	−0.54	−0.70	79
Making ends meet at wave 1									−0.14	−0.26*	
Making ends meet at wave 2									−0.32**	−0.25+	
Satisfaction with partnership in wave 2											
Satisfied										0	563
Not satisfied										0.29	63
Constant	−2.47***	−2.67***	−2.67***	−3.09***	−4.75***	−4.68***	−4.34***	−4.10***	−2.07*	−3.12**	
R^2	0.0257	0.1009	0.1023	0.1043	0.1289	0.1371	0.1501	0.1524	0.1813	0.2287	
N	849	849	849	849	849	849	849	849	847	626	847

Source Austrian GGS 2008/9 and 2012/13, wave 1 and wave 2
Remark Models 6 only include individuals with a partner at wave 2 (either cohabiting or LAT)
Significance levels: $+p < 0.10$; $*p < 0.05$; $**p < 0.01$; $***p < 0.001$

on average in their late twenties when moving together with a partner and in their mid-thirties when separating from their partner, some of the health differences are explained by age differences.

In the final model, poor health at wave 1, age, and financial constraints at wave 2 are significantly related with poor health at wave 2, the arrival of a newborn is associated with good health (Table 9, Model 9). The stepwise model setup allows insights for the association between explanatory variables: As the estimated coefficient for separation becomes almost zero when including economic constraints (Table 9, Models 8 and 9), we might conclude that financial problems after separation are coupled with poor health. Regarding the birth of a newborn: The estimated coefficient for the small group of persons having two newborn children within a period of four years is positive. Although not statistically significant, this is in sharp contrast to the large and highly significant coefficient for the arrival of one newborn child, thus indicating the stress of having two children within a short period of time. Finally, when including individuals with a partner at wave 2 (either cohabiting or LAT), the estimated coefficients for current satisfaction with partnership lie in the expected direction, but are not statistically significant.

We carried out all analyses for ages 25–44 only, thus excluding young adults aged 18–24. As expected, the overall share of persons living with their parents decreased from 24 to 11% and mean self-perceived health became worse (52% rated own health as very good, as compared to 57% for ages 18–44). When excluding young adults—who most often lived in the parental home, especially mean self-perceived health among those living with parents decreased. Nevertheless, in multivariate regressions, the estimated coefficients for household position and control variables are in line with results derived for the age group 18–45, with minor deviations in size and statistical significance.

Discussion

Despite extensive evidence of the broad-ranging impact of single parenthood and family disruption, few studies have examined the relationship between family composition and health, and none have examined the full range of structural and social correlates across two parent families, stepfamilies, and single mother families. Yet, causation has often been a problem given that the majority of available data sets were cross-sectional. There are a few exceptions, including longitudinal studies that find selection to operate alongside divorce effects (Hope et al. 1999; Mastekaasa 1997; Davies et al. 1997). Whether causation or selection are the drivers for the association between health and living conditions can be disentangled only with longitudinal studies capturing these dimensions from youth and early adulthood onwards. The aim of this study has therefore been to provide cross-sectional and longitudinal evidence toward differentiating these effects. According to previous literature and theoretical frameworks, we formulated various expectations on the associations between household position and health.

In line with our *first* expectation, we find a clear association between living together with a partner as compared to not living in a couple context. Individuals living alone and single parents reported bad health significantly more often than those living with a partner and one child. Differences remain, even after controlling for socio-economic conditions. Living together with a partner in young and middle adulthood corresponds to the 'normative life course' and is positively related with self-perceived health.

A *second* important finding is that—if not cohabiting with a partner—having a living apart together partner is positively related with health among men. Thus, it is not only marital status and cohabitation which are associated with health (Horwitz and White 1998; Lillard and Panis 1996), but an LAT partnership was also related with it, especially among men.

Numerous studies have examined mortality as well as health and marital status (Lillard and Panis 1996; Lillard and Waite 1995; Bardage et al. 2005), concentrating on old age, but our study reveals insights for an association between partner status and health already much earlier in life. We might conclude that no, or missed, transitions might be against the norm and associated with poor health. Our results on poor health in non-partnership are to some extent contrary to the well-known idea of the 'de-institutionalization' of the life course that the social and temporal organization of the life course becomes less guided by normative, legal or organizational rules (Elzinga and Liefbroer 2007).

Further evidence in the realm of partnership concerns the quality of the relationship, confirming earlier research (Umberson et al. 2006; Miller et al. 2013). As expected, partnership quality is associated with health, underlining the relevance of psychological well-being for self-perceived health. In addition, the size of the estimated coefficient indicates that these are important determinants for self-perceived health in young and middle adulthood.

Our study provides important insights into health in stepfamilies in the European context. According to research results in the US (Heard et al. 2008; Turney and Carlson 2011), our expectation was that individuals living in patchwork families would report poor health more often. Our results indicate that Austrian women living in complex families rated their health as poor more often than did women cohabiting with a child or children and partner and no pre-union children, either their own or from the partner. People living in patchwork families may experience stress as they are raising their offspring. Stepfamily context and childrearing across households may create ambiguous family boundaries, increase conflict in couple relationships, and diminish the quality and quantity of parental investment in children, all of which may lead to impaired mental health (Boss 1980; Cherlin and Furstenberg 1994; Turney and Carlson 2011). As results are not significant for Austrian men living in a stepfamily context, we find evidence for gender differences with regard to complex families.

The gender gap in life expectancy is a well-known fact in demography, with female life expectancy exceeding that of males (Waldron 2000; Luy and Gast 2014; Caselli et al. 2014). Research on gender differences in mortality and morbidity has mainly focused on older people (Bardage et al. 2005), but our study provides evidence that women evaluate their health worse than men already in young and middle adulthood. In line with previous literature, age and education are positively associated with subjective well-being (Bardage et al. 2005). Moreover, educational and gender specific differences become evident, stemming from both cross-sectional and longitudinal approaches: Poor health in complex families is observed among people with less education, whereas highly educated people in a stepfamily context do not report worse health.

Age and education turned out to be crucial mediators for poor health. For example, we anticipated negative health outcome for mothers of two or more children. In fact, this group reported poor health more often than women with their partner and one child only. But when controlling for age and education, the effect for mothers of two and more children became insignificant. Controlling for socio-economic factors also appreciably reduced the effect for single mothers. The latter is consistent with earlier findings from a study in the US (McLanahan and Sandefur 1994), which asserts that single parent families are not inherently problematic but rather are affected by deprivation in economic, parental, and community resources. The deficits for single mothers are reduced when making ends meet is controlled for. Having a higher education and fewer economic constraints contribute to better health assessments. This suggests that structural disadvantages can help to create health disadvantages for people through the family environment in which they live. Single parents and stepfamilies are not "inherently problematic, but are likely to occur in concert with demographic, economic, psychosocial, and behavioural risk factors" which more directly influence health (Heard et al. 2008, p. 775f).

In the longitudinal approach, the effect of new parenthood turned out to be strong. Our expectations that the arrival of a newborn child has a positive effect on health was confirmed. Nevertheless, the birth of two children within a rather short period of four years tended to be associated with poor health, indicating stressful situations for the new parents. According to existing research, our expectation was that separation harms subjective health in the short- and medium term, which is expressed by lower self-assessed health after separation. Looking into the longitudinal analyses we observe that individuals who changed from a couple-context to a non-couple context within four years reported poor health more often at the second point in time compared to those who changed from a non-couple to a couple-context. But this difference vanished when controlling for age, education, and existence of LAT partnership, indicating at a complex relationship between different life domains and age. A further important result is that the association with age, education, economic constraints, and having no partner became even stronger from a longitudinal perspective. These results confirm our cross-sectional findings and reflect that transitions against the norm (e.g. union dissolution and separation) generate lasting negative health effects. It also implies that such transitions underlie age and socio-structural mechanisms such as education and economic status that are well-known determinants of health (Avendano et al. 2009; Stutzer and Frey 2010).

Some limitations of this study should be mentioned. First, this study is limited to self-perceived health and we are not able to disentangle the various dimensions of self-perceived health in the current study with the data at hand. Self-rated health is, however, the most widely regarded valid and reliable indicator of health status, although we acknowledge the meaning of self-rated health to differ between individuals (Schüz et al. 2011). Self-reported health is a multidimensional and multi-faceted construct (Liang 1986), including—among others—functional status, behavioural factors, and interpersonal resources. It has been suggested that psychological factors in particular can be crucial for self-perceived health. Experiencing depression is a key predictor of self-rated health besides physical symptoms (Schneider et al. 2004; Schüz et al. 2011). As our target population are people in young and middle adulthood, physical impairments might be less important and mental problems might determine to a larger extent the self-perception of health. Scholars have shown that self-assessments of teen and adolescence health are more likely to reflect overall functioning and life difficulties (e.g. participation in sports, school achievement, relations with friends, high Body Mass Index (BMI), depressed mood) than physical symptoms (Mechanic and Hansell 1987; Vingilis et al. 1998). Further evidence on longitudinal data suggests that health ratings seem to become less dependent on one's social well-being and more determined by current health characteristics and behaviours, as individuals transit from adolescence to young adulthood (Heard et al. 2008). Studies have shown the importance of psychological well-being and health behaviours for adolescent self-assessments of health, highlighting the importance of self-esteem, high BMI, and participation in sports or other forms of exercise (Mechanic and Hansell 1987; Vingilis et al. 1998; Heard et al. 2008).

Second, our longitudinal analyses are based on two observations four years apart. It is possible that some respondents might have experienced further changes between waves which are not captured in the current study. Third, the longitudinal sample is slightly biased towards healthy respondents, as dropout was higher among persons reporting poor health at wave 1 (Buber-Ennser 2014).

Despite these limitations, the results have a number of implications for our understanding of differences in health outcomes, and household position and parenthood. *First*, in line with the literature on the relationship between healthy behaviour and its protective effect on health and mortality (Berkman and Glass 2000; Gorman and Sivaganesan 2007), individuals' social ties are apparently an important determinant. Our findings confirm the argument that marriage provides social support (Lillard and Panis 1996), comprising emotional support (family integration, stress reduction) and instrumental support (provision of care), which are associated with reduced health impairments. *Second*, apart from knowledge on marriage and cohabitation—especially at old age—(Scafato et al. 2008), the current study provides evidence that social ties and support gained in new forms of unions such as living apart together are also associated with better subjective health. Third, most studies examining the association between marital status and health and mortality focus on the elderly population, whereas this study provides insights for young and middle adulthood. It is important to consider family and household structure during early and middle adulthood, as it may initiate a health trajectory that can either protect or harm health across the life course (Wadsworth 1997).

Overall, we show that if perceived health varies by household position and parental status, it also varies within household position category according to individuals' living arrangements and actual or missed transitions, such as the moving out of the parental home or the arrival of a newborn. Our findings are conservative, as we are examining a context in which parenting and the division of paid labour and domestic and care work are highly gendered. In gender unequal contexts, social inequalities by education, gender, and entry into various living arrangements may play a major role in who is able to maintain good health and who is not.

Acknowledgements The Austrian GGS was financed by the Federal Ministry of Economy, Family and Youth, the Federal Ministry of Science and Research and the Federal Ministry of Labour, Social Affairs and Consumer Protection. We thank Christian Wegner-Siegmundt, Gabriele Doblhammer, and Jordi Gumà for valuable comments and Werner Richter, Ian Copestake and Renee Lueskow for language editing.

References

Aassve, A., Goisis, A., & Sironi, M. (2012). Happiness and childbearing across Europe. *Social Indicators Research, 108*(1), 65–86. https://doi.org/10.1007/s11205-011-9866-x.

Amato, P. R. (2000). The consequences of divorce for adults and children. *Journal of Marriage and Family, 62,* 1269–1287.

Amato, P. R. (2010). Research on divorce: Continuing trends and new developments. *Journal of Marriage and Family, 72*(3), 650–666. https://doi.org/10.1111/j.1741-3737.2010.00723.x.

Amato, P. R., & Hohmann-Marriott, B. (2007). A comparison of high- and low-distress marriages that end in divorce. *Journal of Marriage and Family, 69*(3), 621–638. https://doi.org/10.2307/4622471.

Aseltine, R. H., Jr., & Kessler, R. C. (1993). Marital disruption and depression in a community sample. *Journal of Health and Social Behavior, 34*(3), 237–251. https://doi.org/10.2307/2137205.

Avendano, M., Jürges, H., & Mackenbach, J. P. (2009). Educational level and changes in health across Europe: Longitudinal results from SHARE. *Journal of European Social Policy, 19*(4), 301–316. https://doi.org/10.1177/1350506809341512.

Ball, K., Burton, N. W., & Brown, W. J. (2009). A prospective study of overweight, physical activity, and depressive symptoms in young women. *Obesity, 17*(1), 66–71. https://doi.org/10.1038/oby.2008.497.

Baranowska, A., & Matysiak, A. (2011). Does parenthood increase happiness? Evidence for Poland. *Vienna Yearbook of Population Research, 9,* 307–325. https://doi.org/10.1553/populationyearbook2011s307.

Bardage, C., Pluijm, S. M. F., Pedersen, N., Deeg, D. J. H., Jylhä, M., Noale, M., et al. (2005). Self-rated health among older adults: A cross-national comparison. *European Journal of Ageing, 2*(2), 149–158. https://doi.org/10.1007/s10433-005-0032-7.

Beaujouan, E. (2011). Second-union fertility in France: Partners' age and other factors. *Population-E, 66*(2), 239–274.

Beaujouan, E., & Bhrolcháin, M. N. (2011). Cohabitation and marriage in Britain since the 1970s. *Population Trends, 145*(3), 35–39.

Beaujouan, E., & Solaz, A. (2013). Racing againt the biological clock? Childbearing and sterility among men and women in second unions. *European Journal of Population, 29*(1), 39–67. https://doi.org/10.1007/s10680-012-9271-4.

Benzeval, M. (1998). The self-reported health status of lone parents. *Social Science and Medicine, 46*(10), 1337–1353. https://doi.org/10.1016/S0277-9536(97)10083-1.

Berghammer, C. (2014). The return of the male breadwinner model? Educational effects on parents' work arrangements in Austria, 1980–2009. *Work, Employment & Society, 28*(4), 611–623. https://doi.org/10.1177/0950017013500115.

Berkman, L. F., & Glass, T. (2000). Social integration, social networks, social support, and health. In L. F. Berkman & I. Kawachi (Eds.), *Social epidemiology* (pp. 137–173). Oxford, New York: Oxford University Press.

Bernardi, L., Ryser, V.-A., & Le Goff, J.-M. (2013). Gender role-set, family orientations, and women's fertility intentions in Switzerland. *Swiss Journal of Sociology, 39*(1), 9–31.

Booth, A., & Amato, P. (1991). Divorce and psychological stress. *Journal of Health and Social Behavior, 32*(4), 396–407. https://doi.org/10.2307/2137106.

Boss, P. G. (1980). Normative family stress: Family boundary changes across the life-span. *Family Relations, 29,* 445–450.

Brockmann, H., & Klein, T. (2004). Love and death in Germany: The marital biography and its effect on mortality. *Journal of Marriage and Family, 66*(3), 567–581. https://doi.org/10.2307/3600213.

Bronte-Tinkew, J., Allison, H., Scott, M. E., & Johnson, D. (2009). Fathering with multiple partners: Links to children's well-being in early childhood. *Journal of Marriage and Family, 71*(3), 608–631. https://doi.org/10.2307/40262905.

Brown, S. L., Bulanda, J. R., & Lee, G. R. (2005). The significance of nonmarital cohabitation: Marital status and mental health benefits among middle-aged and older adults. *The Journals of Gerontology Series B: Psychological Sciences and Social Sciences, 60*(1), S21–S29. https://doi.org/10.1093/geronb/60.1.S21.

Brückner, H., & Mayer, K. U. (2005). De-standardization of the life course: What it might mean? And if it means anything, whether it actually took place? *Advances in Life Course Research, 9,* 27–53. https://doi.org/10.1016/S1040-2608(04)09002-1.

Buber-Ennser, I. (2014). Attrition in the Austrian Generations and Gender Survey: Is there a bias by fertility-relevant aspects? *Demographic Research, 31*(16), 459–496. https://doi.org/10.4054/DemRes.2014.31.16.

Buber-Ennser, I. (2015). Childrearing in Austria: Work and family roles. *Journal of research in Gender Studies, 5*(2), 121–146.

Bumpass, L. L., Ralley, R. K., & Sweet, J. A. (1995). The changing character of stepfamilies: Implications of cohabitation and nonmarital childbearing. *Demography, 32*(3), 425–436.

Caselli, G., Drefahl, S., Wegner-Siegmundt, C., & Luy, M. (2014). *Future mortality in low mortality countries (world population & human capital in the twenty-first century).* Oxford: Oxford University Press.

Castro-Martín, T., Domínguez-Folgueras, M., & Martín-García, T. (2008). Not truly partnerless: Non-residential partnerships and retreat from marriage in Spain. *Demographic Research, 18*(16), 443–468.

Cherlin, A. J., & Furstenberg, F. F., Jr. (1994). Stepfamilies in the United States: A reconsideration. *Annual Review of Sociology, 20,* 359–381. https://doi.org/10.2307/2083370.

Curtis, L. J. (2001). Lone motherhood and health status. *Canadian Public Policy/Analyse de Politiques, 27*(3), 335–356. https://doi.org/10.2307/3552473.

Curtis, L. J., & Pennock, M. (2006). Social assistance, lone parents and health: What do we know, where do we go? *Canadian Journal of Public Health/Revue Canadienne de Sante'e Publique, 97,* S4–S10. https://doi.org/10.2307/41965615.

Davidson, K. (2002). Gender differences in new partnership choices and constraints for older widows and widowers. *Ageing International, 27*(4), 43–60. https://doi.org/10.1007/s12126-002-1014-0.

Davies, L., Avison, W. R., & McAlpine, D. D. (1997). Significant life experiences and depression among single and married mothers. *Journal of Marriage and Family, 59*(2), 294–308. https://doi.org/10.2307/353471.

Dawson, D. A. (1991). Family structure and children's health and well-being: Data from the 1988 national health interview survey on child health. *Journal of Marriage and Family, 53*(3), 573–584. https://doi.org/10.2307/352734.

De Jong Gierveld, J. (2004). Remarriage, unmarried cohabitation, living apart together: Partner relationships following bereavement or divorce. *Journal of Marriage and Family, 66*(1), 236–243. https://doi.org/10.1111/j.0022-2445.2004.00015.x.

Easterlin, R. A. (2006). Life cycle happiness and its sources: Intersections of psychology, economics, and demography. *Journal of Economic Psychology, 27*(4), 463–482. https://doi.org/10.1016/j.joep.2006.05.002.

Elder, G. H. (1995). The life course paradigm: Social change and individual development. In P. G. Moen, G. H. Elder, & K. Lüscher (Eds.), *Examing lives in context. Perspectives on the ecology of human development* (pp. 101–139). Washington: American Psychological Association.

Elzinga, C. H., & Liefbroer, A. C. (2007). De-standardization of family-life trajectories of young adults: A cross-national comparison using sequence analysis. *European Journal of Population, 23*(3–4), 225–250. https://doi.org/10.1007/s10680-007-9133-7.

Evenhouse, E., & Reilly, S. (2012). Multiple-father families and welfare. *Journal of Family Issues, 33*(7), 966–995. https://doi.org/10.1177/0192513x11406496.

Franz, M., & Lensche, H. (2003). Allein erziehend—allein gelassen? Die psychosoziale Beeinträchtigung allein erziehender Mütter und ihrer Kinder in einer Bevölkerungsstichprobe [Single parenthood—left alone? Phychosocial impairments of single mothers and their children in a population sample]. *Zeitschrift für Psychosomatische Medizin und Psychotherapie, 49*(2), 115–138. https://doi.org/10.2307/23870797.

Furstenberg, F. F. (1979). Recycling the family: Perspectives for researching a neglected family form. *Marriage and Family Review, 2,* 1–22.

Galobardes, B., Shaw, M., Lawlor, D. A., Lynch, J. W., & Smith, G. D. (2006). Glossary: Indicators of socioeconomic position (part 1). *Journal of Epidemiology and Community Health, 60*(1), 7–12. https://doi.org/10.2307/40795066.

Goldman, N. (1993). Marriage selection and mortality patterns: Inferences and fallacies. *Demography, 30*(2), 189–208. https://doi.org/10.2307/2061837.

Gorman, B. K., & Sivaganesan, A. (2007). The role of social support and integration for understanding socioeconomic disparities in self-rated health and hypertension. *Social Science and Medicine, 65*(5), 958–975. https://doi.org/10.1016/j.socscimed.2007.04.017.

Guzzo, K. B. (2009). Maternal relationships and nonresidential father visitation of children born outside of marriage. *Journal of Marriage and Family, 71*(3), 632–649. https://doi.org/10.2307/40262906.

Hanappi, D. (2012). *Job insecurity and life satisfaction: Do parents' jobs hurt more?"* Presented at the SCANCOR Seminar, School of Education, February 13, Stanford University, CA.

Hank, K., Deindl, C., & Brandt, M. (2013). Changes in older Europeans' health across two waves of SHARE: Life-course and societal determinants. *Journal of Population Ageing, 6*(1–2), 85–97. https://doi.org/10.1007/s12062-012-9076-6.

Harknett, K., & Knab, J. (2007). More kin, less support: Multipartnered fertility and perceived support among mothers. *Journal of Marriage and Family, 69*(1), 237–253. https://doi.org/10.2307/4622428.

Heard, H. E., Gorman, B. K., & Kapinus, C. A. (2008). Family structure and self-rated health in adolescence and young adulthood. *Population Research and Policy Review, 27*(6), 773–797. https://doi.org/10.2307/41217982.

Hemström, Ö. (1996). Is marriage dissolution linked to differences in mortality risks for men and women? *Journal of Marriage and Family, 58*(2), 366–378. https://doi.org/10.2307/353502.

Heuveline, P., & Timberlake, J. M. (2004). The role of cohabitation in family formation: The United States in comparative perspective. *Journal of Marriage and Family, 66*(5), 1214–1230. https://doi.org/10.2307/3600335.

Holmes, T. H., & Rahe, R. H. (1967). The social readjustment rating scale. *Journal of Psychosomatic Research, 11*(2), 213–218. https://doi.org/10.1016/0022-3999(67)90010-4.

Hope, S., Power, C., & Rodgers, B. (1999). Does financial hardship account for elevated psychological distress in lone mothers? *Social Science and Medicine, 49*(12), 1637–1649.

Horwitz, A. V., & White, H. R. (1998). The relationship of cohabitation and mental health: A study of a young adult cohort. *Journal of Marriage and Family, 60*(2), 505–514. https://doi.org/10.2307/353865.

Idler, E. L., & Benyamini, Y. (1997). Self-rated health and mortality: A review of twenty-seven community studies. *Journal of Health and Social Behavior, 38*(1), 21–37. https://doi.org/10.2307/2955359.

Joung, I. M. A., van de Mheen, H. D., Stronks, K., van Poppel, F. W. A., & Mackenbach, J. P. (1998). A longitudinal study of health selection in marital transitions. *Social Science and Medicine, 46*(3), 425–435. https://doi.org/10.1016/S0277-9536(97)00186-X.

Karlsson, S. G., & Borell, K. (2002). Intimacy and autonomy, gender and ageing: Living apart together. *Ageing International, 27*(4), 11–26. https://doi.org/10.1007/s12126-002-1012-2.

Khalaila, R., & Litwin, H. (2014). Changes in health behaviors and their associations with depressive symptoms among Israelis aged 50+. *Journal of Aging and Health, 26*(3), 401–421. https://doi.org/10.1177/0898264313516997.

Koball, H. L., Moiduddin, E., Henderson, J., Goesling, B., & Besculides, M. (2010). What do we know about the link between marriage and health? *Journal of Family Issues, 31*(8), 1019–1040. https://doi.org/10.1177/0192513X10365834.

Kohler, H.-P., Behrman, J. R., & Skytthe, A. (2005). Partner + children = happiness? The effects of partnerships and fertility on well-being. *Population and Development Review, 31*(3), 407–445. https://doi.org/10.1111/j.1728-4457.2005.00078.x.

Liang, J. (1986). Self-reported physical health among aged adults. *Journal of Gerontology, 41*(2), 248–260.

Lillard, L. A., & Panis, C. W. A. (1996). Marital status and mortality: The role of health. *Demography, 33*(3), 313–327. https://doi.org/10.2307/2061764.

Lillard, L. A., & Waite, L. J. (1995). Til death do us part: Marital disruption and mortality. *American Journal of Sociology, 100*(5), 1131–1156. https://doi.org/10.2307/2782273.

Litwin, H., & Sapir, E. V. (2009). Perceived income adequacy among older adults in 12 countries: Findings from the survey of health, ageing, and retirement in Europe. *The Gerontologist, 49*(3), 397–406. https://doi.org/10.1093/geront/gnp036.

Luy, M., & Gast, K. (2014). Do women live longer or do men die earlier? Reflections on the causes of sex differences in life expectancy. *Gerontology, 60*(2), 143–153.

Marcussen, K. (2005). Explaining differences in mental health between married and cohabiting individuals. *Social Psychology Quarterly, 68*(3), 239–257. https://doi.org/10.1177/019027250506800304.

Marks, N. F. (1998). Does it hurt to care? Caregiving, work-family conflict, and midlife well-being. *Journal of Marriage and Family, 60*(4), 951–966. https://doi.org/10.2307/353637.

Mason, M. A., & Kuhltau, K. (1989). Determinants of child care ideals among mothers of preschool-aged children. *Journal of Marriage and Family, 74*(4), 593–603.

Mastekaasa, A. (1997). Marital dissolution as a stressor: Some evidence on psychological, physical, and behavioral changes during the preseparation period. *Journal of Divorce and Remarriage, 26*(155–183).

McLanahan, S. S., & Sandefur, G. (1994). *Growing up with a single parent: What hurts, what helps*. Cambridge, MA: Harvard University Press.

Mechanic, D., & Hansell, S. (1987). Adolescent competence, psychological well-being, and self-assessed physical health. *Journal of Health and Social Behavior, 28*(4), 364–374. https://doi.org/10.2307/2136790.

Meyer, D. R., Cancian, M., & Cook, S. T. (2005). Multiple-partner fertility: Incidence and implications for child support policy. *Social Service Review, 79*(4), 577–601. https://doi.org/10.1086/454386.

Miller, R. B., Hollist, C. S., Olsen, J., & Law, D. (2013). Marital quality and health over 20 years: A growth curve analysis. *Journal of Marriage and Family, 75*(3), 667–680. https://doi.org/10.2307/23440908.

Myrskylä, M., & Margolis, R. (2014). Happiness: Before and after the kids. *Demography, 51*(5), 1843–1866. https://doi.org/10.1007/s13524-014-0321-x.

Osborne, C., & McLanahan, S. (2007). Partnership instability and child well-being. *Journal of Marriage and Family, 69*(4), 1065–1083. https://doi.org/10.2307/4622508.

Perelli-Harris, B., Berrington, A., Berghammer, C., Keizer, R., Lappegård, T., Mynarska, M., et al. (2014). Towards a new understanding of cohabitation: Insights from focus group research across Europe and Australia. *Demographic Research, 31*(34), 1043–1078.

Perelli-Harris, B., Kreyenfeld, M., Sigle-Rushton, W., Keizer, R., Lappegård, T., Jasilioniene, A., et al. (2012). Changes in union status during the transition to parenthood in eleven European countries, 1970s to early 2000s. *Population Studies, 66*(2), 167–182. https://doi.org/10.1080/00324728.2012.673004.

Perelli-Harris, B., & Lyons-Amos, M. (2015). Changes in partnership patterns across the life course: An examination of 14 countries in Europe and the United States. *Demographic Research, 33*(6), 145–178.

Perrig-Chiello, P., & Knöpfli, B. (2015). *Forschungdossier: Trennung und Scheidung—im Längsschnitt (2012–2014)*. Bern: University of Bern.

Régnier-Loilier, A., Beaujouan, E., & Villeneuve-Gokalp, C. (2009). Neither single, nor in a couple: A study of living apart together in France. *Demographic Research, 21*(4), 75–108. https://doi.org/10.4054/DemRes.2009.21.4.

Ren, X. S. (1997). Marital status and quality of relationships: The impact on health perception. *Social Science and Medicine, 44*(2), 241–249. https://doi.org/10.1016/S0277-9536(96)00158-X.

Ross, C. E., Mirowsky, J., & Goldsteen, K. (1990). The impact of the family on health: The decade in review. *Journal of Marriage and Family, 52*(4), 1059–1078. https://doi.org/10.2307/353319.

Ross, C. E., & Wu, C.-L. (1995). The links between education and health. *American Sociological Review, 60*(5), 719–745. https://doi.org/10.2307/2096319.

Scafato, E., Galluzzo, L., Gandin, C., Ghirini, S., Baldereschi, M., Capurso, A., et al. (2008). Marital and cohabitation status as predictors of mortality: A 10-year follow-up of an Italian elderly cohort. *Social Science and Medicine, 67*(9), 1456–1464. https://doi.org/10.1016/j.socscimed.2008.06.026.

Schneider, B., Rapp, I., Klein, T., & Eckhard, J. (2014). Relationship status and health: Does the use of different relationship indicators matter? *Global Public Health, 9*(5), 528–537. https://doi.org/10.1080/17441692.2014.904917.

Schneider, G., Driesch, G., Kruse, A., Wachter, M., Nehen, H.-G., & Heuft, G. (2004). What influences self-perception of health in the elderly? The role of objective health condition, subjective well-being and sense of coherence. *Archives of Gerontology and Geriatrics, 39*(3), 227–237. https://doi.org/10.1016/j.archger.2004.03.005.

Schüz, B., Wurm, S., Schöllgen, I., & Tesch-Römer, C. (2011). What do people include when they self-rate their health? Differential associations according to health status in community-dwelling older adults. *Quality of Life Research, 20*(10), 1573–1580. https://doi.org/10.2307/41488225.

Stryker, S. (1980). *Symbolic interactionism: A social structural version*. Menlo Park, CA: Benjamin/Cummings.

Stutzer, A., & Frey, B. S. (2010). Recent advances in the economics of individual subjective well-being. *Social Research, 77*(2), 679–714. https://doi.org/10.2307/40972234.

Thomson, E. (1997). *Her, his, and their children: Influence on couple childbearing decisions*. NSFH Working Paper No. 76, University of Wisconsin-Madison: Center for Demography and Ecology.

Thomson, E. (2004). Step-families and childbearing desires in Europe. *Demographic Research, Special Collection, 3,* 117–134. https://doi.org/10.4054/DemRes.2004.S3.5.

Thomson, E. (2014). Family complexity in Europe. *The ANNALS of the American Academy of Political and Social Science, 654*(1), 245–258. https://doi.org/10.1177/0002716214531384.

Thomson, E., Hoem, J. M., Vikat, A., Buber, I., Prskawetz, A., Toulemon, L., et al. (2002). Childbearing in stepfamilies: How parity matters. In E. Klijzing & M. Corijn (Eds.), *Dynamics of fertility and partnership in Europe: Insights and lessons from comparative research* (Vol. II, pp. 87–99). New York and Geneva: United Nations.

Thomson, E., Lappegård, T., Carlson, M., Evans, A., & Gray, E. (2014). Childbearing across partnerships in Australia, the United States, Norway, and Sweden. *Demography, 51*(2), 485–508. https://doi.org/10.1007/s13524-013-0273-6.

Thomson, E., Winkler-Dworak, M., Spielauer, M., & Prskawetz, A. (2012). Union instability as an engine of fertility? A micro-simulation model for France. *Demography, 49*(1), 175–195.

Treviño, R., & Gumà, J. (2013). De la monoparentalidad a la reconstitución familiar: Un análisis a partir de fuentes transversales. *Papers: Revista de Sociologia, 98*(2), 287–309.

Turney, K., & Carlson, M. J. (2011). Multipartnered fertility and depression among fragile families. *Journal of Marriage and Family, 73*(3), 570–587. https://doi.org/10.2307/29789603.

Uhlenberg, P., & Mueller, M. (2003). Family context and individual well-being. In J. T. Mortimer & M. J. Shanahan (Eds.), *Handbook of the life course* (pp. 123–148, Handbooks of Sociology and Social Research). New York: Springer US.

Umberson, D., Williams, K., Powers, D. A., Liu, H., & Needham, B. (2006). You make me sick: Marital quality and health over the life course. *Journal of Health and Social Behavior, 47*(1), 1–16. https://doi.org/10.2307/30040295.

Van de Velde, S., Bambra, C., Van der Bracht, K., Eikemo, T. A., & Bracke, P. (2014). Keeping it in the family: The self-rated health of lone mothers in different European welfare regimes. *Sociology of Health & Illness, 36*(8), 1220–1242. https://doi.org/10.1111/1467-9566.12162.

Vikat, A., Thomson, E., & Hoem, J. M. (1999). Stepfamily fertility in contemporary Sweden: The impact of childbearing before the current union. *Population Studies, 53*(2), 211–225.

Vingilis, E., Wade, T. J., & Adlaf, E. (1998). What factors predict student self-rated physical health? *Journal of Adolescence, 21*(1), 83–97. https://doi.org/10.1006/jado.1997.0131.

Voydanoff, P. (2005). Toward a conceptualization of perceived work-family fit and balance: A demands and resources approach. *Journal of Marriage and Family, 67*(4), 822–836. https://doi.org/10.2307/3600241.

Wadsworth, M. E. J. (1997). Health inequalities in the life course perspective. *Social Science and Medicine, 44*(6), 859–869. https://doi.org/10.1016/S0277-9536(96)00187-6.

Wahrendorf, M., & Siegrist, J. (2010). Are changes in productive activities of older people associated with changes in their well-being? Results of a longitudinal European study. *European Journal of Ageing, 7*(2), 59–68. https://doi.org/10.1007/s10433-010-0154-4.

Waldron, I. (2000). Trends in gender differences in mortality: Relationships to changing gender differences in behaviour and other causal factors. In E. Annandale & K. Hunt (Eds.), *Gender inequality in health* (pp. 150–181). Buckingham: Open University Press.

Witvliet, M. I., Arah, O. A., Stronks, K., & Kunst, A. E. (2014). A global study on lone mothers: Exploring the associations of self-assessed general health with motherhood types and gender inequality in 32 countries. *Women's Health Issues, 24*(2), e177–e185. https://doi.org/10.1016/j.whi.2013.12.001.

Woo, H., & Zajacova, A. (2015). *Examination of age variations in the predivtive validity of self-rated health.* Paper presented at the Population Association of America (PAA) 2015, San Diego,

The Contextual and Household Contribution to Individual Health Status in Germany: What Is the Role of Gender and Migration Background?

Daniela Georges, Daniel Kreft and Gabriele Doblhammer

Introduction

As early as 1997 George Engel postulated the need to consider the multidimensionality of health in the contextual perspective on health, illness, and health care (Engel 1977), yet the meso-structural level of health is often neglected in research. The meso-level is located between state and individual actors and it describes influences of the direct environment, such as families and households. Theoretical approaches and empirical findings highlight that these characteristics are also important determinants of individual health.

It is well known that different types of households result in different morbidity and mortality risks (for a detailed overview, see Hank and Steinbach in this volume). Although, across the studies various indicators are used to reflect the household structure (usually marital status is taken into account, together with the life form, e.g. family structure, parenthood, presence and number of children, partnership status, cohabitation), this finding applies largely independent (Schneider et al. 2014). Our approach is to map this multidimensionality of living arrangements by examining several indicators together.

D. Georges (✉) · D. Kreft · G. Doblhammer
Institute for Sociology and Demography, University of Rostock, Rostock, Germany
e-mail: daniela.georges@uni-rostock.de

D. Kreft
e-mail: daniel.kreft2@uni-rostock.de

G. Doblhammer
e-mail: gabriele.doblhammer@uni-rostock.de

D. Georges · D. Kreft · G. Doblhammer
Rostock Center for the Study of Demographic Change, Rostock, Germany

G. Doblhammer and J. Gumà (eds.), *A Demographic Perspective on Gender, Family and Health in Europe*, https://doi.org/10.1007/978-3-319-72356-3_9

Today private households and families are experiencing a differentiation and pluralisation, wherein the non-family sector (childless couples, living alone, living apart together) is growing and the family sector (couples with children, single parents) is shrinking (Meyer 2006). Meanwhile, in Germany less than half the population lives in a family, that is, with children. The proportion of households with at least three members has been declining for many years (1991: 35.6%, 2014: 24.8%), while 1-person and 2-person households are increasing. As a result, the average household size shrank from 2.27 in 1991 to 2.01 in 2014 (Statistisches Bundesamt 2015a). Life forms such as cohabitation, single parents, living alone, or childless couples do not completely repress the traditional family (married couples with children), but they are becoming increasingly common. We will analyze whether this development is accompanied by increasing health inequalities.

Gender is still a central determinant of health and health inequalities (Oksuzyan et al. 2014; Verbrugge 1989; see Oksuzyan et al. in this volume). Men and women show—at least partly—different mechanisms of health and illness, and they are vulnerable to different diseases (Denton et al. 2004). These differences are also apparent in the context of households and may even be exacerbated by household effects. Within households, social roles and gender norms are produced and reproduced, and usually the set of roles is different for men and women. To what extent this attribution of roles really has an effect on health and well-being, though, depends on the specific composition of the household, the type, strength and direction of relations, and other factors (McIlvane et al. 2007; Lowenstein et al. 2007), and is subject of our investigation.

Against the background of increasing global migration flows (Willekens 2015), the importance of the migration background as a determinant of (health) inequalities is increasing. Today, more than 200 million persons are living outside their country of birth, i.e. they migrated to another country (Willekens 2015). This raises a new cultural diversity within populations, which affects the health situation and demographic characteristics in the countries involved (both in the country of origin as well as in the host country) (Kohls 2012).

Germany has been an immigration country since World War II and is characterized by a large number of people with a migration background: About 20% (16.4 million) of the population in Germany has a migration background (Statistisches Bundesamt 2015a).[1] The largest groups among them are the Turks, who were recruited in the 1960s and 1970s as guest workers, and their descendants, and the Aussiedler,[2] who immigrated after the collapse of the Soviet Union (Statistisches Bundesamt 2015a). These two groups not only differ (more or less; see Section "Why Investigate the Health of Migrants and Distinguish Between

[1]"Migration background" includes all people who immigrated to Germany themselves or are descendants of persons who immigrated to Germany (Statistisches Bundesamt 2015b).

[2]This terms refers to foreign-born persons who hold German citizenship which was not acquired by an act of naturalization, who moved to Germany after 1949 [definition based on Statistisches Bundesamt (2011)].

Different Migration Backgrounds?") from the German host society, but also among themselves. In a health context it can be shown that Turks have increased risks of infectious diseases (Neuhauser and Razum 2008) and lower mental health (Milewski and Doblhammer 2015). By implication, Turkish migrants have disadvantages in healthy life expectancy relative to the German population; especially Turkish women show great disadvantages in life expectancy and healthy life expectancy compared to German women (Carnein et al. 2015). Aussiedler have higher rates of non-natural deaths but lower overall mortality than native Germans (Becher et al. 2007). While it is less common for Aussiedler to have severe diseases, they do suffer more frequently from mental disorders (Becher et al. 2007; Knipper and Bilgin 2009). At the household level, we find that the size and structure of a household depends on the migration background, where households of migrants are more frequently familial, larger, and have more children (Friedrich 2008; Worbs et al. 2013; Wittig et al. 2004; Woellert and Klingholz 2014). Both the household structure and health are therefore subject to a cultural imprint. Against the backdrop that once young migrants also age and are currently reaching ages associated with increasing health risks, the necessity to scrutinize integration and health inequalities in the context of migration background arises.

The direction and intensity of these connections have yet not been examined for Germany. We try to close this gap by analyzing the effects of household structure, namely the generational structure, on individual health. Due to the expected differences between men and women and between different migration backgrounds mentioned, we contextualize this by gender and migration background. Our main research questions are therefore: What is the influence of the household on health? What are the differences between men and women and which of these depend on the migration background? In addition, we conduct a mediator and moderator analysis to answer these questions: What is the impact of economic resources on the household effects? What influence do different characteristics of the household structure have on health in the context of migration background? The results can contribute to a better understanding of meso-level influences on health. They allow us to estimate the impact of changes in the family sector and contribute to a better understanding of health inequalities among migrants. Additionally, they can help identify vulnerable groups and exploit intervention as well as prevention measures in the German case.

Theoretical Perspectives and Findings

Health as an Outcome of Household Production

As George Engel's biopsychosocial model illustrates, illness and health cannot be understood as only individual characteristics, but rather they must be explored in a multilevel context (Engel 1977). This is why it is not effective to consider only

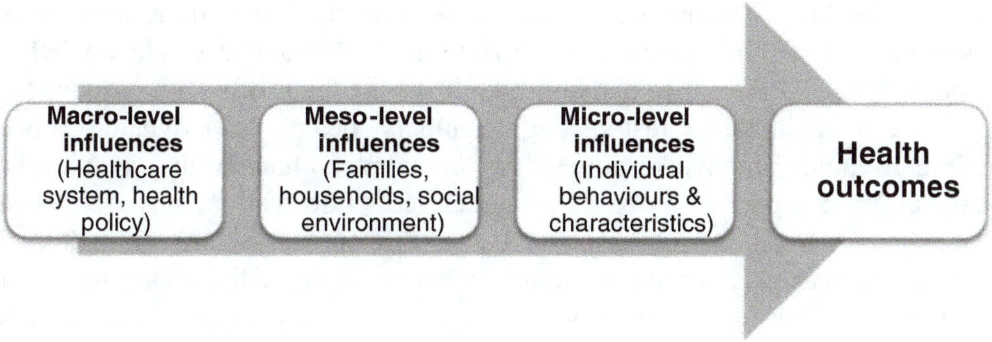

Fig. 1 Multidimensionality of health factors and health outcomes

effects on the individual level; a consideration of other contexts is also required when investigating determinants of health. In addition to individual characteristics, it is necessary to include families and other social organisations as well as healthcare facilities and health policy in order to gain a holistic understanding of health and disease (Holmes et al. 2008). Health outcomes are the result of factors at different levels, as we illustrate in Fig. 1.

Because they yield daily influences, households represent a crucial determinant of health. They set resources and demands and represent a special form of social networks, which are characterised by emotional ties, a specific role allocation, and permanent exchange relations. As a result, household members have similar resources and needs, and thus they show similar health outcomes (Hughes and Waite 2002; Berman et al. 1994). Currently, investigating the household as a determinant of health disparities appears to be particularly exciting, because households, household types, and household structures are becoming increasingly diverse. With increasing life expectancy, intergenerational relationships can last much longer, resulting in new (generational and familial) relationship potentials, e.g. long-term relations between grandparents and their grandchildren and multigenerational households[3] (Arránz Becker and Steinbach 2012). These supposedly positive developments might even so be problematic: particularly the middle ages are in a "sandwich position" between their children and their parents, and are therefore faced with both a double burden as well as competing social role attributions (McIlvane et al. 2007).

In addition to this (partially) unequal distribution of roles, households fulfil the function as an instance of socialisation. They impart values, norms, duties and behaviour patterns, which are also reflected in health aspects. Within households and families, all members are producers of their own and the other members' health (Jacobson 2000), and as a result of exchange relationships, health knowledge is shared, health behaviours are adopted, and a similar perception of health is configured (Jacobson 2000; Settertobulte and Palentien 1996).

[3]Despite the new potential, multigenerational households are rather atypical and tend to be less important; e.g. in Germany the proportion of all households with three or more generations declined from 1.2% in 1991 to 0.4% in 2012 (Hammes 2013).

One of the first conceptual frameworks, developed for the connection between households and health outcomes, is the Household Production of Health (HHPH) approach. The HHPH implies that households are the locus of health production, as they strive to maintain or restore their members' health. In a dynamic process, within households, internal resources (e.g. knowledge about health, health-related behaviours) are linked to external resources (e.g. information, resources, health services), so there is an allocation and adaption of health care strategies. This combination makes households more efficient than individuals and allows short-term responses and interventions, which have a quicker impact than contextual effects. Because health behaviour within a household is thus influenced by both the household itself and external factors, it can be assumed that different households and different types of households react differently given identical conditions, and that they would thus show different health outcomes (Berman et al. 1994). Economic theories, such as the approach of the New Household economics (NHE), expand the HHPH approach through economic aspects. This approach posits that the objectives of households are utility maximization and satisfaction, whereby health outcomes represent one possible source of satisfaction, which competes with other outcomes. Households are assumed to know how to produce health and strive to achieve a maximum of outcomes using available resources. The consideration, which and how many resources are used for which outcome, is a dynamic process. On the one hand, different combinations can result in the same outcomes, and on the other hand, similarly available resources do not necessarily result in equal outcomes (Berman et al. 1994). According to the NHE, health is subject to a large variance and depends heavily on intra-household choices. Statistical multilevel models are suitable and necessary to regard this variance when one investigates the effects of household and individual characteristics (DiPrete and Forristal 1994).

Findings consequently indicate that different types of households and living arrangements are linked to differences in health. In research, the aspect of the household is usually displayed by family demographic parameters, such as marital status (Hughes and Waite 2009). Being married is positively associated with good health outcomes (Joung et al. 1994; Schneider et al. 2014; Williams and Umberson 2004). This protective effect of marriage is largely explained by a better economic position and higher social support, but may as well—at least partially—be driven by differences in living arrangements. It has to be assumed that the living arrangements have an additional, but separate effect on health outcomes (Joung et al. 1994). While living alone is associated with health risks (Manderbacka et al. 2014; Cramer 1993), both partnership and parenthood are protective factors for health (Helbig et al. 2006; Koskinen et al. 2007; Zunzunegui et al. 2001; Kravdal et al. 2012).

According to Ferrer et al. (2005), the magnitude of household influences on health differences itself is dependent on the household composition. For married people without children, this effect of household and family is very pronounced; in this group, 22% of health differences are explained by the family-level effect (Ferrer et al. 2005). Soons and Kalmijn (2009) examined health differences between marriage and cohabitation and found that this effect is explained by the level of institutionalization of cohabitation: In countries where the proportion of cohabitants is higher, the difference is smaller than in countries with a low proportion (Soons and Kalmijn 2009). With regard to the household composition, in Finland it was found that for those living alone, lone parents and cohabitants have a higher amenable mortality, which is attributed to economic disadvantages (Manderbacka et al. 2014). McIlvane et al. (2007) performed an analysis of the impact of the generational composition on self-rated health and found that single parents show low self-rated health. In contrast, living with parents has positive effects and may compensate for other, otherwise unfavourable characteristics, such as a low level of education or being unmarried (McIlvane et al. 2007). A longitudinal analysis of the relationship between living arrangement and different health outcomes was carried out by Hughes and Waite (2002). They state health variances across different living arrangements, where members of married couples living alone or with children show the best health and single mothers have the greatest health disadvantages (Hughes and Waite 2002).

To summarize, the household has a double significance in the production of health. On the one hand, different arrangements are associated with different health risks and health outcomes. On the other hand, further outcomes (e.g. gender roles, distribution of responsibilities, perception of health) are determined within households, which are associated with health differences. However, households are not independent, but are embedded in social conditions, so it should be considered that both the welfare state configuration and cultural norms influence this nexus.

Migration Background and Health in a Household Context

Migrants are people who change their main place of residence for a longer time or permanently to another country in the course of a migration process. They have in common that they have gone through this migration process, which is a phase of disruption and reorientation associated with stress and integration challenges (Neuhauser and Razum 2008). This process characterizes both their own situation and the family development over several generations (Neuhauser and Razum 2008). Due to often precarious employment and income situations as well as lower levels of non-transferable economic and educational assets, migrants more frequently belong to socially disadvantaged classes in the host country. This social deprivation is associated with additional health risks and often also has negative effects on the educational success of children with migration background (Schenk 2007). In addition to socio-economic disadvantages and downward social mobility (Constant and Massey 2005; Schenk 2007), problems such as language barriers, processes of integration, and cultural adaptation can affect migrants negatively, e.g. in terms of health (Neuhauser and Razum 2008). Language barriers, differences in health perception, and a lack of knowledge about the health care system in the host society often results in a limited access of migrants to the formal health care system and a lower utilization of health services[4] (Dias et al. 2008; Helman 2007). The stressful experiences associated with immigration and integration as well as social stigmatization and marginalization enhance this effect (Derose, Escarce and Lurie 2007; Neuhauser and Razum 2008). The health of migrants is thus determined by three aspects: the conditions in the country of origin, the conditions of the migration process, and the conditions in the host country (Spallek and Razum 2007).

However, migrants represent a heterogeneous group and differ in their origin, their cultural backgrounds, their motives to migrate, their duration of stay in the host country, their legal status, their degree of integration, their demographic behaviour, and many other characteristics (Lindert et al. 2008; Norredam 2011; Neuhauser and Razum 2008). They differ both among themselves as well as from the society of origin and the host society. Their decision to migrate is subject to a selection process, and in most cases driven by a positive selection mechanism: compared to non-migrants of the country of origin, migrants are mostly young, educated, and relatively healthy[5] (Ghatak et al. 1996; Razum and Rohrmann 2002). Due to this combination of characteristics, migrants also differ positively from the host society, particularly in their work performance (Ghatak et al. 1996).

Migrants with their own migration experiences (i.e. first generation migrants) underwent their socialisation in their country of origin, which often differs from the host society, and therefore have incorporated different cultural ideas, behaviours, norms, and values. Because migrants often maintain ties with their countries of origin (Haas 2010), these patterns usually persist for a longer time after immigration. Gender norms, family ideals, health related behaviours, and health perception therefore are supposedly strongly influenced by the culture of origin and social policies in the home country. Consequently, it can be assumed, that migrants differ in their health outcomes and in household patterns from the host society, whereby the extent of these differences depends on the magnitude of cultural differences as well as the individual degree of integration.

Although social networks (in the potential host society and the society of origin) are an important aspect in the decision to migrate, migrants often experience a temporary loss of social ties and social capital (Haug 2007). The social capital affects the social embedding and the integration. As a source of control (Coleman 1990), social capital enables access to the labour market and thus affects economic and social outcomes. Using the example of Turks in Germany, Lancee and Hartung (2012) demonstrate that, among migrants, being embedded in inter-ethnic contacts results in advantages in the labour market (Lancee and Hartung 2012). The high importance of social networks among migrants can be inferred from the so-called "Latino Health Paradox". Despite a worse socio-economic profile, Latinos in the US have better health outcomes and lower mortality rates than do Whites, which is

[4]Studies have found that the differences in health risks and health care utilization between immigrants and non-immigrants are equalized with increasing duration of stay (Leclere et al. 1994; Kreft and Doblhammer 2012).

[5]This selection is called the "Healthy-Migrant-Effect" (Kohls 2008).

due to social factors, such as social networks and emotional ties (Viruell-Fuentes and Schulz 2009; Abraído-Lanza et al. 1999). Although this effect of social ties probably has a cultural component and depends on the legal status of migrants in the host country, we suspect transferability to other contexts, for example to the German case. Other studies also show that the family situation and the household structure might have a substituting function for external social ties: If the external social capital is low, the household and family act as a central compensating resource (Haug 2007). Burt's "Closure-Argument" highlights the importance of social networks in the creation of social capital (Burt 2001), whereby a dense family network also increases social capital (Haug 2007).

Thus, there are strong ties between the household context and the migration status. Both are strongly embedded in the cultural context and contribute to the formation of social norms (e.g. gender roles, family ideals, health perception). We therefore follow the assumption that the impact of the household on health is different between migrants and non-migrants.

Gender Differences in Health and Household Context

"The embeddedness of gender in all social relationships may make it impossible to separate gender from the very life circumstances that we examine in order to understand gender patterns in health. (Walters et al. 2002)"

Gender inequalities in health are reported frequently. Men and women not only differ in general in their morbidity and mortality, but also have different determinants for health and illness. For a detailed overview, see Oksuzyan et al. in this volume. This diversity is also reflected in the household context.

In the household context additional gender differences become apparent. The previously presented studies consistently illustrate—as far as they performed gender-specific analyses—a difference of determinants and effect sizes between men and women (Manderbackaet al. 2014; Williams and Umberson 2004; Soons and Kalmijn 2009; Hughes and Waite 2002). The underlying mechanism is that men's health shows a higher dependency on behavioural determinants, while for women social structural and psychosocial determinants are more important. It has to be assumed that household factors have a stronger impact on women's health than on men's health. Gender-based health inequalities thus reflect (among other things) social factors and an unequal distribution of family demands (Denton et al. 2004; Artazcoz 2001), which goes together with the social roles and role allocation within households already described (see Section "Health as an Outcome of Household Production"). Gender or gender-specific role assignments are crucial determinants of health, as they have an influence on how people behave and how they access health services (UN 2010; World Health Organization 2010).

Household and care work are still rather female domains (Oláh et al. 2014). Together with the increasing involvement of women in the labour market, additional burdens arise for women (Geulen 2004). The understanding of gender roles and division of tasks is strongly influenced by social-political standards and cultural norms. Especially in conservative welfare states, the value of the family is quite high and there is a traditional division of tasks, due to which men and women are attributed different roles. Conservative welfare states have low levels of egalitarian participation on the labour market and shared household tasks (Hook 2006; Huschek et al. 2011; Batalova and Cohen 2002). This ideal of the traditional family image is maintained by social policies and thus can promote gender differences in the context of households and health (Esping-Andersen 1990).

Why Investigate the Health of Migrants and Distinguish Between Different Migration Backgrounds?

The need for migration background-specific analyses of health in Germany arises from the special composition of the German population. In 2014, one of every five people in Germany (16.4 million) had a migration background, i.e. they immigrated themselves or are descendants of migrants (Statistisches Bundesamt 2015a). Thus, the number of migrants in Germany is currently at a record high and a growing ethnic and cultural diversity is emerging. Against this backdrop, and due to the close ties between health and migration background, migrants must be considered as a group that is exposed to additional health risks. We carry out an internal differentiation of the migrant population in Germany and consider the two largest groups of migrants—Turkish migrants and Aussiedler—separately, because they differ in many characteristics and health outcomes. In the following analysis, we measure the migration background according to the definition of the German Federal Statistical Office (Statistisches Bundesamt) and consider both the (current and former) nationality and/or country of birth as well as the parents' ancestry. People with a migration background thus are all those who migrated to Germany themselves (first generation migrants), who were born as a foreigner in Germany, or who have at least one parent who immigrated or was born as a foreigner in Germany (second generation migrants) (Statistisches Bundesamt 2011).

Turkish migrants and Aussiedler are the two largest groups of people with a migration background in Germany. In 2014, approximately 3 million Turks lived in Germany, of which about 1.4 million were first generation migrants (Statistisches Bundesamt 2015b). The high number of Turks in Germany is explained by the recruitment of guest workers between the 1950s and the 1970s and subsequent family reunification. Aussiedler are the second large migrant group in Germany, comprising approximately 3 million people. Aussiedler, sometimes called "In-Migrating Ethnic Germans", are descendants of emigrants who moved from Germany to Eastern Europe before the 20th century or persons of German origin who stayed in the former German regions after the 2nd World War (Kreft and Doblhammer 2012). Aussiedler differ from other migrant groups especially in their cultural background and motives to migrate. In their home countries, Aussiedler were a minority and they emigrated to live as Germans among Germans. For Aussiedler, Germany is their cultural home (Janikowski 1999). Due to this German origin, Aussiedler are in the unique situation that they are legally recognized as "Germans by status" and can directly acquire citizenship, which entitles them to participate in the health and welfare system. Aussiedler immigrated from different countries, the majority come from the former Soviet Union (1.4 million), Poland (570,000), Kazakhstan (568,000), and the Russian Federation (555,000) (Statistisches Bundesamt 2015b).

Studies demonstrate significant differences between the host population, Turks, Aussiedler, and other migrant groups in Germany. Regarding health, non-Germans generally are exposed to other and higher health risks; while chronic diseases and cancers are less common among migrants compared to Germans without migration background, they have higher risks of suffering from musculoskeletal disorders, cardiovascular diseases, diabetes, respiratory diseases, and infectious diseases (Neuhauser and Razum 2008). These differences are at least partly explained by poor working and living conditions of non-Germans, and also reflect the relatively high medical standard in Germany[6] (Neuhauser and Razum 2008). More detailed analyses reveal that Turks in Germany have increased morbidity, and especially higher risks for cardiovascular diseases, diabetes, and viral hepatitis (Knipper and Bilgin 2009). This is particularly attributed to an inactive lifestyle and other eating habits (Knipper and Bilgin 2009). Among Turks, eating has a high priority (Rehaag et al. 2012); a bountiful table is a sign of hospitality and although traditional Turkish cuisine is based primarily on vegetables, they are often prepared with copious amounts of oil (Zwick 2007). Aussiedler, on the other hand, exhibit increased risk factors for cardiovascular diseases (e.g. alcohol consumption, obesity, drugs), but seldom have severe diseases. Despite the pooling of risk factors, Aussiedler have surprisingly low rates of mortality (Becher et al. 2007; Wittig et al. 2004; Knipper and Bilgin 2009). Generally, these differences (between the groups of migrants and non-migrants) are more pronounced in women than in men (Worbs et al. 2013). The causes are mainly due to socioeconomic differences, but also cultural differences contribute to this (Neuhauser and Razum 2008).

Turkish migrants in Germany have a low social status on average, e.g. low levels of education and a poor economic situation (Statistisches Bundesamt 2015a; Woellert and Klingholz 2014), and thus bundle characteristics that are associated with health disadvantages (Mielck 2008). On the contrary, the Aussiedler have an advantageous structure in their educational and professional qualification, are usually employed, and thus have a high similarity to the German middle class (Worbs et al. 2013). The proportion of people with a higher education entrance qualification is 43% among Germans,[7] 31% among Aussiedler, and 20% among

[6]E.g., infectious diseases have become very rare in Germany due to medical processes and are now rather diseases of less developed countries (Omran 2005).

[7]In the following descriptions, "Germans" means the German population without a migration background in first or second generation.

Turks; the unemployment rate is 6% among Germans, 9% among Aussiedler, and 16% among Turks (Woellert and Klingholz 2014). The deviating proportions of the Turks are particularly due to the low integration of Turkish women in the education system and the labour market (Woellert and Klingholz 2014; Neuhauser and Razum 2008). Consequently, the housewife ratio, which reflects the proportion of women who stay at home, is markedly higher—49% of Turkish women stay at home but only 17% of Germans and 20% of Aussiedler (Woellert and Klingholz 2014). This demonstrates a still persisting classic distribution of tasks and traditional gender roles among Turks.

The majority of Turks in Germany are very religious, whereas the religious faith is rather understood as a norm than as an individual decision (Wetzels and Brettfeld 2007). Turks are usually Muslims (Haug et al. 2009), and in Islam roles tend to be non-interchangeable and the traditional family ideal is of great importance (Predelli 2004). Aussiedler are usually Christian (83%), and thus have the same confession as the majority of the German population without migration background (Worbs et al. 2013).

Marriage and family life forms have a higher importance among Turks (Sachverständigenkommission 6. Familienbericht 2000), and Turkish migrants show different patterns in their family-formation processes, e.g. marry at an earlier age and have more children (Milewski 2011). Aussiedler, as well, are more likely to be married and to share a household with children than Germans (Worbs et al. 2013). Again, this might be an indicator of the gender roles and family norms of their countries of origin, which are more conservative and traditional than in Germany, especially among Turkish migrants (Huschek et al. 2011; Diehl et al. 2009; de Valk 2008). As a result, the average household size and structure differs between Germans, Turks, and Aussiedler. While Germans live in rather small households (Ø 2.0 persons per household), the household size is larger among Aussiedler (2.3) and especially among Turks (3.1) (Woellert and Klingholz 2014). Familial forms of life, households with many children, and multi-generational households are more common among Turks and Aussiedler (Woellert and Klingholz 2014).

To summarize, there are several differences in many aspects of life between Turks, Aussiedler, and Germans. While Turks differ strongly from Germans—mainly due to their traditional norms—Aussiedler are quite similar to the German population. Aussiedler show—in comparison with Turks—a high degree of integration, which can be attributed to their legal status and their cultural similarity (Woellert and Klingholz 2014). We assume that the decision for or against a specific arrangement is culturally influenced and driven by deviating motivations and thus results in different health-outcomes.

Summary and Hypotheses

The descriptions above illustrate the importance of the household as a determinant of health, whereas the underlying mechanisms are not clear, but embedded in a strong network of individual values, cultural background, and socio-political frameworks. What becomes clear is that the impact of household structures differs across the contexts, for example with regard to gender and migration background. We aim to discover and explain these various mechanisms.

Our analysis is designed to test four hypotheses deduced from the conceptual framework discussed above. First, we test the *family segregation-hypothesis*. There are different patterns in the household formation and different types of households are associated with disparate tasks and resources and finally result in different health risks. Because living in a one generation household, i.e. living alone or living without children, is accompanied by lower levels of family ties, we assume that people in one generation households show health disadvantages. These disadvantages are based particularly on the lack of social support when living alone, the lack of integration into a dense family network, and the positive selection mechanisms into parenthood. We expect, however, a variance according to migration background, resulting from different cultural backgrounds. Because traditional family households are more common among migrants and one generation households tend to contradict the cultural norm, we suspect that living without children is the result of disadvantageous selection among migrants and thus acts more detrimentally among migrants than among non-migrant Germans. Our second hypothesis—*the gender hypothesis*—states that the effect of the household structure is strongly gendered. Due to an allocation of multiple social roles and a high embedding in the household, women's health is stronger and affected by the household composition in a different way than men's health. Due to more traditional gender roles in migrant households we expect this effect to be amplified among migrants. Based on the *mediator hypothesis*, we test whether and how additional characteristics, especially the economic situation, explain health differences by household composition, gender, and migration background. Finally, the *partner hypothesis* hypothesises a positive effect of a partner in the household on health, which is driven by positive health selection into partnership. Due to a higher importance of the traditional family ideal among migrants, we assume that the absence of a partner is more disadvantageous for migrants than for Germans without a migration background. In addition, health related selection forces into partnership may also differ by migration background.

Data and Methods

Data and Variables

Dataset and Analytical Basis: The German Microcensuses 2005 and 2009

We used data from the German Microcensuses 2005 and 2009 (hereafter referred to as Microcensus 2005/2009) which is an annual multi-purpose household survey with a representative sample of one percent of the German population (about 830,000 persons per year). Due to the obligation to provide information to the majority of questions and the presence of information for each member of the household, the Microcensus is highly representative of the German population. The data provide detailed information on the German demographic and labour market structure, including socio-demographic, economic, and household aspects (Statistisches Bundesamt 2015c).

Because the Microcensus is designed as a rotating panel, in which each selected household is annually interviewed over a period of four years, we used two survey years with a distance of four years to ensure that each person is included in the dataset only once. We used the survey years 2005 and 2009 because these combine information about individuals' health status, household context, and migratory background. Pooling the data of the two years increases the number of individuals with a migration background.

Variables

Health Outcomes

The Microcensuses 2005 and 2009 include a health module in addition to the standard programme with a limited set of indicators. In the following analysis, the general health status is measured by the following question: "Have you been ill or had an accidental injury within the last four weeks (before the interview)?" and "How long does/did your illness or your injury last?". In this study all persons with an illness that lasts (lasted) at least four weeks are defined as unhealthy. The time frame of four weeks was chosen in order to exclude persons with short-term illnesses (e.g., the flu or other infections). Because answering the question is optional, the number of cases with missing information is higher than for most of the other variables. Due to missing information in the health variable 69,144 cases [57,053 native Germans (12.64% of the total sample) and 12,091 persons with migration background (2.68%)] have to be excluded from the analysis. In total, 382,113 persons [323,577 native Germans (84.68% of the final sample) and 58,536 migrants (15.32%)] remain in the sample under study.

Variables at the Individual Level

When analysing contextual effects on individual health outcomes, the effects of personal characteristics are controlled for. These individual level variables are sex, age (4 age groups: 30 to <40, 40 to <50, 50 to <60 and 60 to <65 years), family status (single, married, divorced, widowed), presence of a partner in the household, education (low degree = graduation after a maximum of nine classes, medium = ten-class general educational school, high = university entrance qualification), and occupational status [self-employed without employees; self-employed with employees; unpaid family worker; official or judge; employed or soldier; full- and part-time worker (skilled, semi-skilled, and unskilled); non-active population]. One of the key characteristics is the migration background, which includes migration history and ethnic background for first and second generation and thus follows the definition of the Federal Statistical Office (Statistisches Bundesamt 2011). Based on this information, we distinguish between native born Germans, Turks, Aussiedler, and people with a migration background from other countries ("other"). As "native born Germans", we mean all who have no migration background in the first or second generation, i.e. persons who have neither migrated themselves nor have parents who are immigrants in Germany. Turks are identified by current and former nationality: all who have themselves or whose parent(s) had or have Turkish nationality belong to this group. Aussiedler are measured by legal status and represent the group of those whose parent(s) or who themselves is/are registered as Aussiedler. The identification of Aussiedler in the data of the Microcensus is possible on the basis of officially generated information. "Other" includes all persons who have a migration background but are not Turkish or Aussiedler.[8]

Because behavioural factors are strongly linked to health (see e.g. Sturm 2002; World Health Organization 2002), BMI [classified into underweight ($BMI < 18.5$), normal weight ($18.5 \leq BMI \geq 25$), overweight ($25 < BMI \geq 30$), obese ($BMI > 30$), missing information], and smoking habits (never smoked, ex-smoker, smoker, missing) will be controlled for. Additionally, the year of the interview (2005 or 2009) will be included in the models to control for period effects.

Household and Contextual Variables

At the second level, we focus on the household structure and take the number and composition of generations into account: One generation households (1G-HH) comprise persons living alone or as a couple (without children or with children who do not/no longer live in the same household). Two generation households combine a parent and a child generation; we make distinctions for two generations (2G-HH) with one or two children, 2G-HH with three or more children, 2G-HH with (grand)parents. We also created a category for households with three or more generations (3+G-HH). Additionally, we control for the net equivalent income [less than 930 € per month (lowest 20% in the sample); 930 to less than 1400 € (20–50%); 1400 to less than 2110 € (50–80%); more than 2110 € (top 20%)], and analyze the migration background of the household. In contrast to the individual migration background, the migration background of the household provides information about the presence of persons without a migration background. We define three types of households: no migration background (i.e. all persons are non-migrants), mixed households (i.e. households with migrants and non-migrant Germans), and migrant households (all persons with migration background).

[8]A detailed differentiation is not possible and useful due to statistical and definitional problems.

Table 1 Variance inflation factors of the sample, men and women

	Sample	Men	Women
Generation composition	1.18	1.19	1.19
Year of interview	1.01	1.02	1.01
Sex	1.06		
Age group	1.24	1.21	1.32
Family status	1.09	1.07	1.14
Presence of a partner in the same HH	1.13	1.16	1.19
Migration background	2.61	2.60	2.63
Education	1.16	1.15	1.19
Occupational status	1.20	1.22	1.18
BMI	1.03	1.03	1.03
Smoking habits	1.07	1.06	1.05
Equivalent income group	1.24	1.26	1.25
Migration background of the household	2.73	2.72	2.75
Place of residence	1.06	1.06	1.06
Mean VIF	1.34	1.34	1.36
n	382,113	188,108	194,005

Source German Microcensus 2005/2009

Finally, we control for the size of the place of residence (rural with fewer than 20,000 inhabitants; urban with 20,000 inhabitants or more) as an indicator of the contextual embedding and access to health care (Hartley et al. 1994; Bennett et al. 2008).

Pre-regression Diagnostics

The bivariate analysis shows significant statistical correlations between all characteristics and longstanding illness. Covariates are generally not correlated, with the exception of the individual migration background and the household's migration background (Table 1).

Statistical Methods

We modelled the association between health and the observed characteristics by applying multilevel regression models for both sexes combined to account for the dependency of observations on the household-level. Logistic regression models were used to calculate sex specific models. The estimations were performed using the "xtlogit" and "logit" routine in Stata version 14.1.

Sample Under Study

The analyses were restricted to 451,257 individuals between the ages of 30 and 64 living in private households. This specific age groups was chosen because people in this range display a diversity in living arrangements and are typically of an age in which (own) children already or still live at home. Of these, 69,144 individuals were excluded due to missing information about their health status. The two-level regression analysis for both sexes combined were therefore conducted based on 382,113 people at level 1 (individual level), nested within 247,360 households at level 2 (household level). Of these, 323,577 were native born Germans (84.68%), 10,043 were Turkish (2.63%), 13,147 were Aussiedler (3.44%), and 35,346 had a different migration background (9.25%).

The sex specific models included 194,005 women and 188,108 men. The proportion of the migrant groups is similar for both sexes.

Results

Descriptive Statistics

A detailed overview of the sample's composition is given in Table 2.

Longstanding illness is a rather rare phenomenon in our study population. Only 5.47% of the sample have a longstanding illness, where the proportion among women (5.60%) is slightly higher than men (5.34%). People who live in a one generation household (1G-HH) or in a two generation household (2G-HH) with their (grand)parents have worse health than those in other household structures; the proportion of ill persons is 7.30% for both groups. The quota is 3.79% in 2G-HH with one or two children, 3.23% in 2G-HH with three or more children, and 5.28% in households with 3 or more generations (3+G-HH). Turkish people have worst health of all migration backgrounds (8.01% vs. 5.40–5.49%).

In terms of household structure there are differences by migration background and sex. While the majority of native Germans live in 1G-HH (50.08%) followed by 42.68% in 2G-HH with one or two children, 2G-HH with one or two children are the most common composition among the other migrant groups. It is also striking that Turks live in different household structures than Germans, i.e. with three or more children (24.76%) or in 3+G-HH (2.41%). Furthermore, the absence of a partner in the same household is more common among native Germans (26.16%) and least common among Turks (16.17%); the share of persons without a partner among Aussiedler is located between these two groups (20.44%).

We find gender differences to the extent that men live in an 1G-HH (49.22% vs. 46.80%) slightly more frequently than women and slightly less frequently with

Table 2 Characteristics of the sample, men and women

	Sample		Men		Women	
	n	%	n	%	n	%
Longstanding illness						
No	361,199	94.53	178,057	94.66	183,142	94.40
Yes	20,914	5.47	10,051	5.34	10,863	5.60
Generation composition						
1G-HH	183,382	47.99	92,594	49.22	90,788	46.80
2G-HH with one or two children	166,224	43.50	79,792	42.42	86,432	44.55
2G-HH with three or more children	24,914	6.52	12,057	6.41	12,857	6.63
2G-HH with (grand)parents	3524	0.92	1819	0.97	1705	0.88
3+G-HH	4069	1.06	1846	0.98	2223	1.15
Year of interview						
2005	195,681	51.21	96,671	51.39	99,010	51.03
2009	186,432	48.79	91,437	48.61	94,995	48.97
Sex						
Females	194,005	50.77				
Males	188,108	49.23				
Age group						
30 to <40 years	97,679	25.56	48,164	25.60	49,515	25.52
40 to <50 years	127,163	33.28	63,311	33.66	63,852	32.91
50 to <60 years	108,437	28.38	52,925	28.14	55,512	28.61
60 to <65 years	48,834	12.78	23,708	12.60	25,126	12.95
Family status						
Single	68,609	17.96	41,452	22.04	27,157	14.00
Married	264,441	69.20	128,375	68.25	136,066	70.14
Widowed	10,422	2.73	1969	1.05	8453	4.36
Divorced	38,641	10.11	16,312	8.67	22,329	11.51
Presence of a partner in the same HH						
Yes	285,178	74.63	140,130	74.49	145,048	74.77
No	96,935	25.37	47,978	25.51	48,957	25.23
Migration background						
Native Germans	323,577	84.68	159,525	84.81	164,052	84.56
Turkish	10,043	2.63	5172	2.75	4871	2.51
Aussiedler	13,147	3.44	6402	3.40	6745	3.48
Other	35,346	9.25	17,009	9.04	18,337	9.45
Education						
Low	150,914	39.49	77,036	40.95	73,878	38.08
Medium	129,477	33.88	55,996	29.77	73,481	37.88
High	100,718	26.36	54,558	29.00	46,160	23.79

(continued)

Table 2 (continued)

	Sample		Men		Women	
	n	%	n	%	n	%
Missing information	1004	0.26	518	0.28	486	0.25
Occupational status						
Self-employed without employees	17,528	4.59	11,161	5.93	6367	3.28
Self-employed with employees	14,927	3.91	11,259	5.99	3668	1.89
Unpaid family worker	1330	0.35	154	0.08	1176	0.61
Official or judge	15,773	4.13	9270	4.93	6503	3.35
Employed or soldier	139,659	36.55	62,187	33.06	77,472	39.93
Full- or part-time worker	69,372	18.15	46,928	24.95	22,444	11.57
Non-active population	123,524	32.33	47,149	25.06	76,375	39.37
BMI						
Underweight (BMI < 18.5)	5585	1.46	686	0.36	4899	2.53
Normal weight ($18.5 \leq$ BMI ≥ 25)	160,046	41.88	63,410	33.71	96,636	49.81
Overweight (25 < BMI $\geq$ 30)	125,677	32.89	79,641	42.34	46,036	23.73
Obese (BMI > 30)	49,465	12.95	27,673	14.71	21,792	11.23
Missing information	41,340	10.82	16,698	8.88	24,642	12.70
Smoking habits						
Never	173,768	45.48	70,836	37.66	102,932	53.06
Ex-smoker	78,825	20.63	45,359	24.11	33,466	17.25
Smoker	116,285	30.43	65,335	34.73	50,950	26.26
Missing information	13,235	3.46	6578	3.50	6657	3.43
Equivalent income group						
<930 € (lowest 20%)	68,371	17.89	32,019	17.02	36,352	18.74
930 to <1400 € (20–50%)	109,822	28.74	52,511	27.92	57,311	29.54
1400 to <2110 € (50–80%)	107,153	28.04	53,413	28.39	53,740	27.70
>2110 € (top 20%)	71,760	18.78	37,655	20.02	34,105	17.58
Missing information	25,007	6.54	12,510	6.65	12,497	6.44
Migration background of the household						
No migration background	310,811	81.34	152,745	81.20	158,066	81.48
Mixed household	24,534	6.42	12,153	6.46	12,381	6.38
All persons with migration background	46,768	12.24	23,210	12.34	23,558	12.14

(continued)

Table 2 (continued)

	Sample		Men		Women	
	n	%	n	%	n	%
Place of residence						
Rural (fewer than 20,000 inhabitants)	166,103	43.47	82,457	43.83	83,646	43.12
Urban (20,000 inhabitants and more)	216,010	56.53	105,651	56.17	110,359	56.88
Total	382,113	100.00	188,108	100.00	194,005	100.00

Source German Microcensus 2005/2009

children (49.81% vs. 52.33%[9]). Regarding the absence or presence of a partner, there are no striking gender differences.

There are sufficient numbers of cases for all characteristics and the main combinations of characteristics to perform a multilevel regression model and sex-specific logistic regression models.

Gender Differences in Health— Results of Logistic Regression

The results of the logistic regression models are shown in Table 3.

Living in a 1G-HH is accompanied by health disadvantages. This effect applies to both men and women, but is more pronounced for women. Women in 2G-HH with one or two children respectively three or more children and women in 3+G-HH have significantly lower health risks than women in 1G-HH. These group differences exist almost independently of other characteristics, but are reinforced after control for socio-economic characteristics. Women in 2G-HH with three or more children have the best health (OR = 0.45–0.61; $p < 0.001$), followed by women in 3+G-HH (OR = 0.60–0.74; $p = 0.000–0.002$) and women in 2G-HH with one or two children (OR = 0.68–0.71; $p < 0.001$) (Table 3). Among men, health advantages by generation composition appear for those in 2G-HH with children. Those with three or more children have the best health with a reduced risk of illness by 17% ($p = 0.001$), followed by men with one or two children, who have a 13% lower risk ($p < 0.001$). 2G-HH with (grand)parents and 3G-HH do not differ from 1G-HH (Table 3).

When controlling for other characteristics, it became clear that health differences according to migration background exist for women but not for men. Female Aussiedler and women with other migration backgrounds reveal better health than German women: Their risk of poor health is 24% ($p = 0.012$) resp. 20%

[9]The remaining ~1% of men and women live in 2G-HH with (grand)parents.

Table 3 Odds of longstanding illness for men and women: odds ratio and *p*-values from logistic regression

Covariates	Men		Women	
	OR	*p*	OR	*p*
Generation composition (ref. 1G-HH)				
2G-HH with one or two children	0.87	0.000	0.69	0.000
2G-HH with three or more children	0.82	0.001	0.45	0.000
2G-HH with (grand)parents	0.95	0.609	0.88	0.188
3+G-HH	1.04	0.741	0.62	0.000
Year of interview (ref. 2005)				
2009	1.11	0.000	1.15	0.000
Age group (ref. 30 to <40 years)				
40 to <50 years	1.62	0.000	1.72	0.000
50 to <60 years	2.53	0.000	2.39	0.000
60 to <65 years	1.78	0.000	1.77	0.000
Family status (ref. single)				
Married	1.07	0.109	0.84	0.000
Widowed	0.96	0.658	0.81	0.000
Divorced	1.03	0.449	1.11	0.009
Presence of a partner in the same HH (ref. yes)				
No	1.31	0.000	1.42	0.000
Migration background (ref. native Germans)				
Turkish	1.19	0.124	1.01	0.938
Aussiedler	0.93	0.481	0.76	0.012
Other	0.96	0.690	0.80	0.020
Education (ref. low)				
Medium	0.76	0.000	0.87	0.000
High	0.67	0.000	0.73	0.000
Missing information	0.95	0.799	0.90	0.624
Occupational status (ref. employed or soldier)				
Self-employed without employees	1.03	0.686	1.11	0.239
Self-employed with employees	1.01	0.938	1.00	0.970
Unpaid family worker	1.55	0.337	1.89	0.000
Official or judge	1.53	0.000	1.25	0.020
Full- or part-time worker	1.08	0.094	1.21	0.000
Non-active population	6.68	0.000	4.73	0.000
BMI (ref. normal weight; $18.5 \leq BMI \geq 25$)				
Underweight ($BMI < 18.5$)	2.59	0.000	1.70	0.000
Overweight ($25 < BMI \geq 30$)	0.97	0.178	1.21	0.000
Obese ($BMI > 30$)	1.29	0.000	1.76	0.000
Missing information	0.79	0.000	0.94	0.147
Smoking habits (ref. never)				
Ex-smoker	1.47	0.000	1.39	0.000

(continued)

Table 3 (continued)

Covariates	Men		Women	
	OR	*p*	OR	*p*
Smoker	1.15	0.000	1.28	0.000
Missing information	0.70	0.000	0.60	0.000
Equivalent income group (ref. < 930 €; lowest 20%)				
930 to < 1400 € (20–50%)	0.92	0.003	0.84	0.000
1400 to < 2110 € (50–80%)	0.78	0.000	0.78	0.000
>2110 € (top 20%)	0.63	0.000	0.68	0.000
Missing information	0.88	0.008	0.83	0.000
Migration background household (ref. no m.b.)				
Mixed household	1.02	0.799	0.98	0.794
All persons with migration background	1.02	0.851	1.38	0.001
Place of residence (ref. rural; fewer than 20,000 inhabitants)				
Urban (20,000 inhabitants and more)	0.95	0.019	0.99	0.743
Constant	0.01	0.000	0.02	0.000
R^2	0.16		0.12	
Log likelihood	−33,074		−36,731	
n	188,108		194,005	

Source German Microcensus 2005/2009

(p = 0.020) lower (Table 3). The opposite is true for Turkish women: Health disadvantages of Turkish women compared to German women are driven mainly by social status and do remain after controlling for these characteristics (OR = 1.01; p = 0.938). Among men, without controlling for individual socio-economic status, lifestyle factors and contextual/household factors, both migrant groups considered have worse health than do German men. In the model without controlling for these factors, the risk of longstanding illness is 114% higher among Turks ($p < 0.001$) and 14% higher among Aussiedler (p = 0.022). These health differences are fully explained by compositional and structural factors and are attenuated, once controlled for other characteristics (Table 3).

The legal status of a partnership (family status) affects health, but only among women. Living as a female divorcee increases the risk of longstanding illness by 11% (p = 0.009) whereas the health advantage of married women is 16% (p 0.001) and those of the widowed 19% ($p < 0.001$) (Table 3). The effect of a partner in the household is stronger and more consistent than the effect of family status: the absence of a partner increases the risk of poor health both among women (by 42%; $p < 0.001$) and men (by 30%; $p < 0.001$) (Table 3). This partner effect is partly explained by individual socioeconomic differences among men and by contextual characteristics among women, as our stepwise models (results not shown) illustrate.

Finally, we find that women who live in a household consisting of only migrants have worse health. Their risk of illness is increased by 38% (p = 0.001) compared to households with no migration background. For men, this relationship cannot be found.

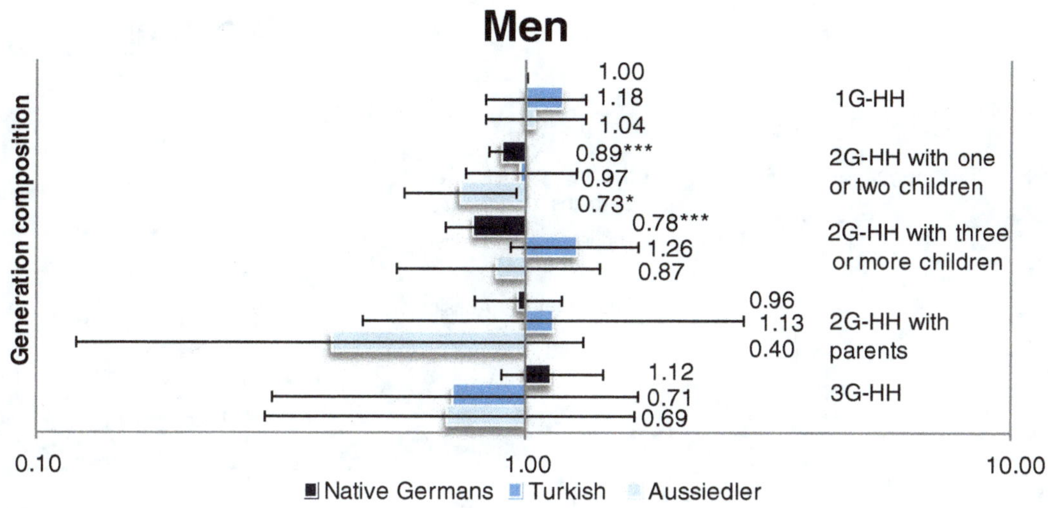

Fig. 2 Household effect according to migration background: odds and 95% confidence intervals of longstanding illness for men.
Note Reference = Native Germans in 1G-HH; logarithmic scale; controlled for all covariates.
Source German Microcensus 2005/2009; n = 188,108; ***$p < 0.001$, **$p < 0.01$, *$p < 0.05$

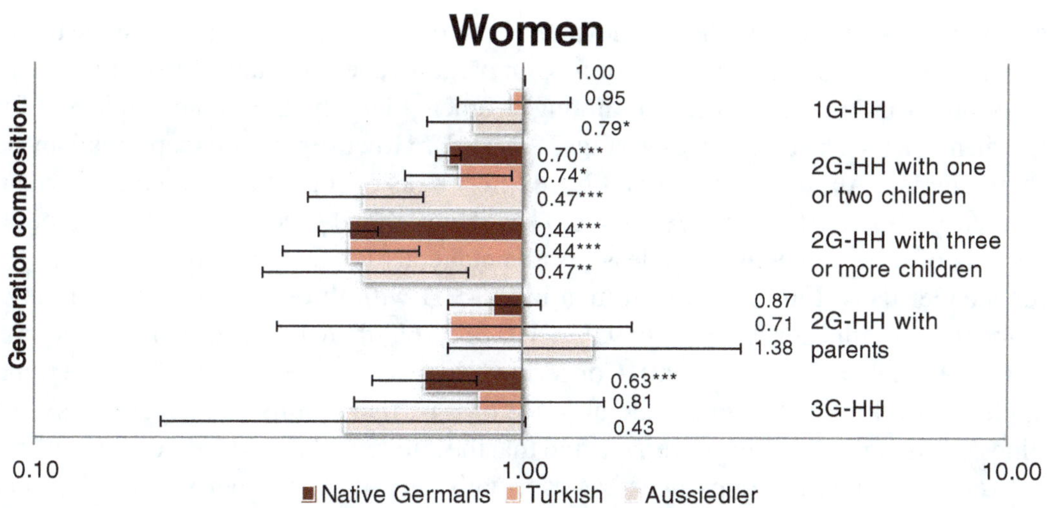

Fig. 3 Household effect according to migration background: odds and 95% confidence intervals of longstanding illness for women.
Note Reference = Native Germans in 1G-HH; logarithmic scale: controlled for all covariates.
Source German Microcensus 2005/2009; n = 194,005; ***$p < 0.001$, **$p < 0.01$,*$p < 0.05$

Our hypotheses suggest that most mechanisms act differently upon migrants and non-migrants. To test this assumption, interaction effects were estimated. Interaction effects indicate an estimation of non-additive effects of (at least) two independent variables on the outcome, assuming that the effect of one variable is influenced by the other variable. We examine the effect of the generation composition and the partner effect and assume that these effects vary among native Germans, Turks, and Aussiedler. Our results do not support this assumption. Among men and women, the effect of the

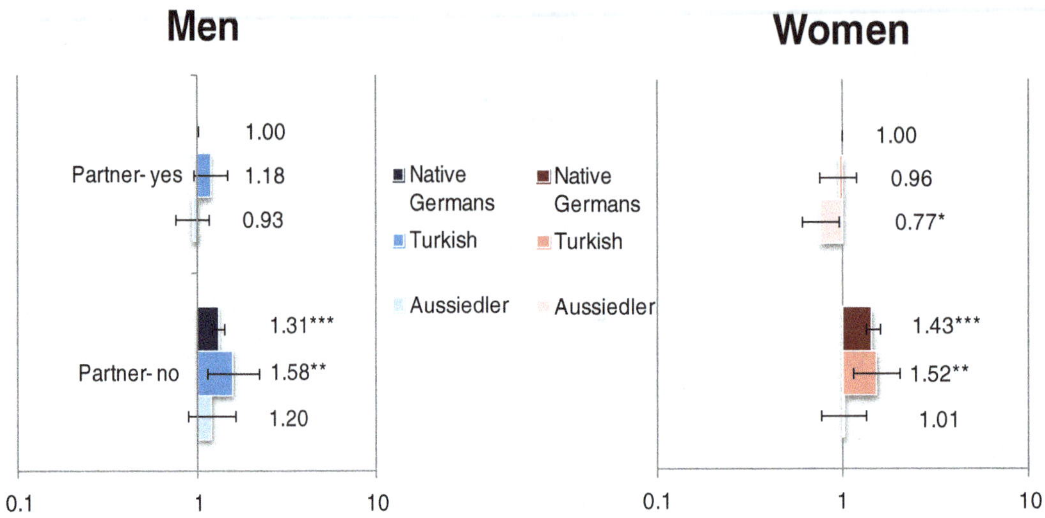

Fig. 4 Partner effect according to migration background: odds and 95% confidence intervals of longstanding illness for men and women.
Note Reference = Native Germans with partner; logarithmic scale; controlled for all covariates.
Source German Microcensus 2005/2009; men: n = 188,108; women: n = 194,005; ***$p < 0.001$, **$p < 0.01$, *$p < 0.05$

generation composition within the household on longstanding illness is the same for all subgroups considered. The generation composition generally causes a shift in health risks and follows—in particular among women—largely the same tendency for Germans, Turks, and Aussiedler (Figs. 2 and 3). However, two exceptions can be found: female Aussiedler in 1G-HH have lower risks of illness compared to German women in 1G-HH (OR = 0.79; $p = 0.043$). Thus, the absence of children or other persons of other generation are less disadvantageous for female Aussiedler than for female Germans (Fig. 3). Turkish men in 2G-HH with three or more children have higher risks of illness (OR = 1.26; 95% CI: 0.93; 1.69) than their German counterparts (OR = 0.78; 95% CI: 0.68; 0.90). Concerning the partner effect, again the same trend applies for all migrant-groups: the absence of a partner results in increased risks of illness. Among women, however, we find that the strength of this negative effect differs between the migrant groups, whereas especially female Aussiedler show a different pattern. Female Aussiedler with a partner have significantly lower risks of illness than German women with a partner (OR = 0.77; $p = 0.019$), and the absence of a partner is not associated with health disadvantages (OR = 1.01; $p = 0.917$) (Fig. 4).

Effects of Household Structure, Migration Background, and Individual Characteristics on Health—Results of Multilevel Regression

The results presented so far are based on gendered logistic regression models. To highlight and understand the variance across households, multilevel regression

Table 4 Odds of longstanding illness: odds ratio and p-values from multilevel regression

Covariates	Model 1		Model 2		Model 3		Model 4		Model 5	
	OR	p	OR	p	OR	p	OR	p	OR	p
Generation composition (ref. 1G-HH)										
2G-HH with one or two children	0.63	0.000	0.72	0.000	0.77	0.000	0.78	0.000	0.75	0.000
2G-HH with three or more children	0.59	0.000	0.67	0.000	0.58	0.000	0.60	0.000	0.55	0.000
2G-HH with (grand)parents	0.95	0.535	0.92	0.342	0.86	0.082	0.87	0.106	0.89	0.198
3+G-HH	0.79	0.010	0.83	0.033	0.76	0.003	0.78	0.008	0.77	0.004
Year of interview (ref. 2005)										
2009	1.14	0.000	1.12	0.000	1.14	0.000	1.12	0.000	1.16	0.000
Sex (ref. Females)										
Males	0.96	0.009	0.97	0.037	1.25	0.000	1.13	0.000	1.12	0.000
Age group (ref. 30 to <40 years)										
40 to <50 years	1.78	0.000	1.85	0.000	1.86	0.000	1.82	0.000	1.84	0.000
50 to <60 years	3.48	0.000	3.87	0.000	3.05	0.000	2.93	0.000	3.01	0.000
60 to <65 years	4.58	0.000	5.33	0.000	2.08	0.000	2.03	0.000	2.13	0.000
Family status (ref. single)										
Married			1.02	0.608	0.98	0.582	0.96	0.233	0.95	0.142
Widowed			0.98	0.734	0.91	0.057	0.86	0.003	0.89	0.021
Divorced			1.22	0.000	1.23	0.000	1.16	0.000	1.14	0.000
Presence of a partner in the same HH (ref. yes)										
No			1.75	0.000	1.60	0.000	1.60	0.000	1.44	0.000
Migration background (ref. native Germans)										
Turkish			2.57	0.000	1.46	0.000	1.48	0.000	1.12	0.232
Aussiedler			1.11	0.039	1.02	0.658	1.03	0.497	0.83	0.028
Other			1.23	0.000	1.02	0.464	1.05	0.117	0.84	0.024

(continued)

Table 4 (continued)

Covariates	Model 1		Model 2		Model 3		Model 4		Model 5	
	OR	*p*	OR	*p*	OR	*p*	OR	*p*	OR	*p*
Education (ref. low)										
Medium					0.76	0.000	0.77	0.000	0.79	0.000
High					0.56	0.000	0.60	0.000	0.67	0.000
Missing information					0.76	0.117	0.90	0.539	0.92	0.639
Occupational status (ref. employed or soldier)										
Self-employed without employees					1.01	0.901	1.01	0.856	0.98	0.750
Self-employed with employees					0.89	0.100	0.90	0.139	0.93	0.293
Unpaid family worker					1.89	0.000	1.99	0.000	1.88	0.000
Official or judge					1.32	0.000	1.32	0.000	1.44	0.000
Full- or part-time worker					1.12	0.001	1.09	0.011	1.02	0.495
Non-active population					7.96	0.000	7.67	0.000	6.78	0.000
BMI (ref. normal weight; 18.5 $\leq$ BMI $\geq$ 25)										
Underweight (BMI < 18.5)							2.05	0.000	2.04	0.000
Overweight (25 < BMI $\geq$ 30)							1.13	0.000	1.11	0.000
Obese (BMI > 30)							1.73	0.000	1.67	0.000
Missing information							0.87	0.000	0.86	0.000
Smoking habits (ref. never)										
Ex-smoker							1.55	0.000	1.58	0.000
Smoker							1.29	0.000	1.27	0.000
Missing information							0.60	0.000	0.59	0.000
Equivalent income group (ref. < 930 €; lowest 20%)										
930 to <1400 € (20–50%)									0.82	0.000
1400 to <2110 € (50–80%)									0.70	0.000

(continued)

Table 4 (continued)

Covariates	Model 1		Model 2		Model 3		Model 4		Model 5	
	OR	*p*	OR	*p*	OR	*p*	OR	*p*	OR	*p*
>2110 € (top 20%)									0.56	0.000
Missing information									0.78	0.000
Migration background household (ref. no m.b.)										
Mixed household									1.00	0.959
All persons with migration background									1.24	0.008
Place of residence (ref. rural; fewer than 20,000 inhabitants)										
Urban (20,000 inhabitants and more)									0.97	0.125
Constant	0.01	0.000	0.01	0.000	0.00	0.000	0.00	0.000	0.01	0.000
lnsig2u	0.88		0.81		0.79		0.76		0.76	
sigma_u	1.55		1.50		1.48		1.46		1.46	
Rho	0.422		0.406		0.400		0.394		0.395	
Log likelihood	−77,299		−76,629		−70,243		−69,612		−69,453	
n	382,113		382,113		382,113		382,113		382,113	

Source German Microcensus 2005/2009

models using pooled data (men and women together) were calculated. Interestingly, the results of the sample reflect mainly the effects among women. We use the results to reveal model changes when stepwise including the covariates and thus to explore possible underlying mechanisms, where the analysis consists of five nested models. The detailed results are shown in Table 4.

The gross effect of the migration background is partly explained and superimposed by other characteristics. Without consideration of socioeconomic characteristics, lifestyle, and contextual factors, native Germans have (only slightly but significantly) better health than Aussiedler (OR = 1.11; $p = 0.039$). The poor health of the Turkish subgroup is particularly striking, as they show a more than 2.5-fold increased risk of illness (OR = 2.57; $p < 0.001$) (Model 2, Table 4). Our full models reveal that the health disadvantage among Turks is primarily explained by worse socioeconomic status and contextual embedding. Considering the socioeconomic status, the risk of illness among Turks is reduced to 1.5-fold of the risk of native Germans (OR = 1.48; $p < 0.001$; Model 4, Table 4), and considering the contextual embedding, there remain no significant health differences between these two groups (OR = 1.12, $p = 0.232$; Model 5, Table 4). Controlling for contextual factors, Aussiedler (OR = 0.83; $p = 0.028$) even have health advantages over native Germans (Model 5, Table 4). The effect of the migration background does not superimpose the effect of the generation composition and is thus an additional risk factor for health outcomes. It also applies to the pooled multilevel model that the effect of the generation structure does not vary according to migration background.

The generation composition of the household is an independent determinant of health outcomes, which is remarkably stable in the model comparison. Persons living in a 1G-HH have worse health compared to the other subgroups. The risk is almost halved among 2G-HH with three or more children (OR = 0.55; $p < 0.001$) and about a quarter lower for 2G-HH with one or two children (OR = 0.75; $p < 0.001$) and for 3+G-HH (OR = 0.77; $p = 0.004$).

Gender effects in terms of long-standing illness vary. As shown in the previous section, men's and women's health is affected by different protective and pathogenic mechanisms. In our baseline model men show slightly better health than women (OR = 0.96; $p = 0.009$; Model 1, Table 4) This health advantage is mainly driven by a conducive socio-economic status; after controlling for this the gender effect is reversed and women show better health (OR = 1.25, $p < 0.001$; Model 3, Table 4). Differences in lifestyle explain some of the gender differences. Taking the lifestyle factors in account, women have a 12–13% lower risk of longstanding illness ($p < 0.001$; Models 4 and 5, Table 4).

The absence of a partner in the same household is a strong and largely independent pathogenic factor associated with an increased risk of illness. Those without a partner in the same household have from a 44% up to a 75% higher risk of longstanding illness ($p < 0.001$; Table 4). This effect is the same across all migrant groups. The risk of divorced people compared to singles is increased by 14% ($p < 0.001$) and that of the widowed is decreased by 11% ($p = 0.021$).

Finally, it is detrimental if all persons in the household have a migration background. This situation results in a 24% increased risk of longstanding illness (p = 0.008; Model 5, Table 4).

Discussion

To our knowledge, our study is one of the first to investigate the influence of the generational composition—a measure of the household structure—on health and to integrate the results in the context of gender and migration background. Not only family characteristics such as marital status and partnership status, which are frequently considered in research, but also the household structure is associated with health. This finding is particularly consistent and robust among women. For women, it applies to all migration backgrounds that living in a one generation household (1G-HH) results in exposure to greater health risks. Living in a two generation household (2G-HH) with three or more children is constantly beneficial and associated with lowest risks of illness. As well, living in a 2G-HH with one or two children is more advantageous than living in a 1G-HH. Our results suggest that this generational structure even results in additional health benefits among female Aussiedler (compared to German women). This link between household structure and health is not explained or offset by other factors and it applies to men as well. However, because men's health is generally less dependent on household characteristics and economic resources than women's health, less robust correlations arise among men. Without controlling for further health related characteristics, health inequalities by migration background are immense, but our analyses indicate that they are mainly driven by socio-economic differences.

Interpretation

Our *family segregation-hypothesis* states that living in a 1G-HH is accompanied by situations of relatively weak family ties—at least within the household—and thus results in health disadvantages. This hypothesis can largely be confirmed, but our assumption, that native Germans and migrants differ in this effect, is not conferred. Our models showed health disadvantages among persons in 1G-HH. Compared to all the other considered subgroups, they constantly have the highest risk of longstanding illness. Among men, the extent of differences between the groups decreases slightly when controlling for other characteristics, among women it even increases. The result, that persons in households with many children (2G-HH with three or more children) have the best health, illustrates the importance of emotional ties and social support within households. This conclusion is consistent with other findings (Zunzunegui et al. 2001; Kravdal et al. 2012), but contradicts those approaches which consider child care a burden and focus the multiple burdens of middle-aged persons (McIlvane et al. 2007; Oláh et al. 2014). Our findings instead indicate that children are a helpful resource. This parenthood-health-interaction, as well as the decision for a specific household type, might be driven by selection effects: in particular, when healthy adults decide to have (many) children and consciously take care of children or other relatives. A detailed analysis of the quality of relationships could be included in subsequent studies. Furthermore, it is conceivable that the effect of the parenthood depends on the age of the children in the household and is different between those with younger and those with older children. As Kravdal et al. (2012) stated, it is likely that parenting and the responsibility for a large household have a positive impact on individual lifestyle and thus result in better health outcomes. However, it should be noted that the group of persons in 1G-HH is composed of three subgroups: those living alone, couples without children, and couples with children that have already moved out of the parental household. 64% of the persons in 1G-HH in our sample live together with a partner. As we controlled for partnership status, we determine the net effect for this group. Our model reference category includes persons in a 1G-HH without a partner in the household. Thus, our findings are consistent with other studies that find that living alone is associated with additional health risks, e.g. due to a higher consumption of alcohol in this group (Cramer 1993) or to differences in access to healthcare providers (Manderbacka et al. 2014). Health disadvantages of couples without children can also be inferred from other studies (e.g. Hughes and Gove 1981). Johnson and Catalano (1981) note that childless married are partly socially isolated and therefore vulnerable to illness; van Balen and Trimbos-Kemper (1993) observe lower levels of well-being among infertile adults. Parents, especially mothers, whose children leave the parental home, sometimes experience a phase of reorientation which is accompanied by feelings of loneliness (Liu and Guo 2007) and negatively affects mental health (Radloff 1980). Persons in 1G-HH thus group unfavourable circumstances and characteristics that may adversely affect health. Considering that persons in 1G-HH partly even have economic benefits (e.g. no costs for child maintenance, couples with "double income and no kids"), our results illustrate the importance of social components and affirm the Social Support Theory (Lakey and Cohen 2000). Furthermore, our results may demonstrate reverse causality, i.e. health selection into childlessness (Gibney 2012).

The *gender hypothesis* states a gendered effect of the household structure, which is greater among people with migration backgrounds. A gender-gradient is evident in the strength of the influence of different household compositions. Among women, the effect is greater and more stable, which was also shown in other studies (Manderbacka et al. 2014; Williams and Umberson 2004; Soons and Kalmijn 2009; Hughes and Waite 2002; Denton et al. 2004; Artazcoz 2001). A higher dependence of women on household characteristics can thus be detected. The result, that living in solely migrant households is disadvantageous only among women, illustrates this effect additionally and is in line with earlier studies (e.g. Haug 2004, 2007). That this effect cannot be proven for men might also represent their greater integration into the labour market, due to which the household is only one of several resources of social capital. The gender hypothesis can be accepted, but there are no differences in the context of migration background. Among migrants the effect of the household structure on health is not any more gendered than among non-migrants.

According to our *mediator hypothesis* additional characteristics, especially the economic situation, are expected to explain health differences by household composition, gender, and migration background. This hypothesis must be rejected in large parts. Our results demonstrate that the socio-economic status is of high importance in the perspective of the migration background; here it explains many of the differences between the groups. However, differences by household composition are generally not explained by structural differences. The socio-economic status itself determines health inequalities, but does not mediate the effect of the generation composition. Of particular importance is how someone positions himself in society, i.e. with regard to education and occupational status. The household's economic situation acts as an additional compensation effect.

Our *partner hypothesis* states a positive effect of a partner in the household, which differs according to migration background. In all considerations the presence of a partner is associated with health benefits and leads to a general shift in health risks, which is in line with existing research (e.g. Koskinen et al. 2007; Joung et al. 1994; Manderbacka et al. 2014). This result may also demonstrate the health-related selection into partnership (Hughes and Gove 1981).

Our hypotheses can largely be confirmed. However, the expected fundamental differences between native Germans and migrants cannot be found. An exception is found for female Aussiedler, for whom living in a 1G-HH as well as the absence of a partner are less disadvantageous than for German women. Supposedly adverse effects are less influential among female Aussiedler. This result especially reflects the generally lower risk of illness among female Aussiedler. Despite this, the basic mechanisms in the production of health, respectively the influence of the household structure on health, are the same for native Germans, Turks, and (male) Aussiedler. One reason for this might be the composition of our sample under study. The migrants in our sample generally have been in Germany for a long time already. Among the Turks, more than 90% have been in Germany for more than 10 years and 70% more than 30 years. Among the Aussiedler, 85% have a duration of stay of longer than 10 years and 25% of longer than 30 years. Our results show that—as explained in Section "Why Investigate the Health of Migrants and Distinguish Between Different Migration Backgrounds?"—Aussiedler have many similarities to the German majority population. Additionally, the results suggest that Aussiedler and Turkish migrants in Germany have strongly adopted values and behaviours of the majority population, which is consistent with Kreft and Doblhammer (2012). We have analyzed whether these findings are also driven by our wide definition of "migration background" (migrants in first and second generation); the differentiated regression models for migrants in first generation largely repeat the previously described findings and underline the robustness of our results.

Our results may reflect selection processes among migrants. The "healthy migrant effect" (Kohls 2008) assumes a positive selection effect, i.e. especially young and healthy persons are likely to migrate.[10] Together with the

[10]However, it is assumed that the health benefits of migrants appear especially shortly after migration and decrease over time (Razum and Rohrmann 2002; Schenk 2007).

"unhealthy-remigration effect" (Razum et al. 1998)—unhealthy migrants are more likely to return to their home countries—the analysis of migrants is possibly biased. So it is conceivable that the migrants in our sample are subject to a positive selection mechanism and thus the effects are underestimated. It should also be kept in mind that Turkish migrants and Aussiedler in Germany are subject to an additional selection process. Due to their health checks in their recruitment as guest workers, at least the first generation of (male) Turkish migrants was selected by health, and Aussiedler are selected by their proximity to German culture. This may have direct and indirect impact on health factors and the integration into society.

Another explanation could be that migrants have greater social resources. In addition to stable family structures, they might be emotionally supported by extended families, social networks, and ethnic communities in times of shortage (Razum and Spallek 2012; Wilkinson and Marmot 2003). Networks across households and/or outside households were not investigated in our study, but could provide further explanations. As Haug (2007) describes, external resources might—along with the household—act as sources of social embeddedness and it seems that this resource is equally compensatory among migrants and non-migrants. The finding that women who live in households without any non-migrants have increased health risks suggests that networks, in particular social contacts with Germans, might counteract health risks and is in line with existing studies (Haug 2004; Lancee and Hartung 2012).

Finally, it should also be questioned whether in fact there are immense differences in value systems, family ideals, and the motivation for the formation of a specific household type between non-migrant Germans and migrants, particularly against the background of a long duration of stay. According to Haas (2010) and Haug (2004), migrants often maintain ties with their countries of origin, which exist and are formative long after migration. Among Turkish migrants, this social capital is rather family-based and kinship based (Haug 2005), which could be detrimental for the social integration and health care utilization and thus might establish an intra-ethnic segmentation (Lue Kessing et al. 2013; Esser 2001). Bearing in mind that Turks and Aussiedler often migrated to reunite their family or—in the case of Aussiedler—to live in their cultural home, this assumption must be questioned. It is conceivable—and supported by our results—that there is a gradual appropriation of cultural peculiarities, which goes together with an adaption of norms and values as well as health risks in the course of stay (Schenk 2007). As in other studies, we conclude that migrants who have been in Germany for a long time adapt behaviours (Milewski 2010, 2011; Berry 1992).

Our results also indicate that there are social structures which compensate for differences at the household level. There are differences in the health structure between Turkish migrants, Aussiedler, and Germans, but these generally do not explain health differences by migration background. One exception are (female) Aussiedler, where it remains partly unclear why they have better health and why their dependence on the household structure follows a different pattern.

Strengths and Restrictions

This study and our results have some restrictions. First of all, the health indicator used must be questioned. Illness is operationalized by longstanding illness. In the questionnaire of the Microcensus, neither a definition of illness is given nor is the severity of illness requested. The time frame of four weeks, which was set as the minimum duration of illness to define a person as ill, is intended to compensate for this weakness. The relatively high item non-response in the health variable might be problematic, as it has to be assumed that non-respondents are in poor health (Goldberg et al. 2001). The consideration of persons living in private households only might lead to an underestimation of ill people, as especially serious illness is often associated with a stay in a health institution and these people are not included in our study.

It should also be questioned whether our indicator reflects the health status for all persons equally or is more relevant to those who are active in the labour market. Because employment rates differ partially between Germans and migrants in Germany, this could cause a bias. Additionally, it should be kept in mind that migrants have fewer chronic diseases and more infectious diseases (see Section "Why Investigate the Health of Migrants and Distinguish Between Different Migration Backgrounds?"), thus this indicator may not completely cover the spectrum of diseases among migrants. Finally, the definitions of health and illness are culturally shaped (Helman 2007) so it is conceivable that Germans, Turkish migrants, and Aussiedler differ in their perception of health and illness and have different patterns in the utilization of health care services and consult physicians more or less frequently. Language barriers among migrants may reinforce this effect and might contribute to a lower awareness of health status among migrants. The fact that the proportion of nonresponse is slightly higher among the migrant groups (18.43% among Turks and 16.05% among Aussiedler) than among the German group (14.99%) indicates uncertainty in answering this question among migrants, but might also reflect a sponsorship-effect (the Microcensus is carried out on behalf of the Federal Statistic Office and this official character could help that respondents answer in the sense of the sponsor or to avoid undesirable answers). Misunderstandings and misinterpretation due to language problems in the interviews with migrants/non-German speakers could be an additional bias.

Second, there are further restrictions on the contextual level. A generalisation of our findings should be verified. Health outcomes, motives for a specific household type, levels of integration, family ideals, and norms are strongly shaped by cultural beliefs, social policies, and other macro structural influences, which means that a transmission of the results, e.g. to other countries, should be part of subsequent studies. Our results reflect the mechanisms in the conservative welfare state of Germany, as well as the cultural values and perceptions of the sub groups analyzed (native Germans, Turks, and Aussiedler in Germany).

Third, with our study design, causality cannot be found, as we carried out a cross-sectional study. We assume that household structures affect health outcomes. This assumption is in line with theoretical approaches (Berman et al. 1994) and longitudinal analyses (Hughes and Waite 2002). However, reverse causality is also conceivable: specific households and generation compositions are formed due to health characteristics. Children and parents might act as a helpful resource, so that living together is chosen more or less deliberately. Likewise, living with parents and/or children might also be driven by economic or health needs and might go together with additional burdens (McIlvane et al. 2007). Overall, the motivations and reasons for a specific living arrangement are quite heterogeneous, so the arrangement-specific impact may be heterogeneous as well. An analysis of the structure of relationships, the quality of relationships, and the exchanges within households appears to be necessary and useful, but this was not initially targeted in our analysis. The necessity to capture the high complexity, multidimensionality, and heterogeneity of health, illness, households, family ties, etc. in a more detailed way is revealed by our gender-specific models and might yield further research suggestions.

Fourth, the classification of generation structures in our analyses is partly imprecise. In particular, the group of the one generation households is rather heterogeneous, as it includes singles and couples who either are childless or whose children have already left the parental home. When using the data of the German Microcensus there is no reliable way to differentiate between these groups, so this is a data problem.

The main strengths of our study are the consideration of different levels that affect health and the modelling of the effect of the generation composition within households on health. The multilevel approach allows us to consider a second level —the household level—and thus to meet the variance across households in health matters, which are postulated by the approaches of the Household Production of Health and the New Household Economics. Our results illustrate this variance and the need for multilevel models. By considering the generation composition, we focus a measurement of the household structure, which will probably gain ground in the future. Already today, we find numerous changes in family and household structures (e.g. the trend towards smaller households, the possibility of coexistence of several generations), which are associated with different health risks and opportunities. This differentiation will also continue in the coming decades, resulting in the need for household to be a level of consideration. By using several household-related characteristics, we can prove that many of these characteristics act independently. Some of the indicators measure similar issues, however, they are not perfectly multicollinear and have an additional effect on health inequalities (e.g. there is a significant correlation between partnership status and the family status ($p < 0.001$), but we find all combinations of characteristics; the proportion of partnerless is 3% among married, 85% among widowed, 76% among divorced, and 73% among singles). What is surprising is the effect of the generation composition, which is stronger and more robust than the effect of the family status, which traditionally is examined as the main indicator for household characteristics. The comparison of men and women as well of the migrant groups shows that this is a largely global effect.

Another major strength of our study lies in the use of a broad database. First, the German Microcensus enables us to identify the household level and to perform stratified analyses. Second, considering the heterogeneity of the migrant population points to an internal differentiation of this group. With our differentiation between the two groups (Turks and Aussiedler) we meet this requirement and thus can make differentiated conclusions for a larger portion of the population in Germany. Finally, due to the obligation to provide information and the sampling, the data of the Microcensus and our analyses are highly representative for the target population examined (the non-institutionalised population in Germany between ages 30 and 64) and provide high accuracy.

Conclusion and Implications

This study provides new insights into the household effect on health and helps to identify health inequalities by migration background and gender. Native Germans, Turks, and Aussiedler differ in their health status, however, these differences are for the most part not due to differences in household composition. Our results indicate that there are effects on the macro level and individual level, which can compensate or superimpose meso-structural disadvantages or differences. Also, we assume that the migrant groups considered, which generally have already been in Germany for a longer time, are well integrated into social structures and have adopted norms, ideals, and health behaviours.

The household structure is significantly associated with health outcomes, whereas persons in 1G-HH (singles, couples without children, those living apart from their families) show health disadvantages. Thus, this group can be identified as particularly vulnerable. Because the influence of the household structure is largely the same for men and women who are Germans, Turks, and Aussiedler, the implication of interventions at the household level appears to reduce health inequalities globally. However, interactions at the family level and household level (e.g. childbearing, health behaviours, allocation of roles, and division of tasks) are a private matter, so connecting factors are difficult to discern. Our analysis clearly shows that women in particular are the beneficiaries of such interventions, as they have a greater dependence on household characteristics and because the household is still a female domain. An establishment of modern role models, a social policy adjustment, and a relief of women in the household could weaken these mechanisms and dependence prospectively.

Additionally, our analysis emphasises the socio-economic situation as a crucial determinant of health, which becomes especially clear in the context of migration background. At first glance, Turks have great health disadvantages and Aussiedler slight disadvantages. These health inequalities among migrants in Germany are mainly driven by their worse economic status. Intervention measures should act on this level as well. The example of Aussiedler in Germany elucidates that a high level of integration into society, the education system, and the labour market also leads to an approximation in individual health outcomes.

References

Abraído-Lanza, A. F., Dohrenwend, B. P., Ng-Mak, D. S., & Turner, J. B. (1999). The Latino mortality paradox: A test of the "salmon bias" and healthy migrant hypotheses. *American Journal of Public Health*. https://doi.org/10.2105/AJPH.89.10.1543.

Arránz Becker, O., & Steinbach, A. (2012). Relations between Grandparents and Grandchildren in the Context of the Family System. *Zeitschrift für Bevölkerungswissenschaft, 37*(3–4), 543–566.

Artazcoz, L. (2001). Gender inequalities in health among workers: The relation with family demands. *Journal of Epidemiology and Community Health*. https://doi.org/10.1136/jech.55.9.639.

Batalova, J. A., & Cohen, P. N. (2002). Premarital cohabitation and housework: Couples in cross-national perspective. *Journal of Marriage and Family*. https://doi.org/10.1111/j.1741-3737.2002.00743.x.

Becher, H., Razum, O., Kyobutungi, C., Laki, J., Ott, J. J., Ronellenfitsch, U., et al. (2007). Mortalität von Aussiedlern aus der ehemaligen Sowjetunion: Ergebnisse einer Kohortenstudie. *Deutsches Ärzteblatt, 104*(23), 1655–1661.

Bennett, K. J., Olatosi, B., & Probst, J. C. (2008). *Health disparities: A rural-urban chartbook*. http://www.cabi.org/cabdirect/FullTextPDF/2009/20093189673.pdf.

Berman, P., Kendall, C., & Bhattacharyya, K. (1994). The household production of health: Integrating social science perspectives on micro-level health determinants. *Social Science and Medicine, 38*(2), 205–215.

Berry, J. W. (1992). Acculturation and adaptation in a new society. *International Migration*. https://doi.org/10.1111/j.1468-2435.1992.tb00776.x.

Burt, R. S. (2001). Structural holes versus network closure as social capital. In N. Lin, K. Cook, & R. S. Burt (Eds.), *Social capital: Theory and research* (pp. 31–56). New York: De Gruyter.

Carnein, M., Milewski, N., Doblhammer, G., & Nusselder, W. J. (2015). Health inequalities of immigrants: Patterns and determinants of health expectancies of Turkish migrants living in Germany. In G. Doblhammer (Ed.), *Health among the elderly in Germany: New evidence on disease, disability and care need* (Beiträge zur Bevölkerungswissenschaft, Vol. 46). Leverkusen: Opladen [u.a.].

Coleman, J. S. (1990). *Foundations of social theory*. Cambridge, MA: Belknap Press of Harvard University Press.

Constant, A. F., & Massey, D. S. (2005). Labor market segmentation and the earnings of German guestworkers. *Population Research and Policy Review* (24), 489–512.

Cramer, D. (1993). Living alone, marital status, gender and health. *Journal of Community & Applied Social Psychology*. https://doi.org/10.1002/casp.2450030102.

de Haas, H. (2010). Migration and development: A theoretical perspective 1. *International Migration Review*. https://doi.org/10.1111/j.1747-7379.2009.00804.x.

de Valk, H. A. G. (2008). Parental influence on work and family plans of adolescents of different ethnic backgrounds in the Netherlands. *Sex Roles*. https://doi.org/10.1007/s11199-008-9464-9.

Denton, M., Prus, S., & Walters, V. (2004). Gender differences in health: A Canadian study of the psychosocial, structural and behavioural determinants of health. *Social Science and Medicine*. https://doi.org/10.1016/j.socscimed.2003.09.008.

Derose, K. P., Escarce, J. J., & Lurie, N. (2007). Immigrants and health care: Sources of vulnerability. *Health Affairs (Project Hope)*. https://doi.org/10.1377/hlthaff.26.5.1258.

Dias, S. F., Severo, M., & Barros, H. (2008). Determinants of health care utilization by immigrants in Portugal. *BMC Health Services Research*. https://doi.org/10.1186/1472-6963-8-207.

Diehl, C., Koenig, M., & Ruckdeschel, K. (2009). Religiosity and gender equality: Comparing natives and Muslim migrants in Germany. *Ethnic and Racial Studies*. https://doi.org/10.1080/01419870802298454.

DiPrete, T. A., & Forristal, J. D. (1994). Multilevel models: Methods and substance. *Annual Review of Sociology, 20,* 331–357.

Engel, G. L. (1977). The Need for a new medical model: A challenge for biomedicine. *Science, 196*(4286), 129–136.

Esping-Andersen, G. (1990). *The three worlds of welfare capitalism*. Princeton, NJ: Princeton University Press.

Esser, H. (2001). *Integration und ethnische Schichtung*. Mannheim. http://edoc.vifapol.de/opus/volltexte/2014/5134/pdf/wp_40.pdf.

Ferrer, R. L., Palmer, R., & Burge, S. (2005). The family contribution to health status: A population-level estimate. *Annals of Family Medicine*. https://doi.org/10.1370/afm.266.

Friedrich, L. (2008). *Wohnen und innerstädtische Segregation von Migranten in Deutschland: Integrationsreport*. Nürnberg.

Geulen, D. (2004). *Sozialisationstheorie interdisziplinär: Aktuelle Perspektiven* (Der Mensch als soziales und personales Wesen, Vol. 20). Stuttgart: Lucius & Lucius.

Ghatak, S., Levine, P., & Price, S. W. (1996). Migration theories and evidence: An assessment. *Journal of Economic Surveys*. https://doi.org/10.1111/j.1467-6419.1996.tb00008.x.

Gibney, S. (2012). OP18 childlessness in Europe: Implications for wellbeing in later life. *Journal of Epidemiology and Community Health*. https://doi.org/10.1136/jech-2012-201753.018.

Goldberg, M., Chastang, J. F., Leclerc, A., Zins, M., Bonenfant, S., Bugel, I., et al. (2001). Socioeconomic, demographic, occupational, and health factors associated with participation in a long-term epidemiologic survey: A prospective study of the French GAZEL cohort and its target population. *American Journal of Epidemiology*. https://doi.org/10.1093/aje/154.4.373.

Hammes, W. (2013). Haushalte und Lebensformen der Bevölkerung: Ergebnisse des Mikrozensus 2012. *Wirtschaft und Statistik*, 782–794.

Hartley, D., Quam, L., & Lurie, N. (1994). Urban and rural differences in health insurance and access to care. *The Journal of Rural Health*. https://doi.org/10.1111/j.1748-0361.1994.tb00216.x.

Haug, S. (2004). Soziale Integration durch soziale Einbettung in Familie. *Verwandtschafts- und Freundesnetzwerke. Zeitschrift für Bevölkerungswissenschaft, 29*(2), 163–192.

Haug, S. (Ed.) (2005). *Aspekte der Integration: Eingliederungsmuster und Lebenssituation italienisch- und türkischstämmiger junger Erwachsener in Deutschland* (1st edn, Schriftenreihe des Bundesinstituts für Bevölkerungsforschung, Bd. 35). Wiesbaden: VS, Verl. für Sozialwiss.

Haug, S. (2007). Soziales Kapital als Ressource im Kontext von Migration und Integration. In J. Lüdicke & M. Diewald (Eds.), *Soziale Netzwerke und soziale Ungleichheit* (pp. 85–111). Wiesbaden: VS Verlag für Sozialwissenschaften.

Haug, S., Müssig, S., & Stichs, A. (2009). *Muslimisches Leben in Deutschland* (1st edn, Forschungsbericht/Bundesamt für Migration und Flüchtlinge, Vol. 6). Nürnberg: Bundesamt für Migration und Flüchtlinge.

Helbig, S., Lampert, T., Klose, M., & Jacobi, F. (2006). Is parenthood associated with mental health? Findings from an epidemiological community survey. *Social psychiatry and psychiatric epidemiology*, https://doi.org/10.1007/s00127-006-0113-8.

Helman, C. (2007). *Culture, health, and illness* (5th ed.). London, New York, NY: Hodder Arnold; Distributed in the United States of America by Oxford University Press.

Holmes, J. H., Lehman, A., Hade, E., Ferketich, A. K., Gehlert, S., Rauscher, G. H., et al. (2008). Challenges for multilevel health disparities research in a transdisciplinary environment. *American Journal of Preventive Medicine*. https://doi.org/10.1016/j.amepre.2008.05.019.

Hook, J. L. (2006). Care in context: Men's unpaid work in 20 countries, 1965–2003. *American Sociological Review*. https://doi.org/10.1177/000312240607100406.

Hughes, M., & Gove, W. R. (1981). Living alone, social integration, and mental health. *American Journal of Sociology, 87*(1), 48–74.

Hughes, M. E., & Waite, L. J. (2002). Health in household context: Living arrangements and health in late middle age. *Journal of Health and Social Behavior, 43*(1), 1–21.

Hughes, M. E., & Waite, L. J. (2009). Marital biography and health at mid-life. *Journal of Health and Social Behavior*. https://doi.org/10.1177/002214650905000307.

Huschek, D., de Valk, H. A., & Liefbroer, A. C. (2011). Gender-role behavior of second-generation Turks: The role of partner choice, gender ideology and societal context. *Advances in Life Course Research*. https://doi.org/10.1016/j.alcr.2011.09.005.

Jacobson, L. (2000). The family as producer of health—An extended grossman model. *Journal of Health Economics*. https://doi.org/10.1016/S0167-6296(99)00041-7.

Janikowski, A. (1999). Berufliche Integration der Aussiedler und Aussiedlerinnen. In R. K. Silbereisen, E.-D. Lantermann, & E. Schmitt-Rodermund (Eds.), *Aussiedler in Deutschland* (pp. 113–142). Wiesbaden: VS Verlag für Sozialwissenschaften.

Johnson, C. L., & Catalano, D. J. (1981). Childless elderly and their family supports. *The Gerontologist*. https://doi.org/10.1093/geront/21.6.610.

Joung, I., van de Mheen, H., Stronks, K., Van Poppel, F. W. A., & Mackenbach, J. P. (1994). Differences in self-reported morbidity by marital status and by living arrangement. *International Journal of Epidemiology*. https://doi.org/10.1093/ije/23.1.91.

Knipper, M., & Bilgin, Y. (2009). *Migration und Gesundheit* (Eine Veröffentlichung der Konrad-Adenauer-Stiftung e.V. und der Türkisch-Deutschen Gesundheitsstiftung e.V). Sankt Augustin, Berlin: Konrad-Adenauer-Stiftung.

Kohls, M. (2008). *Healthy-Migrant-Effect*. Erfassungsfehler und andere Schwierigkeiten bei der Analyse der Mortalität von Migranten: Eine Bestandsaufnahme. Nürnberg.

Kohls, M. (2012). *Demographie von Migranten in Deutschland* (Challenges in public health, Bd. 63). Frankfurt am Main, New York: Lang.

Koskinen, S., Joutsenniemi, K., Martelin, T., & Martikainen, P. (2007). Mortality differences according to living arrangements. *International Journal of Epidemiology*. https://doi.org/10.1093/ije/dym212.

Kravdal, Ø., Grundy, E., Lyngstad, T. H., & Wiik, K. A. (2012). Family life history and late mid-life mortality in Norway. *Population and Development Review*. https://doi.org/10.1111/j.1728-4457.2012.00491.x.

Kreft, D., & Doblhammer, G. (2012). Contextual and individual determinants of health among Aussiedler and native Germans. *Health & Place*. https://doi.org/10.1016/j.healthplace.2012.05.008.

Lakey, B., & Cohen, S. (2000). Social support theory and measurement. In S. Cohen, L. G. Underwood, & B. H. Gottlieb (Eds.), *Social support measurement and intervention: A guide for health and social scientists*. Oxford, New York: Oxford University Press.

Lancee, B., & Hartung, A. (2012). Turkish migrants and native germans compared: The effects of inter-ethnic and intra-ethnic friendships on the transition from unemployment to work. *International Migration*. https://doi.org/10.1111/j.1468-2435.2011.00736.x.

Leclere, F. B., Jensen, L., & Biddlecom, A. E. (1994). Health care utilization, family context, and adaptation among immigrants to the United States. *Journal of Health and Social Behavior, 35* (4), 370–384.

Lindert, J., Schouler-Ocak, M., Heinz, A., & Priebe, S. (2008). Mental health, health care utilisation of migrants in Europe. *European Psychiatry*. https://doi.org/10.1016/S0924-9338(08)70057-9.

Liu, L.-J., & Guo, Q. (2007). Loneliness and health-related quality of life for the empty nest elderly in the rural area of a mountainous county in China. *Quality of Life Research: An international Journal of Quality of Life Aspects of Treatment, Care and Rehabilitation*. https://doi.org/10.1007/s11136-007-9250-0.

Lowenstein, A., Katz, R., & Gur-Yaish, N. (2007). Reciprocity in Parent-child exchange and life satisfaction among the elderly: A cross-national perspective. *Journal of Social Issues*. https://doi.org/10.1111/j.1540-4560.2007.00541.x.

Lue Kessing, L., Norredam, M., Kvernrod, A.-B., Mygind, A., & Kristiansen, M. (2013). Contextualising migrants' health behaviour—A qualitative study of transnational ties and their implications for participation in mammography screening. *BMC Public Health*. https://doi.org/10.1186/1471-2458-13-431.

Manderbacka, K., Peltonen, R., & Martikainen, P. (2014). Amenable mortality by household income and living arrangements: A linked register-based study of Finnish men and women in 2000–2007. *Journal of Epidemiology and Community Health*. https://doi.org/10.1136/jech-2014-204272.

McIlvane, J. M., Ajrouch, K. J., & Antonucci, T. C. (2007). Generational structure and social resources in mid-life: Influences on health and well-being. *Journal of Social Issues*. https://doi.org/10.1111/j.1540-4560.2007.00535.x.

Meyer, T. (2006). Private Lebensformen im Wandel. In Die Sozialstruktur (Ed.), *Deutschlands* (pp. 331–357). Wiesbaden: VS Verlag für Sozialwissenschaften.

Mielck, A. (2008). Soziale Ungleichheit und Gesundheit in Deutschland. *Bundesgesundheitsblatt - Gesundheitsforschung - Gesundheitsschutz*. https://doi.org/10.1007/s00103-008-0465-1.

Milewski, N. (2010). *Fertility of immigrants*. Berlin, Heidelberg: Springer.

Milewski, N. (2011). Transition to a first birth among Turkish second-generation migrants in Western Europe. *Advances in Life Course Research*. https://doi.org/10.1016/j.alcr.2011.09.002.

Milewski, N., & Doblhammer, G. (2015). Mental health among immigrants: Is there a disadvantage in later life? In G. Doblhammer (Ed.), *Health among the elderly in Germany: New evidence on disease, disability and care need* (Beiträge zur Bevölkerungswissenschaft, Vol. 46). Leverkusen: Opladen [u.a.].

Neuhauser, H., & Razum, O. (2008). *Migration und Gesundheit: Schwerpunktbericht der Gesundheitsberichterstattung des Bundes (Gesundheitsberichterstattung des Bundes)*. Berlin: Robert-Koch-Inst.

Norredam, M. (2011). Migrants' access to healthcare. *Danish Medical Bulletin, 58*(10), B4339.

Oksuzyan, A., Shkolnikova, M., Vaupel, J. W., Christensen, K., & Shkolnikov, V. M. (2014). Sex differences in health and mortality in Moscow and Denmark. *European Journal of Epidemiology*. https://doi.org/10.1007/s10654-014-9893-4.

Oláh, L. S., Richter, R., & Kotowska, I. E. (2014). *State-of-the-art report. The new roles of men and women and implications for families and societies. State-of-the-art report* (Families And Societies 11/2014). http://www.familiesandsocieties.eu/wp-content/uploads/2014/12/WP11OlahEtAl2014.pdf.

Omran, A. R. (2005). The epidemiologic transition: A theory of the epidemiology of population change. *Milbank Quarterly*. https://doi.org/10.1111/j.1468-0009.2005.00398.x.

Predelli, L. N. (2004). Interpreting gender in Islam: A case study of immigrant Muslim women in Oslo, Norway. *Gender & Society*. https://doi.org/10.1177/0891243204265138.

Radloff, L. S. (1980). Depression and the empty nest. *Sex Roles*. https://doi.org/10.1007/BF00287233.

Razum, O., & Rohrmann, S. (2002). Der Healthy-migrant-Effekt: Bedeutung von Auswahlprozessen bei der Migration und Late-entry-Bias. *Das Gesundheitswesen*. https://doi.org/10.1055/s-2002-20271.

Razum, O., & Spallek, J. (2012). Erklärungsmodelle zum Zusammenhang zwischen Migration und Gesundheit im Alter. In H. Baykara-Krumme, P. Schimany, & A. Motel-Klingebiel (Eds.), *Viele Welten des Alterns* (pp. 161–180). Wiesbaden: VS Verlag für Sozialwissenschaften.

Razum, O., Zeeb, H., Akgun, H. S., & Yilmaz, S. (1998). Low overall mortality of Turkish residents in Germany persists and extends into a second generation: Merely a healthy migrant effect?*. *Tropical Medicine & International Health*. https://doi.org/10.1046/j.1365-3156.1998.00233.x.

Rehaag, R., Uslucan, H.-H., & Aydin-Canpolat, G. (2012). Kulinarische Praxen als Medium der Identitätsdarstellung deutscher und türkischer Jugendlicher. *Gender*(2), 28–47.

Sachverständigenkommission 6. Familienbericht (2000). *Familien ausländischer Herkunft in Deutschland: Empirische Beiträge zur Familienentwicklung und Akkulturation*. Opladen: Vs Verlag Fur Sozialwisse.

Schenk, L. (2007). Migration und Gesundheit-Entwicklung eines Erklärungs- und Analysemodells für epidemiologische Studien. *International Journal of Public Health*. https://doi.org/10.1007/s00038-007-6002-4.

Schneider, B., Rapp, I., Klein, T., & Eckhard, J. (2014). Relationship status and health: Does the use of different relationship indicators matter? *Global Public Health*. https://doi.org/10.1080/17441692.2014.904917.

Settertobulte, W., & Palentien, C. (1996). Gesundheitserziehung in der Familie. In J. Mansel (Ed.), *Glückliche Kindheit — Schwierige Zeit?* (pp. 102–112). Wiesbaden: VS Verlag für Sozialwissenschaften.

Soons, J. P., & Kalmijn, M. (2009). Is marriage more than cohabitation? Well-being differences in 30 European countries. *Journal of Marriage and Family*(71), 1141–1157.

Spallek, J., & Razum, O. (2007). Gesundheit von Migranten: Defizite im Bereich der Prävention. *Medizinische Klinik (Munich, Germany: 1983)*. https://doi.org/10.1007/s00063-007-1058-8.

Statistisches Bundesamt. (2011). *Fachserie 1 Reihe 2.2 Bevölkerung und Erwerbstätigkeit: Bevölkerung mit Migrationshintergrund. Ergebnisse des Mikrozensus 2009*. Wiesbaden.

Statistisches Bundesamt. (2015a). *Bevölkerung und Erwerbstätigkeit: Haushalte und Familien. Ergebnisse des Mikrozensus 2014*. Wiesbaden.

Statistisches Bundesamt. (2015b). *Bevölkerung und Erwerbstätigkeit. Bevölkerung mit Migrationshintergrund.: Ergebnisse des Mikrozensus*. Wiesbaden.

Statistisches Bundesamt. (2015c). *Erläuterungen zum Mikrozensus*. https://www.destatis.de/DE/ZahlenFakten/GesellschaftStaat/Bevoelkerung/Methoden/Mikrozensus.html. Accessed June 9, 2015.

Sturm, R. (2002). The effects of obesity, smoking, and drinking on medical problems and costs. *Health Affairs*, https://doi.org/10.1377/hlthaff.21.2.245.

UN. (2010). *Global strategy for women's and children's health*. New York.

van Balen, F., & Trimbos-Kemper, T. C. (1993). Long-term infertile couples: a study of their well-being. *Journal of Psychosomatic Obstetrics and Gynaecology, 14*(Suppl), 53–60.

Viruell-Fuentes, E. A., & Schulz, A. J. (2009). Toward a dynamic conceptualization of social ties and context: implications for understanding immigrant and Latino health. *American Journal of Public Health*. https://doi.org/10.2105/AJPH.2008.158956.

Verbrugge, L. M. (1989). The twain meet: Empirical explanations of sex differences in health and mortality. *Journal of Health and Social Behavior, 30*(3), 282–304.

Walters, V., McDonough, P., & Strohschein, L. (2002). The influence of work, househld structure, and social personal and material resources on gender differences in health: an analysis of the 1994 Canadian National Population Health Survey. *Social Science and Medicine, 54*, 677–692.

Wetzels, P., & Brettfeld, K. (2007). *Muslime in Deutschland: Integration, Integrationsbarrieren, Religion und Einstellungen zu Demokrtie*. Berlin: Rechtsstaat und politisch-religiös motivierter Gewalt.

Wilkinson, R. G., & Marmot, M. G. (2003). *Social determinants of health: The solid facts*. Copenhagen: World Health Organization, Regional Office for Europe.

Willekens, F. (2015). Demographic transitions in Europe and the world. In K. Matthijs (Ed.), *Population change in Europe, the Middle-East and North Africa: Beyond the demographic divide* (pp. 13–44, International Population Studies). Burlington: Ashgate Publishing.

Williams, K., & Umberson, D. (2004). Marital status, marital transitions, and health: A gendered life course perspective. *Journal of Health and Social Behavior*. https://doi.org/10.1177/002214650404500106.

Wittig, U., Merbach, M., Siefen, R. G., & Brähler, E. (2004). Beschwerden und Inanspruchnahme des Gesundheitswesens von Spätaussiedlern bei Einreise nach Deutschland. *Das Gesundheitswesen*. https://doi.org/10.1055/s-2004-812799.

Woellert, F., & Klingholz, R. (2014). *Neue Potenziale: Zur Lage der Integration in Deutschland*. Berlin: Berlin Institut f. Bevölkerung u. Entwicklung/Berlin Institute for Population and Development.

Worbs, S., Bund, E., Kohls, M., & Babka von Gostomski, C. (2013). *(Spät-)Aussiedler in Deutschland: Eine Analyse aktueller Daten und Forschungsergebnisse* (Forschungsbericht/

Bundesamt für Migration und Flüchtlinge, Vol. 20). Nürnberg: Bundesamt für Migration und Flüchtlinge.

World Health Organization. (2002). *The world health report 2002—Reducing risks, promoting healthy life*.

World Health Organization. (2010). *Gender, women and primary health care renewal: A discussion paper*. Geneva: World Health Organisation.

Zunzunegui, M. V., Béland, F., & Otero, A. (2001). Support from children, living arrangements, self-rated health and depressive symptoms of older people in Spain. *International Journal of Epidemiology, 30*(5), 1090–1099.

Zwick, M. M. (2007). Migration, Ernährung und Körper - das Beispiel türkischer MigrantInnen in Deutschland. *SIETAR*(2), 13–17.

Health-Risk Behaviour of Women and Men—Differences According to Partnership and Parenthood. Results of the German Health Update (GEDA) Survey 2009–2010

Elena von der Lippe and Petra Rattay

Background

Beginning life with a partner and becoming a parent are major life events for both men and women, bringing important changes. Diverse patterns of partnerships exist, and these exert differing effects on lifestyle. In making the transition to living with a partner, individuals may change existing behaviours or adopt new ones. Furthermore, the status of the relationship (e.g., cohabitation or marriage) may itself affect lifestyle. A marriage disruption may also lead to changes in certain behaviours. Similarly, the transition to parenthood contributes to changes in lifestyle and daily habits, including health behaviours. The number and age of the children in the household may also play a role.

These life changes may translate to a more responsible concern with lifestyle and health, and, according to Backett and Davison (1995), alterations in the evaluation of health behaviours. From the perspective of health behaviour, the transition to marriage exerts a positive influence—in marriage, an enhanced sense of obligation inhibits harmful behaviours and encourages healthy ones (Fuller 2010; Umberson 1987). Parenting similarly increases responsibility and greater self-regulation (Umberson 1987).

E. von der Lippe (✉) · P. Rattay
Robert Koch Institute, Berlin, Germany
e-mail: vonderLippeE@rki.de

P. Rattay
e-mail: RattayP@rki.de

G. Doblhammer and J. Gumà (eds.), *A Demographic Perspective on Gender, Family and Health in Europe*, https://doi.org/10.1007/978-3-319-72356-3_10

Conceptual Framework

Different mechanisms have been proposed for the link between family status and health behaviour. In the first, partnership and parenting positively influence health behaviour through social control and through social support (Brockmann and Klein 2004; Umberson 1987, 1992; Umberson et al. 2010). Social control in particular seems to be an important determinant of health behaviour, affecting health behaviours directly (e.g., sanctions for deviant behaviour, regulation, and physical intervention) and indirectly (e.g., internalisation of norms of healthful behaviour and facilitation of positive health behaviours) (Umberson 1987). There may also be mechanisms by which having a partner and living with children could lead to a decrease in healthy behaviour (e.g., stress caused by combined social roles, social and domestic responsibilities, increased demands on time, or discord in the relationship) (Brown et al. 2009; Eng et al. 2005; Hull et al. 2010; Nomaguchi and Bianchi 2004). A transition to divorce or widowhood could also be detrimental to health because of the loss of social control or social support provided by a partner. Furthermore, it is also noted that many associations are reciprocal (e.g., a stressful relationship may lead to heavy drinking that, in turn, further stresses the relationship).

Another explanation for the link between partnership and health behaviour is that the search for a partner is associated with specific health behaviours. The need to be attractive and to go to places where potential partners might be found may result in behaviours such as increased physical activity, dieting, higher alcohol consumption, and smoking (Rapp and Schneider 2014).

One interesting finding emerging from the research on family status and health behaviour is that the effects of marriage and parenting are different for men and women. Women are more likely to attempt to control the health behaviours of other family members than are men (Fuller 2010). Consequently, marriage is more likely to be associated with social control for men. Additionally, men engage in health-risk behaviours more often, and this may be a focus of social control in marriage (Umberson 1987). Interestingly, women more often report experiencing social control by a parent or a child (Fuller 2010)—it may be that for women, the experience of marriage as a source of social control is relatively diminished in the context of other agents of social control.

A final consideration is the socio-economic situation of women and men, which varies depending on living arrangements. Socio-economic status (SES) could be a mediator in the association of partnership and parenthood with health behaviour. For example, single parents often have a lower SES than do partnered parents, and this may contribute to a higher prevalence of health-risk behaviour. It cannot be assumed, however, that the relationships between partnership and parenthood and health behaviour can be explained entirely by socio-economic and occupational factors (Roos et al. 1998). In the same vein, SES could be a moderator, as SES and family status may interact and show cumulative adverse effects on health behaviour.

Current State of Research

Much of the research on health-risk behaviour has focused on smoking, at-risk alcohol consumption, substance (drug) use, obesity, physical activity, and nutrition. As these behaviours are measured through diverse instruments, the comparison of research findings is not straightforward.

Smoking

Research on smoking has shown that married people have higher success in quitting smoking than do unmarried people (McDermott et al. 2004; Waldron and Lye 1989). The higher smoking cessation rate among married people is usually discussed in the context of the social support provided by marriage (Waldron and Lye 1989) or the development of a more responsible concern with lifestyle and health when living with a partner (Backett and Davison 1995).

The association of smoking cessation with parenthood has been mainly investigated in women. Women are most motivated to stop smoking during pregnancy because of concerns about the health of their baby (McDermott et al. 2004). Many women who plan to become pregnant will stop smoking before pregnancy, while others will quit upon learning they are pregnant (DiClemente et al. 2000). Smoking is also related to the age of the children in the household. Waldron and Lye (1989) found that mothers of preschoolers are less likely to be smokers than are women without children, possibly because of increased smoking cessation during pregnancy. Similarly, Umberson (1992) reported that, in both women and men, having adult children is associated with more cigarette smoking than is having children under the age of 16 years. Interestingly, according to DiClemente et al. (2000), the most influential factor for a postpartum relapse is having a partner who smokes.

The association of smoking cessation with parenthood has been less investigated in men. This is an important omission, given the concerns about the effects of second-hand smoke on fetal and child health (and call for health promotion interventions targeting tobacco consumption in men) (White et al. 2012). Nevertheless, parenthood and preparation for parenthood are to some extent also associated with spontaneous quitting in men (Brenner and Mielck 1993), as indicated by Bottorff et al. (2006), who found expectant and new fathers experienced new discomfort with their smoking (Bottorff et al. 2006).

Alcohol Consumption

The research on at-risk alcohol consumption has focused on the association between drinking behaviour and social roles (Hajema and Knibbe 1998; Kuntsche et al. 2009), among these, mainly the roles of parent, partner, and employee.

Kuntsche et al. (2009) reported that men who live with a partner have a lower risk of heavy drinking than do single men. Similarly, women in a 'traditional' role (i.e., partner and parent) have the lowest risk of alcohol consumption. Kuntsche et al. (2009) also found that the higher the number of social roles the individual holds, the stronger the protective effect of social role on at-risk alcohol consumption. There is the expectation that drinking should not interfere with the adequate performance of social roles. Therefore, the social control on drinking may be stronger among individuals who hold more social roles. Hajema and Knibbe (1998) reported that social controls, including sanctions, may influence drinking behaviour in those with new roles; however, this is not true in the reverse situation of job loss—a reduction of social control (or more leisure time) is not necessarily associated with an increase in drinking.

In addition to the influence of social roles, education seems equally important for at-risk alcohol consumption. Kuntsche et al. (2006) found that type of social welfare system and relative gender equity determines largely how education, employment, and family roles are associated with heavy drinking.

Diet

In general, women follow dietary recommendations more often than men (Abel et al. 1992; Anderson et al. 1994; Robert Koch Institute 2011). Additionally, both married men and women have a healthier diet than do their divorced counterparts (Roos et al. 1998), but the loss of a partner, through divorce or death, appears to influence the dietary habits of men more than those of women (Roos et al. 1998).

The transition to parenthood is generally believed to influence dietary behaviour (Bassett-Gunter et al. 2013; McIntyre and Rhodes 2009). For instance, many parents consume healthy foods in order to act as role models for their children (Bassett-Gunter et al. 2013). An earlier study (Roos et al. 1998) reported that parental status is a determinant of dietary behaviour in women but not in men; however more recently, this pattern has also been observed in men. Bassett-Gunter et al. (2013) found that both new and established fathers report greater intentions to eat healthily than do men without children.

Berge et al. (2011) reported that young adult mothers had poorer dietary intakes compared with women without children. The authors concluded that there may be conflicting factors influencing dietary behaviour in mothers: they may want to model good nutrition but at the same time, have less available time to eat healthily (Berge et al. 2011).

A difference was additionally found between first-time parents and established parents. Olson (2005) showed that first-time mothers make the most consistent positive changes in food choice behaviour, whereas, Bassett-Gunter et al. (2013) found that established mothers have lower intentions to eat healthily compared with new parents and nonparents. The authors concluded that having multiple children negatively affects the motivation of mothers to eat healthily.

It has been suggested that in attempting to understand dietary behaviours in women, a conceptual framework should include a focus on both structural position (educational level and employment status) and family status (partner and parental statuses), whereas in men, the focus should be on educational level and partner status (Roos et al. 1998). Furthermore, Roos et al. (1998) reported that the patterns of association between eating behaviour and family status/structural factors were similar in the various multivariate models that were tested.

Physical Activity

The research on physical activity with regard to marriage and family has usually been grounded on the theory of planned behaviour (Ajzen 1991). For instance, McIntyre and Rhodes (2009) concluded that in women, being physically active and continuing this lifestyle during the transition to motherhood is based on a perception of control, in terms of time, fatigue, social support, and child care. Elsewhere, barriers to physical activity for couples were found to be 'being too tired', 'lacking willpower', 'trouble in sticking to a routine', 'finding planning time', and additionally in women, a 'lack of companions' with whom to exercise (Burke et al. 1999).

Repeated studies have shown that being unmarried, both in men and women, is associated with higher levels of physical activity (Kaplan et al. 2001; Nomaguchi and Bianchi 2004; Umberson 1992); however, in one study using the same data but two different methods to evaluate the association between marriage and physical activity, the authors arrived at two contradictory results—one analysis yielded no association, and the other found that the transition from a single to a married state resulted in significant positive changes in physical activity (King et al. 1998).

Parenthood significantly influences physical activity in women and men. Having young children reduces sport and exercise activities in women (Sternfeld et al. 1999); most often, leisure-time activities are actually replaced by household activities, perhaps due to a change in roles (Bellows-Riecken and Rhodes 2008). Both in men and women, living with young children leads to higher household activity and less sitting time, with a stronger association when there are more children in the household (Candelaria et al. 2012). Nomaguchi and Bianchi (2004) also found that living with small children is associated with less exercise but that the number of children in the household does not influence the time spent in exercise. The explanation given for this negative association between having young children and lower physical activity is that caring for small children is physically and emotionally demanding and leaves parents with little time or energy to exercise (Berge et al. 2011). Notably, as children age, physical activity in mothers increases (Umberson 1992).

The Social Context

Most studies have been conducted in English-speaking countries and are reflective of those societies; as such, the findings may not be generalizable to countries with different social structures. Indeed, the association of partnership, parenthood, and health behaviour has been proposed to be closely connected to the social welfare system of a country (Kuntsche et al. 2006). Deriving from the classic typology of welfare states

(Esping-Andersen 1990), three different family policy regimes can be distinguished in Europe (Gerlach 2008): The Nordic model of family policy focuses on the achievement of gender equity, high participation of women in the labour market, and high compatibility between working and family demands. In contrast, the Anglo-Saxon family policy regime emphasises the role of the market as the central provider of welfare services and is characterised by low social benefits for families (restricted to families in need) and high female employment rates. Finally, the continental European family policy regimes, to which the German regime belongs, are characterised by the promotion of 'traditional' families (i.e., consisting of working men and family-oriented women). In continental European countries, measures to balance work and family efforts between women and men and to increase the employment rate of women are less well established than in the Nordic model of family policy.

In Germany, family policy historically has relied mainly on monetary benefits and tax breaks (e.g., income splitting), which focus primarily on the material security of families. Over the past decade, German family policy has introduced paid parental allowance and promoted the growth of childcare facilities. Nevertheless, the German birth rate remains low and the employment rate of mothers is average compared with that of other European countries.

These differences in family policy may influence the association between family status and health behaviour and suggest that the existing research findings may not be easily generalised to the German context. Because of the paucity of German studies examining the association of the described health behaviours with partnership and parenthood, it was important to investigate these associations in the German population.

Research Questions/Hypotheses

Based on the theoretical background and the previous empirical research, we investigated the following research questions and related hypotheses:

1. Is there an association between health behaviour and either partner or parental status?

   Hypotheses:

   (a) Partnered persons and persons living with children display healthier behaviours than do individuals without a partner or without children, respectively (because of higher levels of social support and social control).
   (b) Parents of preschool-aged children and/or a higher number of children show healthier behaviours than do parents of older children or lower number of children, respectively (because of higher levels of social control).
   (c) Single parents display higher risk behaviour than do partnered parents (because of higher levels of stress and lower levels of social support).

2. Is the association between family status and health behaviour influenced by differences in SES and/or employment status?

Hypothesis:

(d) The association between family status and health behaviour is mediated by the SES and the employment status.

3. Is the association between family status and health behaviour different in women and men?
   Hypotheses:

   (e) The association between partner status and health behaviour is stronger for men than for women (because of higher levels of social control through the partner).
   (f) Women living with children display healthier behaviour than do men living with children (because of higher engagement in parenting, and therefore higher levels of obligations and social control).

Methods

Data

The analysis was conducted using data obtained from the German Health Update (GEDA) survey (Lange et al. 2015), an ongoing, national telephone survey of the health of the adult German population. The repeated cross-sectional GEDA surveys aim to provide current data on health and disease, determinants of health, and the use of health services, for use in national and European health reporting systems, health policy, and public health research (Lange et al. 2015).

For the current analysis, the data sets from the years 2009 and 2010 were merged. The fieldwork for GEDA 2009 was conducted between July 2008 and June 2009, and for GEDA 2010 between September 2009 and July 2010. The data were collected from German-speaking adults living in private households with a land-line connection (Robert Koch Institute 2011, 2012). Sampling involved a two-step process. First, random samples of telephone numbers from the German fixed-line network were generated using the Gabler-Häder method, which assured the inclusion of unregistered and unpublished telephone numbers (Gabler and Häder 1999). Second, the 'last birthday method' was applied for random selection of respondents within a contacted household—the adult household member with the last birthday was selected for the sample. Data collection employed computer-assisted telephone interviewing, and the interviews took approximately half an hour to complete on average. The GEDA study was approved by The Federal Commissioner for Data Protection and Freedom of Information, and verbal informed consent was obtained from all of the participants in advance. A total of 43,312 adults took part in the surveys (cooperation rates: GEDA 2009 = 51.2% and GEDA 2010 = 55.8%).

In the present analysis, we included only men and women who were aged 18–45 at the time of the survey, resulting in a sample size of 20,717 (9070 men and 11,647 women). After cleaning the data for missing information on partner and parental status, we were left with data from a final sample of 20,595 respondents.

Measuring Instruments

Outcomes

The data on tobacco consumption were obtained from the survey question 'Do you smoke regularly or occasionally'? The possible survey answer categories were: 'Yes, regularly', 'Yes, occasionally', 'No, not any more', and 'Never have smoked', and we dichotomised these, collapsing the categories 'regularly' and 'occasionally' into one category (smoking) and the rest in another (nonsmoking).

To define at-risk alcohol consumption, we used the Consumption subscale of the Alcohol Use Disorder Identification Test (AUDIT-C) (Bush et al. 1998). The AUDIT-C is a three-item alcohol screening tool consisting of the questions "How often do you have a drink containing alcohol?", "How many standard drinks containing alcohol do you have on a typical day?", and "How often do you have six or more drinks on one occasion?" The screen assigns test scores to one of three categories: 'never drinker', 'moderate drinker' or 'at-risk alcohol drinker' (Gual et al. 2002; Reinert and Allen 2007). We converted these to a binary variable indicating at-risk alcohol consumption (yes/no) by collapsing the categories 'never drinker' and 'moderate drinker'.

Survey data on fruit and vegetable consumption were used to indicate dietary behaviour. These data were obtained through a set of questions on the number of portions. One portion is defined as a handful of fruit or vegetables. Additionally, the consumption of pure fruit or vegetable juice is counted as maximum one portion consumption per day. This was based on the World Health Organization (WHO) '5-a-day' campaign, which recommends 'a minimum of 400 g of fruits and vegetables per day' (Food and Agriculture Organization 2004). In the current analysis, unhealthy diet was defined as the consumption of fewer than two portions of fruit and vegetables per day.

The data on physical activity were obtained through questions on the frequency (days per week) and duration of physical activity that was strenuous enough to induce sweating or breathlessness. We dichotomised the responses as 'high physical activity' or 'low physical activity', defining high physical activity as a physical activity for at least 30 min per day on five or more days per week (Robert Koch Institute 2011).

Predictors

For the purpose of the analysis of partnership, we categorised survey respondents as 'single' (defined as never married and living alone), 'married or cohabiting', or 'divorced or widowed', collapsing the last category because of the low number of cases. We defined women and men as parents if they lived in the household with at least one child younger than 18 years and we did not differentiate between genetically related, adopted, or step children. We also included data on the number of the children living in the household ('none', 'one', 'two or more') and the age of the youngest child in the household (0–6, 7–10, 11–17 years).

Mediators

We also investigated the possible mediating effects of SES and employment status. SES was calculated using a scale based on level of education, household income, and professional status, with possible scores between 3 and 21 points (Lampert et al. 2013). Respondents with scores in the first quintile were categorised as 'low SES', those with scores in the second to fourth quintiles formed the group of 'middle SES', and those with scores in the highest quintile were categorised as 'high SES' (Lampert et al 2013). Employment status (self-defined) was categorised as 'employed full time', 'employed part time', or 'non-employed'.

Control Variables

Age (18–24; 25–34; 35–44 years), geographic region ('East Germany, including Berlin' or 'West Germany'), self-rated health ('good' or 'poor'), and health limitation ('not limited', 'limited but not severely', or 'severely limited') were selected as control variables in the regression analysis. Both self-rated health and health limitation have been identified as important health indicators in the Minimum European Health Module (EHEMU 2010) and were included in the regression analysis to control for potential health-driven behaviours.

Data Analysis

Logistic regression models were estimated to investigate the association of health-risk behaviour of both women and men with parenthood and partnership. In the first models, we included all respondents from the sample, comparing childless men and women with those who had children. We then included only individuals living with children, to investigate the possible association of health-risk behaviour with the number and age of the children in the household.

Stratifying by sex, we analysed the different outcomes and groups, comparing two models: In Model 1, the control variables were age, region, self-rated health, and health limitation. In Model 2, SES and employment status were additionally included as controls. The comparison between these two models allowed for an investigation of the possible mediating effects of SES and employment status on the association between family status and health behaviour.

To investigate whether associations were significantly different for men and women, we calculated a third model (Model 3) for both sexes, including interaction terms. In the analysis of women and men living with and without children, interactions between sex and partner status, and sex and number of children were estimated. In the analysis of only individuals with children, the interactions between sex and partner status, sex and number of children in the household, and sex and age of the youngest child were estimated. The significance of the interactions was tested using the two-tailed Wald test with significance level at $p < 0.05$.

The analyses used weighted data to correct for distributions according to age, sex, geographic region, and education (Robert Koch Institute 2012). All analyses were performed with the Stata/SE 13 statistical package (StataCorp, College Station, TX, USA) using the survey (svy) module.

The sample characteristics are shown in Table 1.

Results

As seen in Fig. 1, for both women and men, there were differences in health-risk behaviour depending on partner status. The prevalence of smoking was significantly higher in divorced and widowed than in single or married persons. Moreover, married women smoked less often than did single women. In men, however, there were no difference in smoking behaviour between single and the married individuals. Regarding at-risk alcohol consumption, the prevalence was significantly higher in single than in married or divorced/widowed men and women. Married persons showed the lowest prevalence of unhealthy diet; however, the differences were statistically significant only for women. Low physical activity was most often seen in single women, followed by married women; in men, low physical activity was seen least often in divorced/widowed persons, but the differences between the partnership groups were not significant.

Figure 2 shows the differences in health behaviour with respect to the number of children living in the household. There were no differences in the prevalence of current smoking between women and men living without or with only one child in the household, but a significantly lower prevalence was found for women and men living with two or more children. Men and women living without children in the household showed at-risk alcohol consumption more often than did those living with children. Men had an unhealthy diet more often than women, but in both men and women, an unhealthy diet was seen less often with an increasing number of children in the household, although the differences were only significant between men and women living without children and those living with two or more children. Finally, women without children reported low physical activity more often than women with children, regardless of the number of children in the household. In men, however, there were no differences in the prevalence of low physical activity with respect to number of children.

Table 1 Sample structure, stratified by sex

	Women			Men		
	n (un-weighted)	% (weighted)	Missing (un-weighted)	n (un-weighted)	% (weighted)	Missing (un-weighted)
Total	11,647	49.1	0.00%	9070	50.9	0.00%
Outcome variables						
Current smoking	3802	34.8	0.03%	3616	42.8	0.03%
At-risk alcohol consumption	2993	24.3	0.59%	3399	36.3	0.84%
Unhealthy diet	4183	39.0	0.86%	5074	57.8	1.18%
Low physical activity	9179	78.4	1.36%	6757	72.7	0.87%
Predictor/control variables						
Partner status			0.46%			0.76%
Single	3572	28.7		4.110	39.7	
Married/cohabiting	7049	65.5		4.530	57.5	
Divorced/widowed	973	5.8		361	2.8	
Number of children			0.00%			0.00%
0	5496	46.9		6101	62.3	
1	2642	22.8		1248	16.9	
2+	3509	30.3		1.721	20.9	
Age of youngest child			0.00%			0.00%
0–6	3180	52.7		1709	56.8	
7–10	1444	22.9		624	20.0	
11–17	1527	24.4		636	23.1	
Age			0.00%			0.00%
18–24	2418	22.3		2384	22.4	
25–34	3359	31.8		2559	31.6	
35–45	5870	45.9		4127	45.0	

(continued)

Table 1 (continued)

	Women			Men		
	n (un-weighted)	% (weighted)	Missing (un-weighted)	n (un-weighted)	% (weighted)	Missing (un-weighted)
Region			0.00%			0.00%
West Germany	9758	80.5		7631	79.2	
East Germany (incl. Berlin)	1889	19.5		1439	20.8	
Self-rated health			0.08%			0.03%
Very good, good	9869	83.4		8.041	86.6	
Fair, poor, very poor	1769	16.6		1.026	13.4	
Health limitations			0.42%			0.30%
Not limited	9625	82.7		7784	84.4	
Limited but not severely	1560	13.4		963	11.6	
Severely limited	413	3.9		296	4.0	
Socio-economic status			0.21%			0.14%
High	3348	20.1		2981	22.4	
Middle	6973	62.7		5077	60.5	
Low	1302	17.3		999	17.1	
Employment status			0.57%			0.50%
Employed full time	4109	33.0		6713	74.1	
Employed part time	4490	37.7		936	9.8	
Non-employed	2982	29.3		1376	16.1	

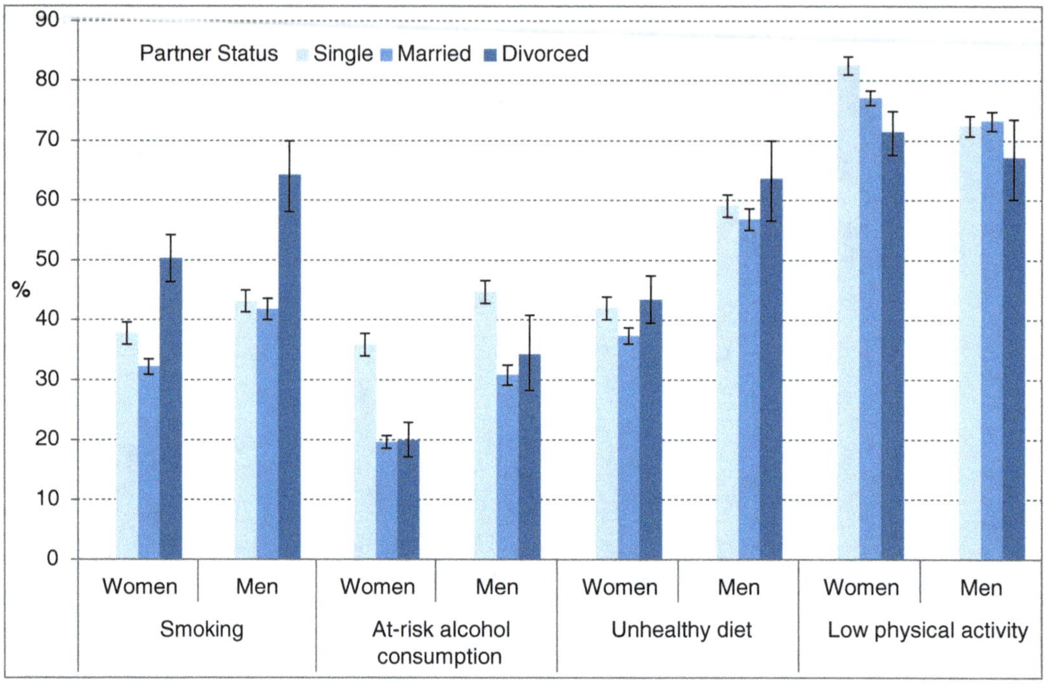

Fig. 1 Proportion of current smoking, at-risk alcohol consumption, unhealthy diet and low physical activity according to partner status, stratified by sex (incl. 95%-CI)

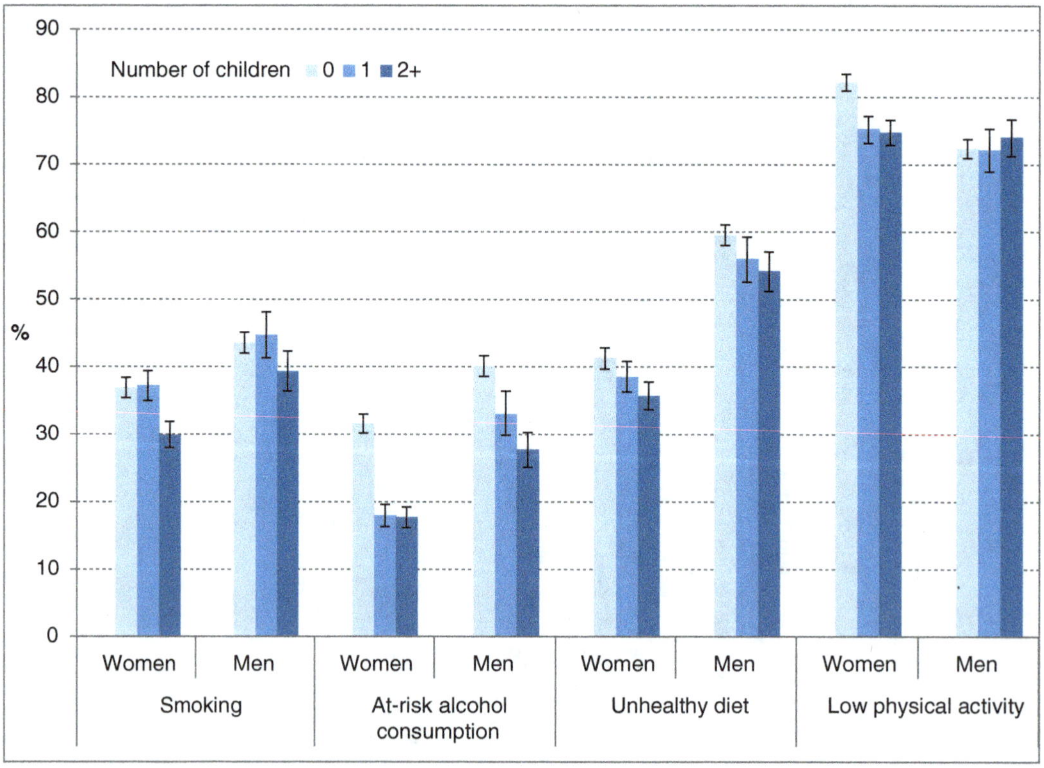

Fig. 2 Proportion of current smoking, at-risk alcohol consumption, unhealthy diet and low physical activity according to the number of children in the household, stratified by sex (incl. 95%-CI)

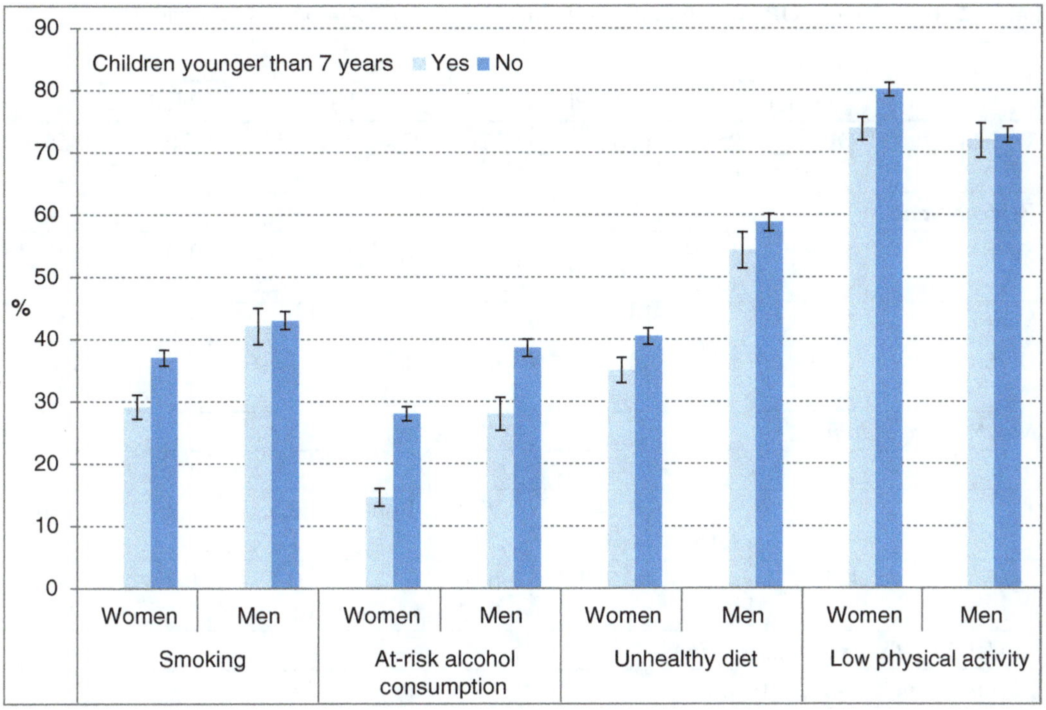

Fig. 3 Proportion of current smoking, at-risk alcohol consumption, unhealthy diet and low physical activity according to the age of the youngest child in the household, stratified by sex (incl. 95%-CI)

Figure 3 presents health-risk behaviour in parents according to the age of the youngest child in the household. Compared with mothers of older children, mothers living with a child younger than 6 years showed a lower prevalence of all health-risk behaviours. In fathers, the same trend was seen for at-risk alcohol consumption and diet, but for smoking and physical activity, no differences were found according to the age of the youngest child.

The results of the regression analysis largely confirmed the descriptive results. With regard to smoking (Table 2), divorced women and men showed significantly higher risks of smoking, even after controlling for age, region, self-rated health, and health limitations (Model 1). The association of health behaviour with the number of children was also confirmed, with a significant reduction in smoking observed only in men and women living with two or more children. The inclusion of SES and employment status in the models (Model 1 vs. Model 2) changed only the relationship, in men, between smoking and living with two or more children, which achieved statistical significance. Finally, analysis of the interactions of partner status and children with sex (Model 3) showed there were no significant differences between women and men in the association of partner and parental status with smoking.

Regression analysis also confirmed the association between at-risk alcohol consumption and partner status found by the descriptive analysis (Table 3), but this was not fully true for the association between at-risk alcohol consumption and

Table 2 Odds ratios (OR) for smoking in women and men, two models compared

	Women				Men			
	Model 1		Model 2		Model 1		Model 2	
Variable	OR	95% CI	OR	95% CI	OR	95% CI	OR	95% CI
Partner status								
Single	1.24**	1.08–1.42	1.17*	1.02–1.34	1.07	0.92–1.25	1.07	0.91–1.25
Married	1		1		1		1	
Divorced	2.05***	1.72–2.43	1.75***	1.47–2.10	2.51***	1.90–3.31	2.32***	1.76–3.06
Number of children								
0	1		1		1		1	
1	1.00	0.87–1.15	1.04	0.90–1.20	1.06	0.88–1.27	0.95	0.80–1.15
2+	0.76***	0.66–0.88	0.79**	0.67–0.92	0.87	0.73–1.03	0.77**	0.64–0.92
Model 3 (both sexes): *interactions*								
Partner status # sex	*p*-value 0.103							
Children # sex	*p*-value 0.733							

Significance level of interactions of partner status and children with sex
OR presented from the models without interactions. Model 1 controlled for age, region, SRH, and health limitations. Model 2 and 3 controlled for age, region, SRH, health limitations, SES, and employment status. $*p < 0.05$; $**p < 0.01$; $***p < 0.001$

number of children in the household—in men, the observed differences lost significance. The inclusion of SES and employment status in the model (Model 1 vs. Model 2) did not substantially change the results. Analysis of the interaction between sex and number of children revealed there were significant differences between men and women in the association of number of children with at-risk alcohol consumption (Model 3), but no significant differences between women and men in the association of partner status with at-risk alcohol consumption (Model 3).

With regard to an unhealthy diet (Table 4), Model 1 showed a significantly higher odds ratio for divorced and widowed women in comparison with married women but not single women (for men, there was a similar tendency, but the results were not significant). After including SES and employment status in the model (Model 1 vs. Model 2), the odds ratio for divorced women lost significance as well. Thus, in women, the association of diet with partner status is to some extent mediated by SES.

After adjusting for age, region, self-rated health, and health limitation, both women and men living with at least two children had a healthier diet than did childless women and men (Model 1); however, for men, the findings changed after inclusion of SES and employment status in the analysis (Model 2). After adjusting

Table 3 Odds ratios (OR) for at-risk alcohol consumption in women and men, two models compared

	Women				Men			
	Model 1		Model 2		Model 1		Model 2	
Variable	OR	95% CI	OR	95% CI	OR	95% CI	OR	95% CI
Partner status								
Single	1.49***	1.30–1.72	1.54***	1.34–1.78	1.42***	1.21–1.65	1.40***	1.20–1.64
Married	1		1		1		1	
Divorced	1.05	0.86–1.28	1.12	0.91–1.37	1.21	0.90–1.64	1.24	0.91–1.67
Number of children								
0	1		1		1		1	
1	0.63***	0.54–0.74	0.66***	0.56–0.77	1.04	0.87–1.26	1.05	0.87–1.27
2+	0.64***	0.55–0.75	0.68***	0.57–0.80	0.86	0.71–1.02	0.88	0.73–1.05
Model 3 (both sexes): *interactions*								
Partner status # sex	*p*-value 0.824							
Children # sex	*p*-value < 0.001							

Significance level of interactions of partner status and children with sex
OR presented from the models without interactions. Model 1 controlled for age, region, SRH, and health limitations. Model 2 and 3 controlled for age, region, SRH, health limitations, SES, and employment status. *$p < 0.05$; **$p < 0.01$; ***$p < 0.001$

for these, living with one child also appeared to be significant and thus, for men, a healthy diet was significantly associated with living with children irrespective of their number. Despite these apparent differences, inclusion of interaction terms in the analysis (Model 3) did not show a significant difference between men and women with regard to the association of diet with partner status and number of children.

After adjusting for age, region, self-rated health, and health limitation, the odds ratios for low physical activity (Table 5) were still lower for divorced and widowed than for married women and men (Model 1); however, in the fully adjusted model (Model 2), there were no longer any differences according to partner status.

The association with the number of children found in the descriptive results was also confirmed in the regression analysis: women with children showed higher odds of physical activity than did those without children, and this remained stable even after adjusting for SES and employment status (Model 2). For men, there were no significant associations with number of children after analysis with either Model 1 or Model 2. The analysis of sex variances showed significant differences between women and men in the association of number of children in the household with physical activity (Model 3).

Table 4 Odds ratios (OR) for unhealthy diet in women and men, two models compared

	Women				Men			
	Model 1		Model 2		Model 1		Model 2	
Variable	OR	95% CI	OR	95% CI	OR	95% CI	OR	95% CI
Partner status								
Single	1.04	0.91–1.18	0.96	0.84–1.10	0.98	0.84–1.15	0.97	0.83–1.14
Married	1		1		1		1	
Divorced	1.29**	1.08–1.53	1.07	0.89–1.27	1.20	0.88–1.64	1.13	0.82–1.57
Number of children								
0	1		1		1		1	
1	0.93	0.82–1.07	0.92	0.80–1.06	0.85	0.71–1.01	0.78**	0.65–0.93
2+	0.83**	0.72–0.95	0.79**	0.68–0.92	0.78**	0.66–0.93	0.73***	0.61–0.86
Model 3 (both sexes): *interactions*								
Partner status # sex	*p*-value 0.555							
Children # sex	*p*-value 0.187							

Significance level of interactions of partner status and children with sex
OR presented from the models without interactions. Model 1 controlled for age, region, SRH, and health limitations. Model 2 and 3 controlled for age, region, SRH, health limitations, SES, and employment status. $^{*}p < 0.05$; $^{**}p < 0.01$; $^{***}p < 0.001$

A further step in the analysis was to narrow the study to only men and women living with children. Here, we included data on the age of the youngest child in the household as well as the number of children.

With respect to tobacco consumption (Table 6), the results show that single mothers had very high odds of smoking compared with their married counterparts; divorced mothers also had higher odds, although not as high as those of single mothers. Divorced fathers had the highest odds of smoking.

Mothers with two children had significantly lower odds of smoking compared with mothers with one child; interestingly, no significant difference was found for mothers with three or more children, although the tendency was similar to that of mothers with two children. For fathers, no significant association was found between the number of children and smoking. Living with children aged 0–6 years showed lower odds of smoking in mothers, but no significant differences were found in fathers. We also did not find mediating effects of SES or employment status on the association between smoking with partner and parental status (there were no changes in the significance levels between Model 1 and Model 2). An analysis of the interaction terms showed there were differences between mothers

Table 5 Odds ratios (OR) for low physical activity in women and men, two models compared

	Women				Men			
	Model 1		Model 2		Model 1		Model 2	
Variable	OR	95% CI	OR	95% CI	OR	95% CI	OR	95% CI
Partner status								
Single	1.13	0.96–1.34	1.17	0.99–1.38	1.16	0.97–1.38	1.12	0.93–1.34
Married	1		1		1		1	
Divorced	0.74**	0.61–0.90	0.82	0.67–1.00	0.71*	0.52–0.99	0.76	0.55–1.05
Number of children								
0	1		1		1		1	
1	0.69***	0.58–0.81	0.66***	0.55–0.79	0.95	0.78–1.16	1.05	0.85–1.29
2+	0.65***	0.55–0.90	0.62***	0.52–0.75	0.99	0.81–1.20	1.10	0.90–1.35
Model 3 (both sexes): *interactions*								
Partner status # sex	*p*-value 0.308							
Children # sex	*p*-value < 0.001							

Significance level of interactions of partner status and children with sex
OR presented from the models without interactions. Model 1 controlled for age, region, SRH, and health limitations. Model 2 and 3 controlled for age, region, SRH, health limitations, SES, and employment status. $^{*}p < 0.05$; $^{**}p < 0.01$; $^{***}p < 0.001$

and fathers in the association of partner status with smoking (Model 3). Sex differences were also observed in the association of age of the youngest child with smoking.

At-risk alcohol consumption was strongly associated with partner status among mothers, with single mothers showing the highest odds (Table 7). No significant differences were found for fathers, despite a visible trend of higher at-risk alcohol consumption in single fathers. We did not find any differences in at-risk alcohol consumption according to the number of the children in the household in either mothers or fathers; however, the age of the youngest child showed significant association in mothers. As with smoking, we did not find a mediating effect of SES or employment status on the relationship between at-risk alcohol consumption and family characteristics (no differences between Model 1 and Model 2). Furthermore, there was no significant difference between mothers and fathers in the association of at-risk alcohol consumption with partner status, number of children, or age of the youngest child (Model 3).

With regard to unhealthy diet (Table 8), in the fully adjusted model (Model 2), we did not find differences according to partner status or number of children in the household, for both mothers and fathers; however, mothers living with children

Table 6 Odds ratios (OR) for smoking in mothers and fathers, two models compared

	Mothers				Fathers			
	Model 1		Model 2		Model 1		Model 2	
Variable	OR	95% CI	OR	95% CI	OR	95% CI	OR	95% CI
Partner status								
Single	2.77***	2.14–3.60	2.26***	1.72–2.97	1.15	0.49–2.70	1.28	0.54–3.05
Married	1		1		1		1	
Divorced	1.96***	1.59-2.41	1.64***	1.32-2.03	3.54***	2.08-6.02	3.22***	1.91-5.46
Number of children								
1	1				1		1	
2	0.83*	0.71–0.97	0.81**	0.69–0.94	0.84	0.69–1.03	0.84	0.68–1.03
3+	0.98	0.77–1.24	0.82	0.64–1.04	0.91	0.67–1.25	0.80	0.58–1.11
Age of the youngest child in the household								
0–6	1		1		1		1	
7–10	1.68***	1.39–2.02	1.46***	1.21–1.78	0.94	0.73–1.21	0.92	0.71–1.19
11+	1.67***	1.37–2.03	1.33**	1.09–1.63	1.10	0.85–1.43	0.99	0.76–1.28
Model 3 (both sexes): *interactions*								
Partner status # sex	*p*-value 0.029							
Children # sex	*p*-value 0.831							
Age of the youngest child # sex	*p*-value 0.002							

Significance level of interactions of partner status and children with sex

OR presented from the models without interactions. Model 1 controlled for age, region, SRH, and health limitations. Model 2 and 3 controlled for age, region, SRH, health limitations, SES, and employment status. $*p < 0.05$; $**p < 0.01$; $***p < 0.001$

Table 7 Odds ratios (OR) for at-risk alcohol consumption in mothers and fathers, two models compared

	Mothers				Fathers			
	Model 1		Model 2		Model 1		Model 2	
Variable	OR	95% CI	OR	95% CI	OR	95% CI	OR	95% CI
Partner status								
Single	1.68**	1.25–2.27	1.84***	1.35–2.50	1.53	0.60–3.88	1.51	0.60–3.80
Married	1		1		1		1	
Divorced	1.11	0.88–1.41	1.22	0.96–1.56	0.71	0.38–1.32	0.73	0.39–1.36
Number of children								
1	1		1		1		1	
2	1.12	0.95–1.32	1.15	0.97–1.36	0.87	0.70–1.07	0.88	0.71–1.09
3+	0.89	0.68–1.17	1.02	0.78–1.33	0.75	0.54–1.08	0.79	0.56–1.11
Age of the youngest child in the household								
0–6	1		1		1		1	
7–10	1.34**	1.09–1.65	1.36**	1.11–1.67	1.06	0.82–1.37	1.06	0.82–1.38
11+	1.38**	1.12–1.70	1.47**	1.19–1.83	1.19	0.92–1.55	1.18	0.90–1.53
Model 3 (both sexes): *interactions*								
Partner status # sex	*p*-value 0.380							
Children # sex	*p*-value 0.121							
Age of the youngest child # sex	*p*-value 0.300							

Significance level of interactions of partner status and children with sex
OR presented from the models without interactions. Model 1 controlled for age, region, SRH, and health limitations. Model 2 and 3 controlled for age, region, SRH, health limitations, SES, and employment status. $^{*}p < 0.05$; $^{**}p < 0.01$; $^{***}p < 0.001$

older than 10 years had higher odds of unhealthy diet. The comparison between Model 1 and Model 2 showed that SES and employment status mediated the relationship between nutrition and living with children aged 7–10 years as well as, in women, the association of nutrition and being single. Analysis of the interaction terms showed no significant differences between mothers and fathers in the association of partner and parental status with an unhealthy diet (Model 3).

The fully adjusted models for physical activity (Table 9) showed that divorced mothers had high odds of physical activity, as did mothers living with at least three children. For fathers, no differences in physical activity were found according to partner status or number of children. The age of the youngest child was not significantly associated with physical activity in mothers. Adjustment for SES and

Table 8 Odds ratios (OR) for unhealthy diet in mothers and fathers, two models compared

	Mothers				Fathers			
	Model 1		Model 2		Model 1		Model 2	
Variable	OR	95% CI	OR	95% CI	OR	95% CI	OR	95% CI
Partner status								
Single	1.50**	1.15–1.95	1.25	0.95–1.65	0.57	0.25–1.31	0.63	0.27–1.47
Married	1		1		1		1	
Divorced	1.16	0.94–1.43	0.97	0.78–1.20	1.24	0.68–2.29	1.29	0.68–2.44
Number of children								
1	1		1		1		1	
2	0.94	0.81–1.08	0.89	0.77–1.03	0.96	0.79–1.17	0.98	0.80–1.20
3+	1.15	0.92–1.44	0.93	0.74–1.17	0.96	0.71–1.30	0.92	0.67–1.24
Age of the youngest child in the household								
0–6	1		1		1		1	
7–10	1.23*	1.03–1.47	1.06	0.89–1.27	0.95	0.75–1.20	0.93	0.73–1.18
11+	1.52***	1.26–1.82	1.25*	1.03–1.51	1.21	0.94–1.55	1.11	0.86–1.44
Model 3 (both sexes): *interactions*								
Partner status # sex	*p*-value 0.160							
Children # sex	*p*-value 0.529							
Age of the youngest child # sex	*p*-value 0.709							

Significance level of interactions of partner status and children with sex
OR presented from the models without interactions. Model 1 controlled for age, region, SRH, and health limitations. Model 2 and 3 controlled for age, region, SRH, health limitations, SES, and employment status. $*p < 0.05$; $**p < 0.01$; $***p < 0.001$

employment status (Model 2) led to significance in the relationship between age of the youngest children and physical activity in men: fathers living with a child aged 7–10 years showed lower odds of physical activity than did fathers living with younger or older children. The comparison between Model 1 and Model 2 showed no other mediating effects of SES and employment status. Analysis of the interaction terms (Model 3) showed no significant differences between mothers and fathers in the associations of physical activity with partner status, number of children, or the age of the youngest child.

Table 9 Odds ratios (OR) for low physical activity in mothers and fathers, two models compared

	Mothers				Fathers			
	Model 1		Model 2		Model 1		Model 2	
Variable	OR	95% CI	OR	95% CI	OR	95% CI	OR	95% CI
Partner status								
Single	1.07	0.78–1.46	1.18	0.85–1.62	0.67	0.27–1.65	0.57	0.21–1.59
Married	1		1		1		1	
Divorced	0.68**	0.54–0.86	0.74*	0.59–0.94	0.95	0.51–1.79	1.06	0.54–2.07
Number of children								
1	1		1		1		1	
2	1.02	0.87–1.21	1.00	0.85–1.18	0.96	0.76–1.22	0.97	0.77–1.23
3+	0.67**	0.53–0.85	0.72**	0.56–0.91	0.93	0.65–1.32	1.06	0.73–1.53
Age of the youngest child in the household								
0–6	1		1		1		1	
7–10	0.98	0.80–1.20	1.02	0.83–1.25	1.29	0.97–1.72	1.36*	1.01–1.82
11+	0.93	0.76–1.15	1.01	0.81–1.25	0.84	0.63–1.13	0.95	0.70–1.27
Model 3 (both sexes): *interactions*								
Partner status # sex	*p*-value 0.213							
Children # sex	*p*-value 0.135							
Age of the youngest child # sex	*p*-value 0.184							

Significance level of interactions of partner status and children with sex
OR presented from the models without interactions. Model 1 controlled for age, region, SRH, and health limitations. Model 2 and 3 controlled for age, region, SRH, health limitations, SES, and employment status. *$p < 0.05$; **$p < 0.01$; ***$p < 0.001$

Discussion

The four health-risk behaviours in the current study were found to be differently associated with partnership and parenthood. The association of partnership and parenthood with health behaviour is not homogeneous and cannot be explained through only one mechanism, such as social control or social support. The clearly health detrimental behaviours, i.e., smoking and at-risk alcohol consumption, seem to be more strongly associated with partnership and parenthood than are nutrition and physical activity.

Our work suggests that partner status is strongly associated with smoking in both men and women, irrespective of parenthood, which is consistent with findings from other studies (McDermott et al. 2004; Waldron and Lye 1989). The provision of social support for quitting smoking and the social control against relapse is usually given as the explanation for the positive effect of marriage on smoking (Klein et al. 2013). In our study, we were unable to distinguish the smoking habits of the partner, but results from previous work show that living with a smoker is correlated with relapse of smoking (Kahn et al. 2002) and is a barrier to quitting (McDermott et al. 2006). Thus, the protective effect of marriage may be available only when the partner also does not smoke. The slight correlation between smoking and parenthood (especially of two children) could be understood in the terms of increased responsibility to protect children. According to McDermott et al. (2006), parents have the responsibility to protect children from passive smoking and, as well, of positive role modelling to protect children from becoming smokers themselves. This seems to be valid, particularly for women with young children.

We also found that single men and women have significantly higher at-risk alcohol consumption than do their married counterparts. These results confirm findings of other studies (Hajema and Knibbe 1998; Kuntsche et al. 2006). It has been previously argued that decreased consumption within marriage is likely to be an effect of decreased exposure to situations where drinking is considered appropriate and not an effect of selection within this group (Hajema and Knibbe 1998). Thus, the transition to marriage and parenthood has been seen as a constraint on drinking behaviour (Paradis 2011). Yet in the current study, the association with parenthood was only found in women. Similarly, a strong sex difference in the associations of heavy drinking and social roles was also found in Germany, by Kuntsche et al. (2006) in a comparison of several industrialised countries. Often, social stratification is considered to be more important for men, whereas family roles are more important for women (Kuntsche et al. 2006). Thus, differences between women and men in health behaviours may be primarily a function of differences in the social roles occupied by men and women (Nomaguchi and Bianchi 2004). This could explain the relationship between parenthood and heavy drinking in mothers; however, this seems to be valid only for mothers with at least one preschool-aged child, as mothers with older children also show higher odds of heavy drinking. The constraint of parental roles thus seems to have a relative short-term effect. These results are in line with the suggestion that mothers tend to feel more guilty about going out for drinks because of the social pressure to always be "on call" for their children (Paradis 2011), and this could be especially the case for mothers with preschool-aged children.

We also found a healthy diet to be strongly associated with living with children but independent of the number of children in the household (especially in men). These findings are consistent with findings of previous research (Bassett-Gunter et al. 2013; Condon et al. 2004). It is generally considered that parenthood motivates individuals to eat healthily because parents perceive themselves to be role models for their children (Bassett-Gunter et al. 2013; Patrick and Nicklas 2005). Previous findings that women have less intention to eat healthily with an increase in the number of the children in the household (Bassett-Gunter et al. 2013; Hung 2007) could not be confirmed in our analysis; however, in women, there is a relationship with the age of the children in the household. The finding that mothers with older children eat less healthily could mean that role modelling is mainly valid for young children. Another consideration is that fruit and vegetable consumption is only one element of good nutrition—no other dietary measure was available in the dataset (e.g., sugar or fat intake). Yet, Yannakoulia et al. (2008) showed that in relation to marital status, there may be different patterns of healthy dietary behaviour.

With regard to physical activity, we found that mothers are more active than women without children, but a similar difference was not found in men. It is usually considered that parents play a substantial role in the development of physical activity patterns in their children (Gustafson and Rhodes 2006), and in Germany it may be that this role falls under the purview of mothers. Unfortunately, in our analysis, we were unable to differentiate between leisure-time activity and household activity. Other research has shown that with entry to parenthood, leisure-time activity is replaced by household activity because of a change in roles (Candelaria et al. 2012; Grace et al. 2006; Scharff et al. 1999; Sternfeld et al. 1999). As mothers usually engage more often in the care of children, their physical activity related to child-care (e.g., spending time on the playground or carrying the child) may be an important influence lacking in fathers. Sitting time is lower for both mothers and fathers compared with nonparents, but again, this finding is more prevalent among women (Candelaria et al. 2012). This too is likely related to the increased household activity in households with children. A similar argument was given by Burton and Turrell (2000), who concluded that in general, the physical activity of men and women is different and that parenthood may have a greater effect on physical activity in mothers than on fathers. Interestingly, other studies have shown a reduction in physical activity in mothers, especially in mothers of young children (Candelaria et al. 2012; Hull et al. 2010). These contradictory results may have been related to differences in the definition of physical activity (as opposed to sporting activity) and the methods used to measure physical activity.

Returning to our hypothesis on the mediating effect of SES and employment status, we conclude that the associations between health behaviour and family status can be explained to a limited extent by SES and employment status. This is consistent with the finding of Roos et al. (1998) that family status (partnership and parenthood) and structural factors (educational level and employment) are independently associated with nutrition.

Our hypotheses regarding sex differences in the association of family status and health behaviour remain unconfirmed—sex differences are not as strong as expected. Contrary to previous findings (Umberson 1992), we found no sex differences in the relation of partner status with any health behaviour. This could be attributable to changes in social roles in Germany in recent decades, as women are now more active in the labour market and men, to some degree, in household activities. Nevertheless, the birth of a child (especially the first) does seem to lead to a return to traditional family patterns (Federal Ministry for Family Affairs, Senior Citizens, Women and Youth 2011), as evidenced by the strong differences in health behaviour seen between women and men living with and without children. Further, the relationship between age of the youngest child and health behaviour suggests that during pregnancy and first years of parenthood, women in particular are willing to stop harmful health behaviours, such as smoking and at-risk alcohol consumption but that as children grow, this willingness seems to decrease (Waldron and Lye 1989). Longitudinal studies are needed to validate this hypothesis.

Strength and Limitations

The strength of our study was the use of a large sample that was representative of the German population. The size of the sample allowed the study of specific subgroups. Also, the large set of indicators included in the GEDA survey allowed a deep analysis.

The main limitation of our analysis was our reliance on cross-sectional data. This means that we were unable to study changes over time or to make inferences about causality in the relationship between health behaviour and partner and parental status. Thus, it could be that partnership and parenthood influence health behaviour (causality) and that health behaviour also influences the partnership and parenthood experience (selectivity) (Hank and Steinbach in this book), but this will have to be investigated elsewhere. Another limitation is that the data on health behaviour were self-reported and therefore subject to social desirability bias. This may have been truer for women and men with children than for those living without children, especially regarding smoking and at-risk alcohol consumption. Finally, we only had data on parents with children living in the household, and therefore our findings reflect only these parents—parents who were not living with their children (because of a separation/divorce or after leaving the parental home) could not be identified in our data.

Further Research

A further step would be to test the moderating effects of SES and employment status. We were unable to do this with our data because of the relatively low number of cases, especially for lone fathers. Future research should also include diverse populations (for instance immigrants) in order to investigate the relationship between family status and health behaviour within different demographic groups. Furthermore, international comparisons, using the same or similar outcome and predictor variables, are needed to understand the potential variations between the different welfare states and social settings (see Hank and Steinbach in this volume). In addition, there is a need for trend analysis to explore possible changes in the association of health behaviour with family roles over time. Last but not least, only analyses with longitudinal data offer the possibility of investigating selection and causality effects in the association between health behaviour and partner and parental status.

Conclusion

Understanding the associations between family status and health behaviour can help the identification of appropriate target groups for health promotion and prevention programs, to support healthy lifestyle at all life stages. Both partnership and, especially, parenthood positively correlate with most of the studied health behaviours. In particular, the period around pregnancy, birth, and the first years with a child seems to be a 'teachable moment' during which women are willing to change their behaviour (McBride et al. 2003); however this beneficial effect on health behaviour seems to be temporary. This knowledge suggests that health agencies should develop policies and programs to support the maintenance of healthy behaviour in women after their children have grown or have left the household, or after disruption of a partnership. Furthermore, a more gender-equal focus in health promotion might increase men's involvement in lifestyle change (Edvardsson et al. 2011).

References

Abel, T., McQueen, D. V., Backen, K., & Currie, C. (1992). Patterns of unhealthy eating behaviours in a middle aged Scottish Population. *Scottish Medical Journal, 37*(6), 170–174. https://doi.org/10.1177/003693309203700604.

Ajzen, I. (1991). The theory of planned behavior. *Organizational Behaviour and Human Decision Processes, 50*(2), 179–211. https://doi.org/10.1016/0749-5978(91)90020-T.

Anderson, A. S., Macintyre, S., & West, P. (1994). Dietary patterns among adolescents in the west of Scotland. *British Journal of Nutrition, 71,* 111–122.

Backett, K. C., & Davison, C. (1995). Lifecourse and lifestyle: The social and cultural location of health behaviours. *Social Science & Medicine, 40*(5), 629–638. https://doi.org/10.1016/0277-9536(95)80007-7.

Bassett-Gunter, R. L., Levy-Milne, R., Naylor, P. J., Symons Downs, D., Benoit, C., Warburton, D. E. R., et al. (2013). Oh baby! motivation for healthy eating during parenthood transitions: A longitudinal examination with a theory of planned behavior perspective. *International Journal of Behavioral Nutrition and Physical Activity, 10,* 88.

Bellows-Riecken, K. H., & Rhodes, R. E. (2008). A birth of inactivity? A review of physical activity and parenthood. *Preventive Medicine, 46*(2), 99–110. https://doi.org/10.1016/j.ypmed.2007.08.003.

Berge, J. M., Larson, N., Bauer, K. W., & Neumark-Sztainer, D. (2011). Are parents of young children practicing healthy nutrition and physical activity behaviors? *Pediatrics, 127*(5), 881–887. https://doi.org/10.1542/peds.2010-3218.

Bottorff, J. L., Oliffe, J., Kalaw, C., Carey, J., & Mroz, L. (2006). Men's constructions of smoking in the context of women's tobacco reduction during pregnancy and postpartum. *Social Science & Medicine, 62*(12), 3096–3108. https://doi.org/10.1016/j.socscimed.2005.11.058.

Brenner, H., & Mielck, A. (1993). Children's exposure to parental smoking in West Germany. *International Journal of Epidemiology, 22*(5), 818–823. https://doi.org/10.1093/ije/22.5.818.

Brockmann, H., & Klein, T. (2004). Love and death in Germany: The marital biography and its effect on mortality. *Journal of Marriage and Family, 66*(3), 567–581.

Brown, W. J., Heesch, K. C., & Miller, Y. D. (2009). Life events and changing physical activity patterns in women at different life stages. *Annals of Behavioral Medicine, 37*(3), 294–305. https://doi.org/10.1007/s12160-009-9099-2.

Burke, V., Giangiulio, N., Gillam, H. F., Beilin, L. J., Houghton, S., & Milligan, R. A. K. (1999). Health promotion in couples adapting to a shared lifestyle. *Health Education Research, 14*(2), 269–288. https://doi.org/10.1093/her/14.2.269.

Burton, N. W., & Turrell, G. (2000). Occupation, hours worked, and leisure-time physical activity. *Preventive Medicine, 31*(6), 673–681. https://doi.org/10.1006/pmed.2000.0763.

Bush, K., Kivlahan, D. R., McDonell, M. B., Fihn, S. D., Bradley, K. A., & for the Ambulatory Care Quality Improvement, P. (1998). The audit alcohol consumption questions (audit-c): An effective brief screening test for problem drinking. *Archives of Internal Medicine, 158*(16), 1789–1795. https://doi.org/10.1001/archinte.158.16.1789.

Candelaria, J. I., Sallis, J. F., Conway, T. L., Saelens, B. E., Frank, L. D., & Slymen, D. J. (2012). Differences in physical activity among adults in households with and without children. *Journal of Physical Activity and Health, 9*(7), 985–995.

Condon, J. T., Boyce, P., & Corkindale, C. J. (2004). The first-time fathers study: A prospective study of the mental health and wellbeing of men during the transition to parenthood. *Australian and New Zealand Journal of Psychiatry, 38*(1–2), 56–64.

DiClemente, C. C., Dolan-Mullen, P., & Windsor, R. A. (2000). The process of pregnancy smoking cessation: Implications for interventions. *Tobacco Control, 9*(suppl 3), iii16–iii21. https://doi.org/10.1136/tc.9.suppl_3.iii16.

Edvardsson, K., Ivarsson, A., Eurenius, E., Garvare, R., Nystrom, M. E., Small, R., et al. (2011). Giving offspring a healthy start: Parents' experiences of health promotion and lifestyle change during pregnancy and early parenthood. *BMC Public Health, 11,* 936. https://doi.org/10.1186/1471-2458-11-936.

EHEMU. (2010). European Health Expectancy Monitoring Unit. The Minimum European Health Module.

Eng, P. M., Kawachi, I., Fitzmaurice, G., & Rimm, E. B. (2005). Effects of marital transitions on changes in dietary and other health behaviours in US male health professionals. *Journal of Epidemiology and Community Health, 59*(1), 56–62. https://doi.org/10.1136/jech.2004.020073.

Esping-Andersen, G. (1990). *The three worlds of welfare capitalism.* Princeton, NJ: Princeton University Press.

Federal Ministry for Family Affairs Senior Citizens Women and Youth (Ed.). (2011). *Neue Wege—Gleiche Chancen. Gleichstellung von Frauen und Männern im Lebensverlauf. Erster Gleichstellungbericht* [New ways—Equal chances. Equal treatment of women and men in life-course perspektive. First report on equality of treatment]. Berlin: Federal Ministry for Family Affairs, Senior Citizens, Women and Youth.

Food and Agriculture Organization. (2004). *Joint FAO/WHO Workshop on Fruit and Vegetables for Health (September 1–3, 2004; Kobe, Japan).* Retrieved from http://www.who.int/dietphysicalactivity/publications/fruit_vegetables_report.pdf?ua=1.

Fuller, T. D. (2010). Relationship status, health, and health behavior: An examination of cohabiters and commuters. *Sociological Perspectives, 53*(2), 221–246.

Gabler, S., & Häder, S. (1999). Generierung von Telefonstichproben mit TelSuSa [Generating telephone samples using TelSuSa]. *ZUMA-Nachrichten, 44,* 138–143.

Gerlach, I. (2008). Sozialstaatskonzeptionen und Familienpolitik. In Bundeszentrale für politische Bildung (Ed.), *Informationen zur politischen Bildung (Heft 301): Familie und Familienpolitik.* Bonn: Bundeszentrale für politische Bildung.

Grace, S., Williams, A., Stewart, D., & Franche, R. (2006). Healthpromoting behaviours through pregnancy, maternity leave, and return to work: Effects of role spillover and other correlates. *Women and Health, 43,* 51–71.

Gual, A., Segura, L., Contel, M., Heather, N., & Colom, J. (2002). AUDIT-3 and AUDIT-4: Effectiveness of two short forms of the alcohol use disorders identification test. *Alcohol and Alcoholism, 37*(6), 591–596. https://doi.org/10.1093/alcalc/37.6.591.

Gustafson, S., & Rhodes, R. (2006). Parental correlates of physical activity in children and early adolescents. *Sports Medicine, 36*(1), 79–97. https://doi.org/10.2165/00007256-200636010-00006.

Hajema, K.-J., & Knibbe, R. A. (1998). Changes in social roles as predictors of changes in drinking behaviour. *Addiction, 93*(11), 1717–1727. https://doi.org/10.1046/j.1360-0443.1998.931117179.x.

Hull, E. E., Rofey, D. L., Robertson, R. J., Nagle, E. F., Otto, A. D., & Aaron, D. J. (2010). Influence of marriage and parenthood on physical activity: A 2-year prospective analysis. *Journal of Physical Activity & Health, 7*(5), 577–583.

Hung, C. (2007). The psychosocial consequences for primiparas and multiparas. *Kaohsiung Journal of Medical Sciences, 23,* 352–360.

Kahn, R. S., Certain, L., & Whitaker, R. C. (2002). A reexamination of smoking before, during, and after pregnancy. *American Journal of Public Health, 92*(11), 1801–1808. https://doi.org/10.2105/AJPH.92.11.1801.

Kaplan, M. S., Newsom, J. T., McFarland, B. H., & Lu, L. (2001). Demographic and psychosocial correlates of physical activity in late life. *American Journal of Preventive Medicine, 21*(4), 306–312. https://doi.org/10.1016/S0749-3797(01)00364-6.

King, A., Kiernan, M., Ahn, D., & Wilcox, S. (1998). The effects of marital transitions on changes in physical activity: Results from a 10-year community study. *Annals of Behavioral Medicine, 20*(2), 64–69. https://doi.org/10.1007/BF02884450.

Klein, T., Rapp, I., & Schneider, B. (2013). The influence of couples' living arrangements on smoking habits and body weight. *Comparative Population Studies—Zeitschrift für Bevölkerungswissenschaft, 38*(3), 673–694.

Kuntsche, S., Gmel, G., Knibbe, R. A., Kuendig, H., Bloomfield, K., Kramer, S., et al. (2006). Gender and cultural differences in the association between family roles, social stratification, and alcohol use: A European cross-cultural analysis. *Alcohol and Alcoholism, 41*(suppl 1), i37–i46. https://doi.org/10.1093/alcalc/agl074.

Kuntsche, S., Knibbe, R. A., & Gmel, G. (2009). Social roles and alcohol consumption: A study of 10 industrialised countries. *Social Science and Medicine, 68*(7), 1263–1270.

Lampert, T., Kroll, L., Müters, S., & Stolzenberg, H. (2013). Messung des sozioökonomischen Status in der Studie "Gesundheit in Deutschland aktuell" (GEDA). *Bundesgesundheitsbl, 56,* 131–143.

Lange, C., Jentsch, F., Allen, J., Hoebel, J., Kratz, A. L., von der Lippe, E., et al. (2015). Data resource profile: German health update (GEDA)—The health interview survey for adults in Germany. *International Journal of Epidemiology*. https://doi.org/10.1093/ije/dyv067.

McBride, C. M., Emmons, K. M., & Lipkus, I. M. (2003). Understanding the potential of teachable moments: The case of smoking cessation. *Health Education Research, 18*(2), 156–170. https://doi.org/10.1093/her/18.2.156.

McDermott, L., Dobson, A., & Owen, N. (2006). From partying to parenthood: Young women's perceptions of cigarette smoking across life transitions. *Health Education Research, 21*(3), 428–439. https://doi.org/10.1093/her/cyl041.

McDermott, L., Dobson, A., & Russell, A. (2004). Changes in smoking behaviour among young women over life stage transitions. *Australian & New Zealand Journal of Public Health, 28*(4), 330–335. https://doi.org/10.1111/j.1467-842X.2004.tb00439.x.

McIntyre, C. A., & Rhodes, R. E. (2009). Correlates of leisure-time physical activity during transitions to motherhood. *Women Health, 49*(1), 66–83. https://doi.org/10.1080/03630240802690853.

Nomaguchi, K. M., & Bianchi, S. M. (2004). Exercise time: Gender differences in the effects of marriage, parenthood, and employment. *Journal of Marriage and Family, 66*(2), 413–430. https://doi.org/10.1111/j.1741-3737.2004.00029.x.

Olson, C. M. (2005). Tracking of food choices across the transition to motherhood. *Journal of Nutrition Education and Behavior, 37*(3), 129–136. https://doi.org/10.1016/S1499-4046(06)60267-4.

Paradis, C. (2011). Parenthood, drinking locations and heavy drinking. *Social Science and Medicine, 72*(8), 1258–1265.

Patrick, H., & Nicklas, T. A. (2005). A review of family and social determinants of children's eating patterns and diet quality. *Journal of the American College of Nutrition, 24*(2), 83–92.

Rapp, I., & Schneider, B. (2014). Unterscheiden sich Partnerschaftseffekte auf die Sportaktivität nach dem Gesundheitszustand? In S. Becker (Ed.), *Aktiv und Gesund?* (pp. 379–391). Wiesbaden: Springer Fachmedien Wiesbaden.

Reinert, D. F., & Allen, J. P. (2007). The alcohol use disorders identification test: An update of research findings. *Alcoholism: Clinical and Experimental Research, 31*(2), 185–199. https://doi.org/10.1111/j.1530-0277.2006.00295.x.

Robert Koch Institute (Ed.). (2011). *Daten und Fakten: Ergebnisse der Studie «Gesundheit in Deutschland aktuell 2009»* [Data and facts: Results of the «German Health Update» study 2009]. Beiträge zur Gesundheitsberichterstattung des Bundes. Berlin: Robert Koch Institute.

Robert Koch Institute (Ed.). (2012). *Daten und Fakten: Ergebnisse der Studie «Gesundheit in Deutschland aktuell 2010»* [Data and facts: Results of the «German Health Update» study 2010]. Beiträge zur Gesundheitsberichterstattung des Bundes. Berlin: Robert Koch Institute.

Roos, E., Lahelma, E., Virtanen, M., Prättälä, R., & Pietinen, P. (1998). Gender, socioeconomic status and family status as determinants of food behaviour. *Social Science and Medicine, 46* (12), 1519–1529.

Scharff, D. P., Homan, S., Kreuter, M., & Brennan, L. (1999). Factors associated with physical activity in women across the life span: Implications for program development. *Women Health, 29*(2), 115–134. https://doi.org/10.1300/J013v29n02_08.

Sternfeld, B., Ainsworth, B. E., & Quesenberry, C. P., Jr. (1999). Physical activity patterns in a diverse population of women. *Preventive Medicine, 28*(3), 313–323. https://doi.org/10.1006/pmed.1998.0470.

Umberson, D. (1987). Family status and health behaviors: Social control as a dimension of social integration. *Journal of Health and Social Behavior, 28*(3), 306–319.

Umberson, D. (1992). Gender, marital status and the social control of health behavior. *Social Science and Medicine, 34*(8), 907–917.

Umberson, D., Crosnoe, R., & Reczek, C. (2010). Social relationships and health behavior across the life course. *Annual Review of Sociology, 36*(1), 139–157. https://doi.org/10.1146/annurev-soc-070308-120011.

Waldron, I., & Lye, D. (1989). Family roles and smoking. *American Journal of Preventive Medicine, 5*(3), 136–141.

White, C., Oliffe, J. L., & Bottorff, J. L. (2012). Fatherhood, smoking, and secondhand smoke in North America: An historical analysis with a view to contemporary practice. *American Journal of Men's Health, 6*(2), 146–155. https://doi.org/10.1177/1557988311425852.

Yannakoulia, M., Panagiotakos, D., Pitsavos, C., Skoumas, Y., & Stafanadis, C. (2008). Eating patterns may mediate the association between marital status, body mass index, and blood cholesterol levels in apparently healthy men and women from the ATTICA study. *Social Science & Medicine, 66*(11), 2230–2239. https://doi.org/10.1016/j.socscimed.2008.01.051.

Fertility Histories and Health in Later Life in Italy

Cecilia Tomassini, Giorgio Di Gessa and Viviana Egidi

Background

As stated in the first chapter of this volume, numerous studies in the past have considered the associations between fertility history (in terms of fertility quantum and tempo) and mortality and different health indicators (Green et al. 1988; Westendorp and Kirkwood 1998; Doblhammer 2000; Alonso 2002; Grundy and Tomassini 2005, 2010; Hank 2010; Grundy and Read 2015) for women and, less frequently, for men (Grundy and Tomassini 2006; Grundy and Kravdal 2008). The literature on this topic suggests that there are several potential mechanisms that may cause associations between fertility histories and health in later life, including selection into parenthood, direct biological factors, as well as indirect effects such as the relative costs and benefits of childrearing. Pregnancy and childbirth may have physiological consequences on long term morbidity: breast cancer, for example, has been found to be positively associated with being childless and with later motherhood and negatively associated with early pregnancy (Amir et al. 2010). Motherhood after age 35 was found to be both positively and negatively associated with health. For instance, late motherhood was found to be positively associated with poor health indicators after age 50 (e.g. including diabetes, hypertension, vision difficulties, impaired physical mobility, higher mortality) (Alonso 2002), but in other studies it was negatively associated with presence of limiting long standing

C. Tomassini (✉)
Department of Economics, University of Molise, Campobasso, Italy
e-mail: cecilia.tomassini@unimol.it

G. Di Gessa
Department of Global Health & Social Medicine, King's College London, London, UK
e-mail: giorgio.di_gessa@kcl.ac.uk

V. Egidi
Department of Statistics, Sapienza University of Rome, Rome, Italy
e-mail: Viviana.Egidi@uniroma1.it

G. Doblhammer and J. Gumà (eds.), *A Demographic Perspective on Gender, Family and Health in Europe*, https://doi.org/10.1007/978-3-319-72356-3_11

illnesses (Doblhammer 2000; Grundy and Tomassini 2005). These differences seem to vary by cohort, and this can explain the inconsistence of the results found in the literature. For example, later motherhood today is linked to fertility techniques that may have negative consequences on health (e.g. breast cancer) although the literature mainly rejects this association (Salhab et al. 2005).

Selection may play an important role when considering health and mortality after the reproductive period: women aged 50 and older are selected for premature mortality (for example linked to childbearing itself as maternal mortality), even if this is becoming increasingly rarer for modern populations. Childlessness in the past may have been related to poor health: women with health problems tended not to get married and not to have children. At the same time being able to conceive a child at earlier or later ages may be an indicator of overall good health status and slower ageing (Doblhammer and Oeppen 2003). This is true also for younger cohorts, even if the proportion of people who rationally choose to remain childless is higher than in the past.

It has been also argued that health may also be affected by other psychological factors such as stresses and role changes. On the socio-economic side, personal and family income may be reduced by the costs of childbearing. Early pregnancies may hamper education and work careers and therefore have an impact on future socio-economic status and, directly and indirectly, on health (Fletcher and Wolfe 2009).

In order to disentangle all these different mechanism and pathways, some studies have considered men and women separately, as women are expected to experience the physiological consequences of pregnancy and childbirth while both sexes should be affected by the psychological and economic components of the association.

Additionally, considering different types of health outcomes may provide an interesting insight on the mechanisms that link selected indicators of fertility quantum and tempo and health, helping to identify the process underlined in this association. Furthermore, to our knowledge, no studies have examined this association in the context of a familialistic country such as Italy. Most studies have been based on countries in Northern and Central Europe, where intergenerational exchanges are less frequent and children leave the parental home early, and where the hypothesised psychological factors may be less strong. The notion of the familialistic culture has been used in the past to explain the strong family ties existing in southern Europe (Reher 1998) where, for example, intergenerational co-residence tends to continue until children leave the parental home to get married; and even then they normally live close to their parents (Tomassini et al. 2003). In a familialistic country with strong family ties, frequent contact between generations may play a significant role in enhancing the role of parenthood against childlessness, especially for the subjective indicators of health. Additionally it should be stressed that familialistic countries are characterised by the unbalanced division of house and care work (Anxo et al. 2011): women's multiple roles may affect (positively for the "role enhancing theory" or negatively for the "role strain model") the perception of their health status.

From a demographic point of view, Italy is characterised by sharp declining fertility: the TFR for cohorts born around 1930 was around 2.3, while it declined to 1.6 for those born around 1960. The proportion of childless women is less than 20% for all cohorts considered in this study. Southern Italy is characterised by a higher and earlier level of fertility: on average, for cohorts born in the 30s, Southern women had one more child compared to their Central and Northern counterparts. Additionally more than half of Southern women had three or more children compared to a quarter in Central and Northern Italy (Santini 1995). Italy is also characterised by a high level of late fertility: 40% of births occurred after age 30 in Northern and Central Italy for the 1930 cohort and 37% for the 1960 cohort (in the South 45 and 30% respectively). These trends continue, even in presence of a further decline in the total fertility rate: in 2013, around 8% of births occur after age 39 (ISTAT 2015) compared to less than 4% in England and Wales (ONS 2015). Such trends may indicate how Italian later mothers are less selected in terms of "slower ageing" compared to other countries.

In this chapter, we focus on women and men aged 50 and over with complete fertility histories using two nationally representative surveys. Using different data sources allows us not only to consider different outcomes in health, but also to provide a rich picture of the associations between health and fertility indicators. Our main aim is to examine the association of fertility quantum (for all respondents) and fertility quantum and tempo (for parents only) with several indicators of the health status. These relations are analysed by taking different socio-economic indicators into consideration in order to control for these confounding factors.

Methods

To explore the associations between fertility histories indicators and health we use data from two sources of data. It is not common to collect information both on fertility histories and current (or past) health status in Italy. The only exceptions are the two datasets we use in this chapter.

The first dataset is the Italian Survey on Family and Social Relations (ISF), carried out by the Italian Institute of Statistics in 2009. This cross-sectional survey has a very high response rate (above 80%) and investigates several aspects of family and social networks. From the original sample of around 60,000 individuals we selected respondents aged 50 and over (N = 17,973) with completed fertility histories. The large sample size and the high response rate are the strong points of this source of data, even if the health variables collected are few and no references to early life socio-economic conditions are included in the questionnaire.

The second are data from the Survey of Health, Ageing and Retirement in Europe (SHARE), a multidisciplinary ongoing longitudinal survey of individuals aged 50 and over living in Austria, Belgium, Switzerland, Germany, Denmark, Spain, France, Italy, Greece, the Netherlands, and Sweden. Specific details of sampling frames and methodology, weighting strategies, and questionnaires have been reported elsewhere (Börsch-Supan et al. 2008; Börsch-Supan and Jürges 2005; Schröder 2011). The first wave of SHARE took place in 2004/05 with later waves conducted biennially. Waves 1, 2, 4 and 5 collected data on the respondents' current living conditions and health. Information about the respondents' life histories were collected only in wave 3 (SHARELIFE, 2008/09), when no additional households were sampled; histories were therefore only collected from respondents who participated in either wave 1 or 2. Given our interest in the histories and the baseline characteristics, the data from waves 4 and 5 were not relevant. In order to assess the relationship between fertility history indicators and health, we used the pooled baseline interviews of Italian respondents aged 50 and older from waves 1 and 2 (N = 3709) for whom information on their fertility history had been collected (N = 2383, i.e. 64% of the pooled sample of initial interviews). SHARE was used as it collects all the information needed for these kinds of studies (fertility histories and present and past health indicators), but the low response rate and the small sample size may not produce stable results.

Outcome Variables

Our key health outcomes were self-rated health (SRH), depressive symptoms, and various measures of functional limitations. In the ISF survey, SRH was measured by the WHO question (De Bruin et al. 1996) adopting a 5-point ordinal scale (very good, good, fair, poor, and very poor), whereas in SHARE self-rated health was measured—in both waves—using the first question of the SF-36 scale (Ware 2000) in which the response options are slightly different (excellent, very *good*, *good*, *fair*, or *poor*). In our study, the five SRH items were dichotomised into 'poor' (the last two categories of the ISTAT survey and the last of SHARE) versus better health. The 'fair' category of the WHO scale was aggregated with positive evaluations because of its Italian translation, which has more of a positive connotation (Egidi and Spizzichino 2006). Even if the two scales are not directly comparable, we wanted to confirm the directions of the effects of the socio-demographic and fertility characteristics on self-perception of health.

Functional limitations were measured through a series of indicators targeting situations in which health disorders and conditions had impacted people's usual activities. First, both ISF and SHARE respondents were asked whether they had experienced "limitation in activities people usually do because of health problems for at least the past six months". This single-question item is a validated measure, which approximately captures global activity limitations (Jagger et al. 2010). We categorised respondents as limited regardless of severity of the limitation. SHARE respondents were also asked to fill in two functional limitations scale focusing on different aspects of functional independence: the Activity of Daily Living (ADL) (Katz et al. 1963) and the Instrumental Activity of Daily Living (IADL) scales (Lawton and Brody 1969). In the first case, respondents were asked whether they experienced any difficulties with specific everyday activities that are essential for self-care due to a physical, mental, emotional, or memory problem. Respondents who reported at least one difficulty with basic activities of daily living (activities considered by SHARE are: bathing or showering, dressing, eating, getting in or out of bed, walking across a room, using the toilet) were considered to have an ADL limitation. In the second case, the scale is mainly oriented to social limitations gathering information on more complex activities more related to social life (activities considered by SHARE are: using a map, preparing meals, shopping for groceries, using the telephone, managing medications, maintaining the home, managing finances). Respondents who reported difficulties in at least one of these activities were considered to have an IADL limitation.

SHARE also adopted the EURO-D 12-item scale, a depression symptoms scale especially designed for the mental health evaluation of older European people, the validity and reliability of which has been demonstrated against a variety of relevant clinical assessments (Castro-Costa et al. 2008; Prince et al. 1999). Respondents were asked whether they had experienced any depressive symptoms, such as feeling guilty or being irritable, recently or in the month prior to interview. Those who reported four or more depressive symptoms on the EURO-D scales were classified as reporting depressive symptoms (Prince et al. 1999).

Measures of Interest

A series of categorical indicators capturing the participants' recall of fertility experiences throughout life were used. In both surveys, participants were asked whether they ever had a biological child, including those who lived for a short time. Those who did were then asked how many children they ever had, including any who died since birth. We distinguished between those who had no biological children, one child, two (as reference category), three, and four or more. For respondents who had at least one biological child regardless of whether the child was still alive or not (i.e. "mothers" and "fathers"), we constructed two dichotomous indicators to capture the timing of births. Taking into account both the year in which each biological child was born and the current year of birth of the parent, we created dummy variables indicating whether the respondent became a parent before the age of 20 and 24 (for mothers and fathers respectively) or after the age of 39.

Other Covariates

On the basis of the existing literature, we identified characteristics known to be associated with health and accordingly controlled for the following characteristics: age, level of education, marital status, geographical area, wealth, income, and labour market participation. Age was recoded into three categories (50–64; 65–75, and 75 and older). Educational qualifications were grouped into three categories: low, mid, and high education, where low level of education is defined as pre-primary or primary level of education, and high refers to upper secondary level of education or above. For marital status, we distinguished between people who were "married or cohabiting", "divorced, separated, or never married", or "widowed". We decided to group the never married with those who are separated or divorced because the number of them with children is very low and it is possible that they used to live with a cohabiting partner. Preliminary analyses were also carried out considering marital history indicators such as the total number of marriages, binary indicators of previous widowhood and divorce, as well as the age at or the length of the latest marital disruption. All these indicators were not significant; therefore, we present results on the marital status at the time of the interview only. Three geographical areas were considered (North, Centre, and South) based on the statistical partition proposed by the Italian National Institute of Statistics (www.istat.it). Wealth was measured using a dichotomised indicator of whether the respondent owned his or her house or not (regardless of whether they were mortgage-free). Similarly, economic resources were measured using a dichotomised indicator of whether the respondent perceived that their household was able to make ends meet with great difficulty or not. Employment history was measured by distinguishing between respondents who have/had ever done any paid work and those who never worked. As an additional control variable for the Italian familialistic context, we introduced in the model a variable measuring whether parents had weekly contact with their children. Our hypothesis was to test if family closeness buffers the association found between indicators of fertility histories and subjective health.

No measures of previous health conditions were asked in the ISF, whereas SHARE collected several indicators of participants' recall of health in childhood (defined as by when respondents were born up to and including when they were 15 years old). In particular, we considered an indicator of early life poor health if respondents missed school for more than one month, whether they recall being confined to bed or home for more than one month, or whether they were in hospital for a month or more because of a health condition during childhood. Moreover, SHARE asks questions about the respondents' socio-economic conditions during childhood, and we considered two proxies of these conditions using information on whether the respondents were living with both natural parents at the age of 10, and whether they had enough books to fill one shelf or one or more bookcases in the household.

Statistical Analysis

Our analyses of cross-sectional relationships between fertility history and health consisted of two steps. First, we assessed the impact of the number of biological children ever born on health among all baseline respondents, controlling for demographic and socio-economic factors. Second, restricting the analyses to mothers and fathers, we also controlled for the timing of births. Among SHARE respondents only, we also accounted for health at childhood in subsequent models. Given the binary nature of the outcome variables, we used binomial logistic regression analyses. All analyses on the ISF data were performed using SPSS, weighted by our standardisation of the coefficient provided by ISTAT. All analyses on the SHARE data were performed using Stata (Stata Corp 2013), and adjusted for the survey design effects. No weights were available for the pooled sample used in this study; however, all characteristics relevant for weighting were controlled for in the multivariate analyses.

Results

Descriptive Statistics

Table 1 shows the distribution of demographic, socio-economic, fertility, and health characteristics at baseline of both ISF and Italian SHARE respondents. Overall, about 40% of respondents in both surveys had two children, with slightly higher percentages of adults with three or more children among Italian SHARE respondents. Among parents, one in six fathers and one in 16 mothers had at least one child when they were 40 or older. In both surveys, about seven percent of the respondents became fathers and mothers before the age of 24 and 20 respectively. Male respondents in both surveys were more likely to report better health compared to women for all the variables considered. As for the indicators of socio-economic and health conditions at childhood among SHARE respondents, no gender differences were found, with about 10% of respondents who recalled missing school or spending one month or more confined in bed or in the hospital for one month or more because of a health condition. Table 1 also shows that SHARE respondents were more likely to be younger, married, and from the Centre or South of Italy compared to ISF respondents.

Associations Between Number of Children and Health Indicators—All Respondents

Figure 1 shows results from logistic regression models, which investigated associations between number of children and SRH, limitations, and depressive symptoms, controlling for socio-economic and demographic characteristics. Full details of the associations are shown in Table 2. For reasons of space, results for SRH and global activity limitations are presented only for IFS respondents.

Table 1 Percentage distribution of demographic, socio-economic, fertility and health variables included in SHARE and ISF

All respondents	ISF respondents		SHARE respondents	
	Men (N = 8232)	Women (N = 9741)	Men (N = 1091)	Women (N = 1292)
50–64	52.8	46.5	51.7	59.9
65–74	26.5	26.1	34.9	27.3
75+	20.7	27.4	13.4	12.8
Married or cohabiting	78.8	57.4	89.4	77.1
Divorced/separated/never married	14.8	13.9	7.0	6.1
Widowed	6.4	28.7	3.6	16.8
Low education	37.3	53.2	47.3	59.7
Medium education	27.8	21.1	23.0	17.2
High education	34.9	25.7	29.7	23.1
Home owner	80.2	77.8	82.3	80.1
Household meets end with great difficulty	66.6	38.7	19.9	21.7
In paid work (currently or ever)	92.2	52.1	95.3	67.1
North	47.4	47.2	37.6	39.0
Centre	20.4	20.6	26.0	24.7
South	32.2	32.2	36.4	36.3
Self-rated Health = Poor	12.4	17.1	7.9	11.1
With any LLI	31.6	39.1	32.1	44.3
With 1+ ADL limitations			6.1	9.6
With 1+ IADL limitations			8.2	16.3
With depressive symptoms			20.5	41.3
No children	13.6	12.8	10.5	10.1
1 child	19.9	21.5	18.0	17.1
2 children	39.6	39.2	40.9	39.2
3 children	15.5	17.3	19.7	20.5
4+ children	6.6	9.2	10.9	13.3
Never missed school, in bed, or in hospital for 1+ month in childhood			91.6	89.7
Living with both natural parents at 10			89.8	90.2
Books filled 1+ shelf in HH			23.2	25.7
Parents only	**(N = 7122)**	**(N = 8485)**	**(N = 976)**	**(N = 1160)**
Age first < 20 (24 for men)	8.9	7.6	7.3	6.6
Late parenthood	16.1	6.0	17.3	6.2

Sources SHARE 2004/05, 2006/07 and SHARELIFE 2008/09; ISF 2009. Weighted results

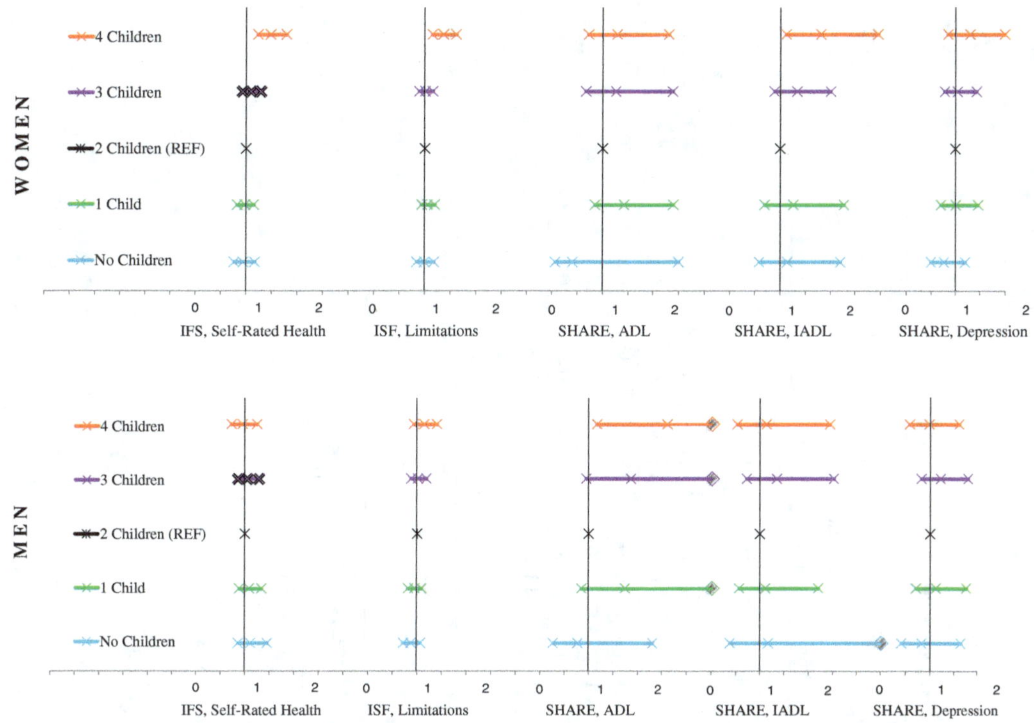

Fig. 1 Odds ratios and 95% confidence intervals, from the logistic model for health indicators for all respondents aged 50 and over. Controlling for age, marital status, education, region, housing tenure, and household income satisfaction

Regardless of the health outcome considered, Fig. 1 shows no significant differences between both male and female respondents who are childless or only had one child and those who had two children (the reference category). Similarly, no significant associations were found between having had three children and health, the only exception being male respondents who were marginally more likely to report ADL limitations ($p < 0.10$). However, having had four or more children is associated with an increased likelihood of reporting poor health, particularly among female respondents. In particular, women who gave birth to four or more children were significantly more likely to report poor SRH, global activity limitations, and IADL limitations compared to those who had two children. Men with four or more children were significantly more likely to report ADL limitations. No significant associations between the number of children and depressive symptomatology were found. Associations with other baseline covariates were broad, as would be expected from previous studies. Older respondents were significantly more likely to report poor health, global limitations, and depressive symptoms; those with higher educational levels were significantly less likely to report poor SRH, global limitations, ADL and IADL limitations, and depressive symptoms compared to those with the lowest education level. There was also a reverse association among the perception of economic resources available, employment history (particularly among men), and health disadvantage. Similarly, results suggest that respondents who were not currently married were more likely to report poor SRH and limitations; similarly,

Table 2 Men's and Women's health by baseline socioeconomic and demographic characteristics, and number of children

	ISF				SHARE					
	SRH = poor		Limitations		1+ ADL limitations		1+ IADL limitations		Depressive symptoms	
	Men	Women	Men	Women	Men	Women	Men	Women	Men	Women
65–74	2.01**	1.88**	2.20**	2.22**	2.88**	2.49**	3.33**	1.74*	1.07	1.20
75+	5.35**	4.19**	5.84**	5.78**	7.58**	4.56**	9.22**	5.03**	1.49	1.87**
Separated/divorced/never married	1.34*	1.76**	1.30**	1.39**	2.31$^+$	1.82	1.09	1.43	0.95	1.14
Widowed	1.49**	1.37**	1.35**	1.50**	1.54	1.27	1.09	1.45*	3.50**	1.29
Medium education	0.71**	0.58**	0.71**	0.71**	0.78	0.74	0.55$^+$	0.52**	0.66*	0.92
High education	0.55**	0.50**	0.55**	0.62**	0.48*	0.71	0.30**	0.25**	0.36**	0.66*
Home owner	0.86$^+$	0.85*	1.01	0.96	0.73	0.80	0.86	1.19	0.71*	0.89
In paid work/retired from work	0.30**	0.95	0.35**	0.80**	0.22**	0.91	0.20**	1.26	0.45*	0.79
HH meets ends	0.45**	0.56**	0.60**	0.61**	1.55	0.75	1.09	0.70$^+$	0.64*	0.65**
Centre	1.22*	1.49**	1.12	1.24**	0.90	1.55	1.33	2.27*	1.04	1.13
South	1.60**	1.56**	1.24**	1.36**	0.63	1.70*	1.55	2.19*	0.97	1.08
No children	1.11	0.94	0.87	0.99	0.78	0.40	1.17	1.14	0.82	0.76
1 child	1.08	0.97	0.94	1.05	1.74	1.41	1.11	1.25	1.11	1.00
3 children	1.05	1.10	1.01	1.00	1.85$^+$	1.25	1.34	1.33	1.21	1.04
4+ children	0.94	1.47**	1.13	1.35**	2.60*	1.27	1.13	1.80*	0.96	1.29
Constant	0.33**	0.12**	1.00	0.40**	0.09**	0.06**	0.14**	0.07**	1.21	1.08
N	8232	9741	8232	9741	1079	1258	1079	1258	1078	1258

Odds Ratios and significance levels
Source SHARE 2004/05. 2006/07, and SHARELIFE; ISF 2009. Weighted data
$^{**}p < 0.01$, $^{*}p < 0.05$, $^{+}p < 0.10$

widowed men and women were respectively more likely to report depressive symptoms and IADL limitations. Finally, respondents from the South of Italy were more likely to report poor SRH, global limitations, and—among women—ADL and IADL limitations compared to those who live in the North of Italy.

Associations Between Quantum and Tempo Fertility Indicators and Health Indicators Among Parents

Figure 2 shows results from logistic regression models which, restricting analyses to parents only, investigated associations between fertility quantum and tempo and SRH, limitations, and depressive symptoms, controlling for socio-economic and demographic characteristics. As before, results for SRH and global activity limitations are presented only for IFS respondents. Full details of the associations are shown in Table 3.

When restricting analyses to respondents who have had at least one child, Fig. 2 shows that for all five outcomes having had one or three children was not associated with health. However, again there was some evidence to suggest that women who had four or more children were significantly more likely to report poor SRH, global

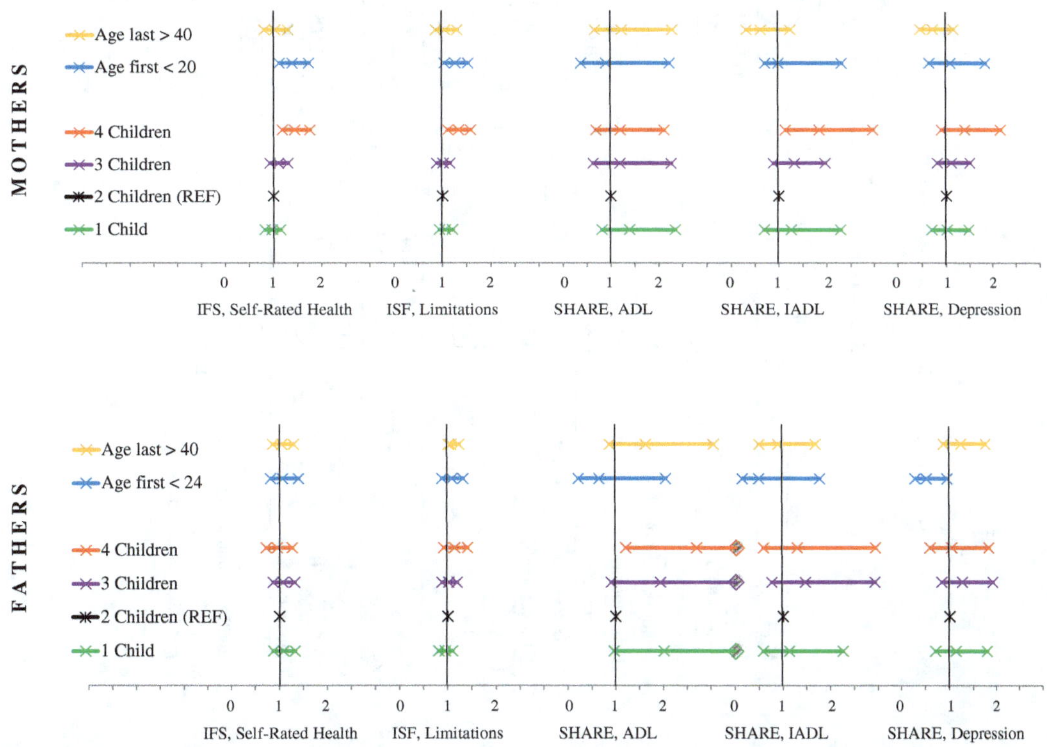

Fig. 2 Odds ratios and 95% confidence intervals, from the logistic model for health indicators for all parents aged 50 and over. Controlling for age, marital status, education, region, housing tenure, and household income satisfaction

Table 3 Fathers' and Mothers' health by baseline socioeconomic and demographic characteristics, by number of children and by fertility history

	ISF				SHARE					
	SRH = poor		Limitations		1+ ADL limitations		1+ IADL limitations		Depressive symptoms	
	Men	Women	Men	Women	Men	Women	Men	Women	Men	Women
65–74	1.95**	2.09**	2.16**	2.28**	2.83*	2.49**	3.58**	1.79**	0.99	1.22
75+	5.09**	4.82**	5.63**	6.45**	6.66**	4.41**	10.6**	5.03**	1.44	1.77**
Separated/divorced/never married	1.55**	1.80**	1.29*	1.45**	1.29	3.76*	0.76	1.81	0.99	1.05
Widowed	1.55**	1.36**	1.32*	1.45**	1.48	1.31	1.45	1.39⁺	5.50**	1.29
Medium education	0.74**	0.61**	0.72**	0.74**	0.83	0.77	0.45*	0.52**	0.63*	0.94
High education	0.56**	0.55**	0.54**	0.66**	0.39*	0.55	0.24**	0.25**	0.36**	0.72
Home owner	0.84⁺	0.83*	1.0	0.96	0.69	0.84	0.89	1.18	0.79	0.86
In paid work/retired from work	0.31**	1.02	0.36**	0.85**	0.27*	0.88	0.25**	1.21	0.49⁺	0.75⁺
HH meets ends	0.44**	0.58**	0.60**	0.61**	1.60	0.82	1.14	0.69⁺	0.61**	0.62**
Centre	1.15	1.55**	1.08	1.28**	1.00	1.58	1.22	2.09*	1.02	1.09
South	1.56**	1.59**	1.22**	1.43**	0.57	1.87*	1.37	2.23*	0.86	1.00
1 child	1.08	0.97	0.94	1.05	2.00⁺	1.38	1.12	1.25	1.12	1.01
3 children	1.06	1.09	1.01	1.00	1.92⁺	1.18	1.46	1.31	1.25	1.09
4+ children	0.94	1.42**	1.12	1.31**	2.67*	1.18	1.28	1.82*	1.02	1.38
Age first < 20 (24 for men)	1.05	1.37**	1.06	1.24*	0.63	0.88	0.46	0.96	0.49*	1.06
Age last > 40	1.02	1.00	1.03	1.02	1.59	1.19	0.86	0.58	1.19	0.68
Constant	0.34**	0.10**	0.99	0.35**	0.07**	0.06**	0.12**	0.07**	1.15	1.21
N	7122	8485	7122	8485	960	1126	960	1126	959	1126

Odds Ratios and significance levels

Source SHARE 2004/05 and 2006/07 and SHARELIFE; ISF 2009. Weighted data

$^{**}p < 0.01$, $^{*}p < 0.05$, $^{+}p < 0.10$

activity limitations, and IADL limitations compared to those who had two children, whereas men were more likely to report ADL limitations. No significant associations between four or more children and depressive symptoms were found.

As for the indicators which capture the timing of births, results suggest that becoming a parent at the age of 40 or older was not associated with any of the health indicators, for neither fathers nor mothers. On the other hand, mothers who gave birth before the age of 20 were significantly more likely to report poor SRH and global activity limitations compared to women who became mothers at older ages. No associations were found between early parenthood and functional limitations. However, male respondents who became fathers at 23 or younger were less likely to report depressive symptoms compared to those who had their first child later at older ages.

Conclusions and Discussion

There are several striking results from our analysis. Unlike other studies, our findings do not show childlessness to be associated with any problems in the health indicators used in this chapter. There are no disadvantages for those without children and therefore, in the context of a familialistic country, without potential social support from children. Selection may have played a role here, if we hypothesised that only the fittest childless people survived to older age. However, given that for the cohorts born after the 30s the progression rate to parity one was quite high (Santini 1995), and that mortality levels in Italy for these generations were not higher compared to other Western countries (Human Mortality Database 2015), selection itself cannot entirely explain such findings.

As previous studies have shown, having four or more children has an important impact on poor self-rated health, presence of limiting illnesses, and IADL limitations among older women, and on ADL limitations among older men. These results do not shed a clear light on the pathways (physiological vs psychological) that may link fertility histories and health; however, they do suggest that high parity may have negative consequences on health, especially for women. As shown in other studies (Grundy and Tomassini 2005; Christensen et al. 1998), not only do women with high parity more frequently rate their health as poor or declared mild or severe limiting illnesses, but they also seem to suffer problems with IADL. Because IADLs, unlike ADLs, include the social dimensions of functional limitations (such as shopping for groceries, managing finances, or maintaining the home) rather than the mere functional ones, this female disadvantage suggests that high parity women may have spent their lives with fewer external activities in addition to their family responsibilities. This may be linked to the presence of many children itself as well as to a more traditional and deprived environment, and it is possible that this relative disadvantage continues in later life. It is also possible that the unbalanced gender division in traditional Italian families in performing family work may play a significant role in female disadvantage related to high parity (Anxo et al. 2011).

When parents are considered, early motherhood has the same significant negative effect on self-rated health and presence of functional limitations as shown in previous studies, while it is protective for men regarding depression. One possible explanation for the latter result may be because younger fathers become grandfathers earlier in life and this role has beneficial consequences on men's mental health (Di Gessa et al. 2015). This result may suggest that the association of fertility behaviour and psychological health is not as strong for women compared to the other health indicators used in this chapter, as found in other previous studies (Hank and Wagner 2013).

In order to expand our results, we also tested whether marital histories may have affected the associations found with the fertility indicators. Introducing in the model variables such as the total number of marriages, binary indicators of previous widowhood and divorce, as well as the age at or the length of the latest marital disruption change the relationship nor the strength of the associations. All such variables were never significant, suggesting that, in this context, the actual marital status is more important than marital histories for health and health related indicators. Furthermore, only among SHARE respondents, we repeated the same analyses also controlling for health and socio-economic conditions at childhood in subsequent models. The results (reported in Tables 4 and 5) showed that only the indicator of early life poor health was significantly associated with current health for all the outcomes considered except IADL limitations; such associations were significant only among women and mothers. However, even accounting for early life conditions, the direction and strength of associations between participants' fertility experiences throughout life and the outcomes of interest did not change.

We also considered, as a fertility history indicator, the occurrence of close births, defined as giving birth to two children, including twins, in less than two consecutive calendar years, but the variable was never significant for the health dimensions we considered in both samples. Some previous studies have found a negative association between closely spaced birth (including twins) and health (Grundy and Tomassini 2005), suggesting potential physiological harm or an additional load of stress for parents, but this effect was not found for any of the health indicators used in this study, suggesting no parental strain due to rearing more than one young child at once.

Another effort to clarify the relations between fertility quantum and tempo and health was introducing the model interactions between age groups and geographic area and number of children. We hypothesised that, for example, the effect of early motherhood and high parity on health could be positive among older cohorts of women from the South, given that among such groups higher and earlier fertility were more accepted and common compared to the rest of the country. We found a significant positive effect of the interaction between early pregnancies and living in the South only among mothers, while the main effect of both variables remained significant. This result may suggest that the consequences of early pregnancy on later life health might be less strong in Southern Italy, confirming our hypothesis.

Another peculiar characteristic of Italy is the potential influence of the quantity and quality of family exchanges on different aspects of health. Our results (not shown) indicate that even controlling for the quantity of contacts between mothers

Table 4 Men's and Women's health by baseline socioeconomic and demographic characteristics, early-life characteristics, and number of children

	SHARE									
	SRH = poor		Limitations		1+ ADL limitations		1+ IADL limitations		Depressive symptoms	
	Men	Women	Men	Women	Men	Women	Men	Women	Men	Women
No children	0.34*	0.57	0.79	0.98	0.79	0.40	1.19	1.11	0.81	0.73
1 child	1.06	1.16	1.13	1.43^{+}	1.75	1.40	1.10	1.25	1.08	0.99
3 children	1.25	1.02	0.89	0.97	1.88^{+}	1.23	1.35	1.29	1.21	1.03
4+ children	1.58	0.76	1.12	1.27	2.61*	1.23	1.14	1.76*	0.98	1.27
Missed school, in bed, or in hospital for 1 + month in childhood	1.37	1.67*	1.15	1.68*	1.43	1.85*	1.20	1.33	1.19	1.73**
Not living with both natural parents at 10	0.67	0.77	1.04	0.99	0.70	0.87	0.84	1.01	0.95	0.96
Books filled less than 1 shelf in HH	0.51^{+}	0.83	0.85	0.92	1.16	0.84	0.90	0.64	0.70	0.84
N	1079	1258	1079	1258	1079	1258	1079	1258	1078	1258

Odds Ratios and significance levels

Source SHARE 2004/05, 2006/07, and SHARELIFE. Controlling for age, marital status, education, home tenure, work status, perception of economic resources available, and geographic area. Weighted data

$^{**}p < 0.01$, $^{*}p < 0.05$, $^{+}p < 0.10$

Table 5 Fathers' and Mothers' health by baseline socioeconomic and demographic characteristics, early-life characteristics, number of children, and fertility history

	SHARE									
	SRH = poor		Limitations		1+ ADL limitations		1+ IADL limitations		Depressive symptoms	
	Men	Women	Men	Women	Men	Women	Men	Women	Men	Women
1 child	1.16	1.18	1.18	1.39^{+}	2.00^{+}	1.37	1.11	1.25	1.08	1.00
3 children	1.23	0.98	0.93	0.94	1.92^{+}	1.16	1.48	1.28	1.25	1.08
4+ children	1.57	0.72	1.22	1.21	2.67*	1.16	1.30	1.78*	1.04	1.36
Age first < 20 (24 for men)	0.66	1.58	0.59^{+}	1.04	0.64	0.87	0.46	0.93	0.47*	1.03
Age last > 40	1.01	0.89	0.94	0.84	1.58	1.24	0.86	0.58	1.21	0.69
Missed school, in bed, or in hospital for 1 + month in childhood	1.23	1.66*	0.94	1.52*	1.21	1.88*	1.37	1.21	1.21	1.56*
Not living with both natural parents at 10	0.67	0.95	1.10	0.98	0.80	0.91	0.89	0.84	0.81	0.94
Books filled less than 1 shelf in HH	0.56	0.80	0.84	0.87	1.11	1.06	0.95	0.71	0.65	0.83
N	960	1126	7122	1126	960	1126	960	1126	959	1126

Odds Ratios and significance levels

Source SHARE 2004/05, 2006/07, and SHARELIFE. Controlling for age, marital status, education, home tenure, work status, perception of economic resources available, and geographic area. Weighted data

$^{**}p < 0.01$, $^{*}p < 0.05$, $^{+}p < 0.10$

and children, such close relations do not affect the association between high parity and health, suggesting that the potential physiological consequences of multiple pregnancies on women's health may not be buffered by close relations with children.

Although our study provides additional light on the relationship between parenthood and health at later life, it also has limitations. First, our analysis is based on cross-sectional data, and it is therefore possible that health problems may have prevented men and women from having any or additional children. Interestingly, however, we have not found any negative effect of being childless or with parity 1 on any indicators of health as in previous studies, suggesting that if reverse pathways (i.e. poor health preventing having any or additional children) shaped such associations, these were not significant.

Second, selection may act differently for different socio-economic groups and for different cohorts. For the older cohort, high parity was associated with lower socio-economic status and with the South of Italy (Santini 1995), but we are not able to control for those variables at the time of birth of the child. Still these results hold when considering current socio-economic indicators. Furthermore, selection by death may bias our sample and could explain why in our study we did not find any disadvantage associated with childlessness among women; however, as mortality before age 50 is very low in Italy (Human Mortality Database 2015), this source of distortion should be minimal.

Third, this study used data from two different sources, IFS and SHARE. Even though the distributions of the variables of interest seem to be relatively comparable across both datasets, the demographic and socio-economic distributions of SHARE respondents differ considerably, with SHARE respondents being younger, more likely to be married, with low education, and from the Centre-South of Italy compared with IFS participants. This may be due to a combination of initial low response rate of the SHARE survey, longitudinal attrition, and the fact that no weights were available for the pooled sample used in this study (Di Gessa 2011). Our research is based on complete case analyses of SHARE, and does not consider how sample attrition might potentially bias associations (Fitzgerald et al. 1998).

This study has tried to provide additional insights in the relation between fertility histories indicators and health in the context of a familialistic country such as Italy. In addition to the physiological justification that may explain the differences found between men and women for the detrimental effect on ADL of high parities, a more complicated link may be hypothesised. The negative effect of high parity on IADL for women may indicate a socially deprived environment for women with more children which the variables included in the questionnaires are not able to capture. Furthermore, in a familialistic country women are exposed to a greater overload of unpaid work (house chores and care activities), both during adult and later life. Both factors may explain the female disadvantage in terms of high parity and early motherhood. Because these characteristics are becoming rarer among younger cohorts (in 2013 only 0.4% of the births occurred to teenagers mothers compared to 4.7% in England and Wales), we hypothesised that these factors will not play a major role in younger cohorts.

References

Alonso, A. (2002). Long term health consequences of delayed childbirth: NHANES III. *Women's Health Issues, 12,* 37–45.

Amir, E., Freedman, O. C., Seruga, B., & Evans, G. D. (2010). Assessing women at high risk of breast cancer: A review of risk assessment models. *Journal of the National Cancer Institute, 102*(10), 680–691.

Anxo, D., Mencarini, L., Pailhé, A., Solaz, A., Tanturri, M. L., & Flood, L. (2011). Gender differences in time use over the life course in France, Italy, Sweden, and the US. *Feminist Economics, 17*(3), 159–195.

Börsch-Supan, A., & Jürges, H. (2005). *The survey of health, aging, and retirement in Europe—methodology*. Mannheim: Research Institute for the Economics of Aging.

Börsch-Supan, A., Brugiavini, A., Jürges, H., Kapteyn, A., Mackenbach, J., Siegrist, J., & Weber, G. (2008). First results from the survey of health, ageing and retirement in Europe (2004–2007). In *Starting the longitudinal dimension*. Mannheim: Mannheim Research Institute for the Economics of Aging (MEA).

Castro-Costa, E., Dewey, M., Stewart, R., Banerjee, S., Huppert, F., Mendonca-Lima, C., et al. (2008). Ascertaining late-life depressive symptoms in Europe: An evaluation of the survey version of the EURO-D scale in 10 nations. The SHARE project. *International Journal of Methods in Psychiatric Research, 17*(1), 12–29. https://doi.org/10.1002/mpr.236.

Christensen, K., Gaist, D., Jeune, B., & Vaupel, J. (1998). A tooth per child? *Lancet, 352,* 204.

De Bruin, A., Picavet, H. S. J., & Nossikov, A. (1996). *Health interview surveys. Towards international harmonization of methods and instruments* (p. 58). European Series: WHO Regional Publications.

Di Gessa, G. (2011). *'Active ageing' and health: An exploration of longitudinal data for four European countries*. Ph.D. thesis. (Ph.D.), London School of Hygiene & Tropical Medicine, London.

Di Gessa, G., Glaser, K. F., & Tinker, A. M. (2015). The health impact of intensive and nonintensive grandchild care in Europe: New evidence from SHARE. *Journals of Gerontology Series. B, Psychological Sciences and Social Sciences*. https://doi.org/10.1093/geronb/gbv055.

Doblhammer, G. (2000). Reproductive history and mortality later in life: A comparative study of England and Wales and Austria. *Population Studies, 54,* 169–176.

Doblhammer, G., & Oeppen, J. (2003). The effect of frailty and mortality selection on the Peerage. *Proceedings the Royal Society Series B Biological Sciences, 270,* 1541–1547.

Egidi V, & Spizzichino D. (2006). Perceived health and mortality: A multidimensional analysis of ECHP Italian data. *Genus, LXII*(3–4).

Fitzgerald, J., Gottschalk, P., & Moffit, R. (1998). An analysis of sample attrition in panel data: The Michigan panel study of income dynamics. *The Journal of Human Resources*, 33(2) (Special Issue: Attrition in Longitudinal Surveys), 251–299.

Fletcher, J. M., & Wolfe, B. L. (2009). Education and labor market consequences of teenage childbearing: Evidence using the timing of pregnancy outcomes and community fixed effects. *Journal of Human Resources, 44,* 303–325.

Green, A., Beral, V., & Moser, K. (1988). Mortality in women in relation to their childbearing history. *British Medical Journal, 297,* 391–395.

Grundy, E., & Kravdal, Ø. (2008). Reproductive history and mortality in late middle age among Norwegian men and women. *American Journal of Epidemiology, 167,* 271–279.

Grundy, E., & Read, S. (2015). Pathways from fertility history to later life health: Results from analyses of the English longitudinal study of ageing. *Demographic Research, 32,* 107–146.

Grundy, E., & Tomassini, C. (2005). Fertility history and health in later life: A record linkage study in England and Wales. *Social Science and Medicine, 61,* 217–228.

Grundy, E., & Tomassini, C. (2006). Fatherhood history and later life health and mortality in England and Wales: A record linkage study. *Social Biology, 53*(3-4), 189–205.

Grundy, E, & Tomassini, C. (2010). Marital history, health and mortality among older men and women in England and Wales. *BMC Public Health, 10*.

Hank, K. (2010). Child bearing history, later-life health, and mortality in Germany. *Population Studies, 64,* 275–291.

Hank, K., & Wagner, M. (2013). Parenthood, marital status, and well-being in later life: Evidence from SHARE. *Social Indicators Research, 114,* 639–653.

Human Mortality Database. (2015). http://www.mortality.org/.

ISTAT. (2015). Retrieved July 6, 2015 from http://dati.istat.it/.

Jagger, C., Gillies, C., Cambois, E., Van Oyen, H., Nusselder, W., Robine, J.M., & EHLEIS Team. (2010). The Global Activity Limitation Index measured function and disability similarly across European countries. *Journal of Clinical Epidemiology*, 63(8):892–899.

Katz, S., Ford, A. B., Moskowitz, R. W., Jackson, B. A., & Jaffe, M. W. (1963). Studies of illness in the aged: The index of ADL: A standardized measure of biological and psychosocial function. *Journal of the American Medical Association, 185*(12), 914–919.

Lawton, M. P., & Brody, E. M. (1969). Assessment of older people: Self-maintaining and instrumental activities of daily living. *The Gerontologist, 9*(3), 179–186.

ONS. (2015). Birth summary tables, England and Wales, 2013 Statistical Bulletin retrieved from https://www.ons.gov.uk.

Prince, M., Reischies, F., Beekman, A., Fuhrer, R., Jonker, C., Kivela, S., et al. (1999). Development of the EURO-D scale: A European, Union initiative to compare symptoms of depression in 14 European centres. *The British Journal of Psychiatry, 174*(4), 330–338. https://doi.org/10.1192/bjp.174.4.330.

Reher, D. (1998). Family ties in Western Europe: Persistent contrasts. *Population and Development Review, 24,* 203–234.

Salhab, M., Al Sarakbi, W., & Mokbel, K. (2005). In vitro fertilization and breast cancer risk: A review. *International Journal of Fertility and Women's Medicine, 50*(6), 259–266.

Santini, A. (1995) *Continuità e discontinuità nel comportamento riproduttivo delle donne nel dopoguerra*. In Working paper, 53, Dipartimento di Statistica, Università di Firenze.

Schröder, M. (2011). *Retrospective data collection in the survey of health, ageing and retirement in Europe. SHARELIFE methodology*. Mannheim: Mannheim Research Institute for the Economics of Aging (MEA).

Tomassini, C., Wolf, D., & Rosina, A. (2003). Parental housing assistance and parent-child proximity in Italy. *Journal of Marriage and the Family, 65,* 700–715.

Ware, J. E. J. (2000). SF-36 health survey update. *Spine, 25,* 3130–3139.

Westendorp, R., & Kirkwood, T. (1998). Human longevity at the cost of reproductive success. *Nature, 396,* 743–746.

The Effect of Current Family Situation on Slow Walking Speed at Old Age

Gabriele Doblhammer, Steffen Peters, Debora Rizzuto and Anna-Karin Welmer

Introduction

Walking (or gait) speed is an important measure of health and frailty among the elderly (Bergman et al. 2007; Studenski et al. 2011; Cooper et al. 2014). Slow walking speed is related to increased mortality (Studenski et al. 2011) and to an increased risk of dementia (Welmer et al. 2014). Together with other deficits in physical function it predicts falls, especially in people with global cognitive impairment (Welmer et al. 2016). The relationship between fast walking speed and health is rooted in more healthy behaviors, lower cardiovascular risk factors, and lower levels of inflammatory markers (Elbaz et al. 2013). Furthermore, slow walking speed, is strongly related to slow processing speed, an early sign of deteriorating cognitive functioning (Welmer et al. 2014). Given its strong predictive power in terms of health it is advantageous in that it can be easily assessed by non-professionals (Atkinson et al. 2007). Turning to the demographic and social correlates of walking speed, a gender difference has been observed, with men

G. Doblhammer (✉)
German Center for Neurodegenerative Disease (DZNE), Bonn, Germany
e-mail: gabriele.doblhammer@uni-rostock.de

S. Peters
Rostock Center for the Study of Demographic Change, Rostock, Germany
e-mail: steffen.peters@uni-rostock.de

D. Rizzuto · A.-K. Welmer
Department of Neurobiology, Care Sciences and Society, Karolinska Institutet, Aging Research Center, Stockholm, Sweden
e-mail: Debora.Rizzuto@ki.se

A.-K. Welmer
e-mail: Anna-Karin.Welmer@ki.se

G. Doblhammer and J. Gumà (eds.), *A Demographic Perspective on Gender, Family and Health in Europe*, https://doi.org/10.1007/978-3-319-72356-3_12

outperforming women particularly at old ages (Weber 2016; also see the chapter of Oksuzyan et al.). Recent studies (Weber 2016; Welmer et al. 2013) have demonstrated a strong social gradient in walking speed, with the highly educated men and women always walking faster than their less educated counterparts. This advantage, however, diminishes at higher ages. Little is known about the relationship between walking speed and family situation, another important determinant of health at old age. This study thus sets out to provide a longitudinal perspective of the predictive power of the current family situation, measured in terms of partnership and parenthood, on slow walking speed.

This book contains several chapters which analyze myriad family effects and in the following we refer to them. Partnership and parenthood have strong positive and negative effects on health over the whole life course (Hank and Steinbach). The European comparative study by Doblhammer and Gumà shows that during mid-life the differences in health by family status were larger among women than among men; as also confirmed by the studies of Georges, Kreft and Doblhammer, and Ennser-Buber and Hanappi. Furthermore, the differences were related to life-style factors such as smoking, at-risk alcohol consumption, unhealthy diet, and physical exercise as demonstrated by the study of von der Lippe and Rattay. At old age there is a general consensus that it is particularly men who benefit from living with a partner and being married (Hank and Steinbach), while the effects for elderly women are less clear. There seem to be strong positive and negative effects of parenthood on health for women, less so for men, independent of the particular characteristics of their partnership biography (Tomassini, Di Gessa and Egidi).

In the following we will briefly summarize these findings, as these provide an important background for our own study, first turning to partnership, then to parenthood, and finally discussing possible pathways of these associations.

Partnership

While the positive effects of partnership and the selection into partnership have been widely documented (particularly those of marriage), the negative effects have been investigated only recently, with the exception of changes in partnership status such as divorce or widowhood (Hank and Steinbach). Such changes have been shown to have gendered effects, e.g. divorce leads to comparatively better health among men and worse health among women. Marital biographies seem to have a stronger impact on slowly developing health conditions such as chronic disease and functional limitations, while current partnership status seems to impact strongly on mental health. The latter seems to be particularly dependent on satisfaction with the partnership and its reciprocity (Hank and Steinbach).

Parenthood

A series of studies have shown that parents of two to three children experience the best health among the elderly, particularly among women, less so among men, independent of the definition of health (Hank and Steinbach; Tomassini, Di Gessa, and Egidi). However, these studies have also pointed out that for women a high number of children results in worse physical and mental health and in higher mortality from cardiovascular disease, and, for both genders, early parenthood appears to be detrimental for later physical health outcomes. A high number of children and early parenthood may be related to economic strain, worse partnership quality, and role overload for (single) parents. The effects of early motherhood depended on the social environment, and its negative effect was less strong in societies where early fertility was more common and socially accepted. The health differences according to number of children were independent of the partnership and fertility biography. Whether childlessness has a negative effect on health at old age is still unclear, as studies come to mixed conclusions. Tomassini, Di Gessa and Egidi find no health disadvantage for the childless in Italy, yet Hank and Steinbach reviewed studies which showed a clear disadvantage in various European countries. On the other hand, they also point out that there is evidence that childless men and women experience less depressive symptoms than parents.

Pathways

Most studies stressed that children and a partner are an important resource at old age in terms of providing care, reducing psychosocial stress, and increasing overall well-being (Hank and Steinbach; Tomassini, Di Gessa, and Egidi). They also pointed out that being a parent at midlife may have positive effects on health behavior (von der Lippe and Rattay). Health detrimental behaviours, such as smoking and at-risk alcohol consumption, seem to be more strongly associated with partnership and parenthood than with poor diet and physical inactivity. The risk of a relapse after quitting smoking is higher if the partner also smokes, while the presence of young children reduces the risk of smoking for women. Single men and women are more likely to have at-risk alcohol consumption, thus the transition to marriage and parenthood has been suggested as a constraint on drinking behaviour. The extent of physical activity is very different in men and women, and parenthood seems to have more effect on the physical activity of mothers than of fathers. Whether the extent of physical activity of mothers is compromised by their children is, however, still unresolved, with some studies finding a decline and others an increase (von der Lippe and Rattay).

Social status explains some of the relationship between family situation and health but by far not all (Doblhammer and Gumà). In this context, an important pathway is related to financial difficulties, mainly among single mothers and mothers living in consensual unions and stepfamilies (Doblhammer and Gumà, Buber-Ennser and Hanappi).

Reverse Causation

Studies dealing with the relationship between health and family status must always account for the possibility of health selection into partnership and parenthood (Hank and Steinbach). Thus, one always needs to account for reverse causation, meaning that an individual's poor health could lead to living single, to losing the partner due to divorce or widowhood, or to staying childless. This becomes even more important at old age when the partners tend to become more equal in their health despite an increasing variability in health profiles with age. Thus, the family status of an individual may to some extent be determined by the health of the partner and the "contagion" or poor health among partners (Giannantoni and Egidi). In our own analysis we try to account for such health selection effects by introducing a time dimension between the characteristics of an individual and the outcome variable walking speed. In other words, we use the characteristics from a previous wave to predict the walking speed in a follow-up wave.

Aims and Hypotheses

Considering all of the various negative and positive effects that partnership and parenthood can have, gives rise to the question of the net-effect of the current family situation at old age. If the current family situation primarily reflects the availability of support, a higher number of family members should result in better health. On the contrary, if possible positive and negative influences of a partner and children prevail at old age, the number of family members is not necessarily positively correlated with good health. In addition, the relationship may be gender specific. Over the whole life course the distribution of paid and unpaid work within households is gender specific (see the chapter by Oláh et al.), which may influence the health behaviour. Also the values and norms in terms of health behaviour that govern the role models for mothers and fathers are gender specific (see the chapter by von der Lippe and Rattay). At old age, women are the main familial care providers to their partners (Revenson et al. 2015) and are thus exposed to the negative effects of the caregiver burden to a larger extent than men. At the same time, men are mainly at the receiving end of care provision due to their lower life expectancy.

Despite the presence of positive and negative effects of partnership and parenthood on health over the whole life course, we assumed that the availability of possible familial resources of help is the decisive factor at old age. Thus, we hypothesized that those living with a partner and who had had children would have the best walking performance and would maintain it for a longer period, due to the health selection into partnership and parenthood as well as due to protective effects. On the contrary, the childless without a partner would fare worst. The other groups (with either partner or children) would fare intermediately. This should be true for both genders, yet even more so for men because women are the main care providers at old age and thus are at the giving rather than the receiving end of help.

Study Population

Study population: We used the Swedish National Study on Aging and Care in Kungsholmen (SNAC-K)—a part of Stockholm (Lagergren et al. 2004). The sample included persons aged 60 years and older, living in private or institutional households. The sample was randomly selected by specific age cohorts. To reduce attrition during the follow-up, eleven age cohorts were chosen with different intervals: six-year intervals in the younger age groups (60–78 years old), and three-year intervals in the older groups (>78 years old). The two youngest and the four oldest age groups were oversampled. The baseline survey was conducted in 2001–2004 and follow-ups were performed every 6 years for younger cohorts (60–78 years) and every 3 years for older cohorts (78+ years). Data was collected at the research center or at participants' homes through interviews, clinical examinations, and testing by trained staff. The following Fig. 1 shows the structure of the study population and the final analysis sample of our study.

A total of 5111 people were initially selected for participation; of those 200 died before start of the study, 262 had no contact information, 32 had moved, 23 did not speak Swedish, and 4 were deaf. Of the remaining 4590 people, 3363 (73.3%) participated in the baseline examination. At baseline (BL), the study population (Fig. 1, top) of 1782 respondents below age 78 (young), and 1581 persons aged 78 years and above (old). Of the young, 157 died before the six-year follow-up (6YFU) and 229 had either moved or refused to participate any more, resulting in 1396 respondents, all of whom have information at baseline and in the follow-up. Of the old, 437 died and 152 dropped out due to other reasons. Thus, 992 persons were re-examined at the first follow-up after three years (3YFU). Of these, 662 also participated in the 6YFU, as 249 people had died between the 3YFU and the 6YFU and another 81 persons didn't participate for other reasons.

To arrive at the analytical sample (Fig. 1, bottom), we excluded all participants who were unable to walk at the baseline examination or who did not participate in any of the follow ups. This resulted in an analytical sample of 2097 persons (Fig. 1, bottom) (1323 young and 774 old participants at BL). Of the young, all the 1323 persons participated in the 6YFU. Of the old, 774 were re-examined in the 3-year follow-up, and 575 participated in the 6YFU.

Slow walking speed (Seeman et al. 1994): Respondents who considered themselves to be normal or fast walkers were requested to walk a distance of 6 meters;

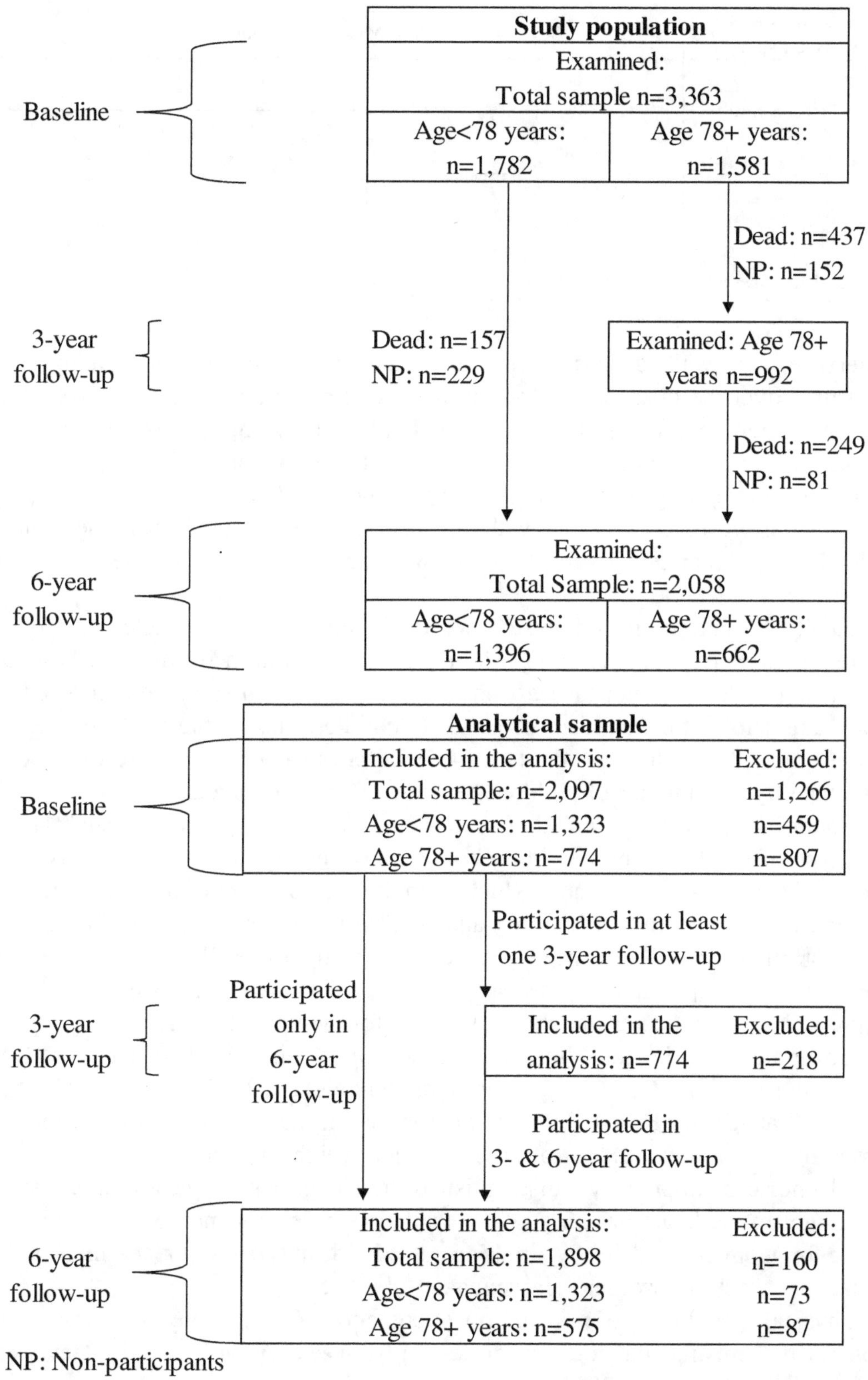

Fig. 1 Study population and analytical sample. *Source* SNAC-K data 2004–2010, own calculations

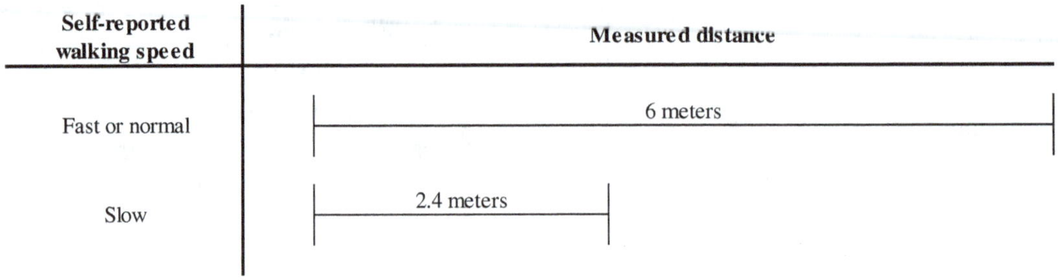

Fig. 2 Measurement of walking speed

otherwise, they walked 2.4 m. Previous studies demonstrated that walking speed measured over the distances 2.4 and 6 m are comparable (Bohannon 2008). Time was measured in seconds (Fig. 2). We divided the sample into fast and slow walkers using the median (Total: 1 m/s; men: 1 m/s; women 0.85 m/s).

Change in walking speed: The change was measured between the follow-up and the previous wave. Those with a walking speed decrease of more than one standard deviation (as compared to the baseline walking speed) were defined as having experienced a decline.

Family Situation: In a first step we distinguished two characteristics of the current family situation: (1) living with a partner or not in the same household, and (2) having children or not (at least one child). In a second step, we combined this information to distinguish four groups: (1) childless, no partner; (2) childless, in partnership; (3) children, no partner; (4) children, in partnership. We did not differentiate by the number of children because of small numbers.

Control variables: We included socio-demographic characteristics such as age, sex, type of residence (private household versus nursing home); a pre-constructed index of socio-economic status which combined information about income, education as years of formal schooling, and blue/white collar occupation. In addition, we controlled for walking speed at baseline (less than one SD from the average), and the follow-up time (3-year and 6-year) in the Level and Change Models, expressed as an indicator variable at the two follow-up occasions.

Covariates: We included important life-style and health characteristics. Body mass index with BMI $\leq$ 25: normal/underweight, >25–30: overweight, >30: obesity (Launer and Harris 1996). We combined normal and underweight into one group due to the low number of cases of underweight participants.

Alcohol consumption: we distinguished the categories no/occasional consumption, light-to-moderate drinking (1–14 drinks per week for men or 1–7 drinks per week for women), and heavy drinking ($\geq$=15 drinks per week for men or >=8 drinks per week for women) (Jarvenpaa et al. 2005).

Physical activities: we used the questions about medium physical activity and combined them into the four categories daily, weekly/monthly, rarely/never, not specified (Rydwik et al. 2013).

The number of chronic diseases: chronic diseases were diagnosed by a physician on the basis of clinical examination and patient history. A disease was defined as chronic if it was of prolonged duration, left residual disability, worsened quality of life, or required a long period of care, treatment, or rehabilitation (Calderon-Larranaga et al. 2016).

Depression: we selected three items from the Montgomery-Åsberg Depression Rating Scale (Montgomery and Asberg 1979) and combined them into one variable indicating the presence of sadness, pessimistic thoughts, and feelings of loneliness.

Modelling Strategy and Statistical Analysis

We performed two types of GEE-regressions (Ziegler 2011) with binary outcome variables and logistic link functions. (1) In the "Level Models" we predicted slow walking speed in the follow-up by the characteristics of the previous wave. This implies that for individuals below age 78, all of whom had one follow-up after six years, only one outcome measurement was included in the model and that the characteristics from the BL were used as predictors of the walking speed in the 6YFU. People aged 78 and above in principle had two follow-ups, and the characteristics from the BL were used as predictors for walking speed in the 3YFU, and the characteristics from the 3YFU were used as predictors for walking speed in the 6YFU. Thus, each individual contributed a maximum of two outcome measurements and one outcome measurement in the case of death, attrition, or missing value. (2) In the "Change Models" we explored the decline in walking speed between two waves using the characteristics from the first of the two waves as predictors. Similar to above, characteristics from the BL were used to predict the change in walking speed for those below age 78 until the 6YFU, and they can only be included once in the model. For those aged 78 and above the characteristics of the BL predicted the change in walking speed by the 3YFU, and the characteristics of the 3YFU predicted the change by the 6YFU, and they can be included in the model a maximum of two times. In both model types we used an indicator variable to account for the different length of the follow-up periods.

The within-person residual covariance matrix was evaluated with the unstructured correlation structure. To establish the gross-effect of the (change in) family position, we ran sex-specific models controlled for age, the respective design variables, and the walking speed at the previous wave. We refer to these models as Model 1. We then explored the interaction effect between the partnership and the child variables using the category *childless, no partner* as the reference category. We depict the gradient of the relationships in two figures. To explore possible interdependencies of the current family situation with other health characteristics, we introduced additional variables (Model 2: type of residence & SES; Model 3: Model 2 + BMI, alcohol consumption and physical activity; Model 4: Model 3 + number of chronic morbidities, depression, Model 5: Model 4 + alcohol consumption and physical activity + number of chronic morbidities, depression). All models were estimated separately for the two sexes. All calculations were performed in Stata 12.1, (StataCorp, TX, USA).

Results

Slow walking speed (Table 1): Among those who were able to walk, walking speed at baseline ranged between 0.13 and 2 m/s, with a mean of 1.13 m/s (±0.36 m/s). We used this information as a control variable in both the Change and the Level Models. In the Level Models, walking speed ranged between 0 and 3 m/s and the median was 1 m/s: 1181 of the individuals were below the median and, thus, considered slow walkers. In the Change Models the mean change in walking speed was −0.13 m/s with a SD of 0.30 m/s (median: −0.12 m/s); 512 individuals (20%) had a decline of more than one SD to the negative.

Family position (Table 2): For our main variable of interest, which is family position, as well as the other control variables, we explored the distributions at baseline (BL) and at the 3YFU. At BL, about 15% of the respondents were *childless without a partner*, which increased to almost 18% in the 3YFU. Only 5% at BL (3% in the 3YFU) were *childless and with a partner*, while 35% (BL) and 42% (3YFU) had *children but no partner*. At BL, the vast majority (41%) had *children and was living with a partner*, which decreased to 29% in the 3YFU.

Covariates (Table 2): 64% (BL) of the respondents were female, which increased to 69% in the 3YFU. Only about 1% was living in nursing homes (3% in the 3YFU). The vast majority had high SES (91% BL, 85% 3YFU), reflecting the highly socially selected population in Kungsholmen. Only 12% were obese, the vast majority had under/normal weight or were pre-obese. Only 22% were heavy drinkers (BL & 3YFU), at BL 50% were light-to-moderate drinker, in the 3YFU the majority were no/occasional drinkers. At BL, 46% rarely/never did any physical activity, in the 3YFU this was 57%. The respondents were rather healthy in terms of physical and mental health: 25% had no chronic diseases at BL (13% at 3YFU); the majority had one or two chronic diseases. At baseline, 50% had signs of depression, at the 3YFU 53%.

Table 1 Walking speed at baseline, and as outcome variables in the Level and Change Models

Sample overview						
Walking speed baseline (control variable)	Outcome level models			Outcome change models		
Min./max.: 0.13–2 m/s	Min./max.: 0–3 m/s			Min./max.: −1.39–1.01 m/s		
Mean/SD: 1.13 ± 0.36 m/s	Mean/SD: 0.95 ± 0.40 m/s			Mean/SD: −0.13 ± 0.30 m/s		
Median: 1.2 m/s	Median: 1 m/s			Median: −0.12 m/s		
		N	%		N	%
Outcome binary-coded	≥ Median	1372	53.74	Decline > 1 SD	2041	79.95
	<Median	1181	46.26	Decline ≤ 1 SD	512	20.05
Total		2553	100.00		2553	100.00

Table 2 Characteristics of the analysis population

Variable	Category	Baseline		3-year follow-up	
		N	%	N	%
Age groups	60	589	28.09	–	–
	66	420	20.03	–	–
	72	314	14.97	–	–
	78	322	15.36	–	–
	81	147	7.01	233	51.10
	84	126	6.01	88	19.30
	87	72	3.43	67	14.69
	90+	107	5.10	68	14.91
Sex	Male	762	36.34	141	30.92
	Female	1335	63.66	315	69.08
Family position	Childless, no partner	314	14.97	80	17.54
	Childless, in partnership	112	5.34	15	3.29
	Child(ren), no partner	727	34.67	191	41.89
	Child(ren), in partnership	854	40.72	130	28.51
	Not specified	90	4.29	40	8.77
Type of residence	Tenant/owner	2068	98.62	442	96.93
	Residential care home	29	1.38	14	3.07
SES	Low	27	1.29	10	2.19
	Middle	155	7.39	57	12.50
	High	1915	91.32	389	85.31
BMI	Under-/normal weight	917	43.73	159	34.87
	Pre-obesity	867	41.34	150	32.89
	Obesity	270	12.88	56	12.28
	Not specified	43	2.05	91	19.96
Alcohol	No or occasional	593	28.28	208	45.61
	Light-to-moderate	1048	49.98	147	32.24
	Heavy drinking	456	21.75	101	22.15
Physical activity	Daily	116	5.53	24	5.26
	Weekly/monthly	683	32.57	92	20.18
	Rarely/never	959	45.73	261	57.24
	Not specified	339	16.17	79	17.32
Chronic diseases	0	528	25.18	60	13.16
	1	631	30.09	119	26.10
	2	456	21.75	130	28.51
	3+	482	22.99	147	32.24
Depression	No	1046	49.88	240	52.63
	Yes	1051	50.12	216	47.37

(continued)

Table 2 (continued)

Variable	Category	Baseline		3-year follow-up	
		N	%	N	%
Walking speed baseline	>1 SD from average in the negative	296	14.12	104	22.81
	Less than 1 SD or higher than average	1801	85.88	352	77.19
Duration between predictor and outcome	3 years	720	34.33	456	100
	6 years	1377	65.67		
Total		2097	100.00	456	100.00

Multivariate Analyses

We first discuss the results from the Level Models, which explored the predictors of current slow walking speed. Model 1 shows the gross effect of the current family situation, Model 5 the effect corrected for confounding variables and covariates.

For both sexes combined, the presence of children significantly reduced the risk of slow walking speed but living with a partner did not have any statistically significant influence (Table 3). However, the latter result significantly depended on gender. Living in a partnership did not change the risk of slow walking speed for men (Table 3, Model 1 and Model 5), but appeared to be detrimental for the walking speed of women, particularly when controlled for other health related characteristics. Having children was associated with a lower likelihood of slow walking speed for both men and women, however the association was only significant for both sexes combined. (Model 1 and Model 5).

The interaction effect between partner and children confirmed the sex-specific results (Fig. 3). For men we found a clear negative gradient: the more family resources, the lower their risk of slow walking speed. The risk of slow walking speed was highest for the *childless, living without a partner* and it was lowest for those *with children, living in a partnership*; For women no clear and statistically significant gradient emerged, despite the larger sample size. Children tended to be beneficial, but living in a partnership tended to increase the risk of slow walking speed, counterbalancing the positive effect of children. The risk of slow walking speed was highest for the *childless, living in a partnership.*

Among men, SES and residency accounted for some but not all of the advantage of the partnered with children (Table 4: Model 2), but their advantage was attenuated when life-style (Table 4: Model 3) and morbidity information (Table 4: Model 4) were included. Among women no significant differences existed. The most pronounced tendency was the disadvantage of the childless women living in partnership. None of the confounding variables nor of the health related covariates could account for their particularly slow walking speed .

Table 3 Odds ratios of logistic regression main effects models for partnership and children on the risk of slow walking speed (Level Models)

Characteristics	Model 1		Model 5	
	OR	*p*-value	OR	*p*-value
Total[a]				
In partnership (ref.: no partner)	0.98	0.88	1.13	0.38
Child (ref.: childless)	0.73	0.03	0.73	0.04
Men				
In partnership (ref.: no partner)	0.73	0.16	0.82	0.41
Child (ref.: childless)	0.64	0.09	0.74	0.35
Women				
In partnership (ref.: no partner)	1.22	0.24	1.42	0.05
Child (ref.: childless)	0.81	0.23	0.79	0.19

Model 1: controlled for age, design variables
Model 5: controlled for age, design variables, type of residence & SES, BMI, alcohol consumption & physical activity, number of chronic morbidities, depression
[a]Controlled for age, sex, design variables

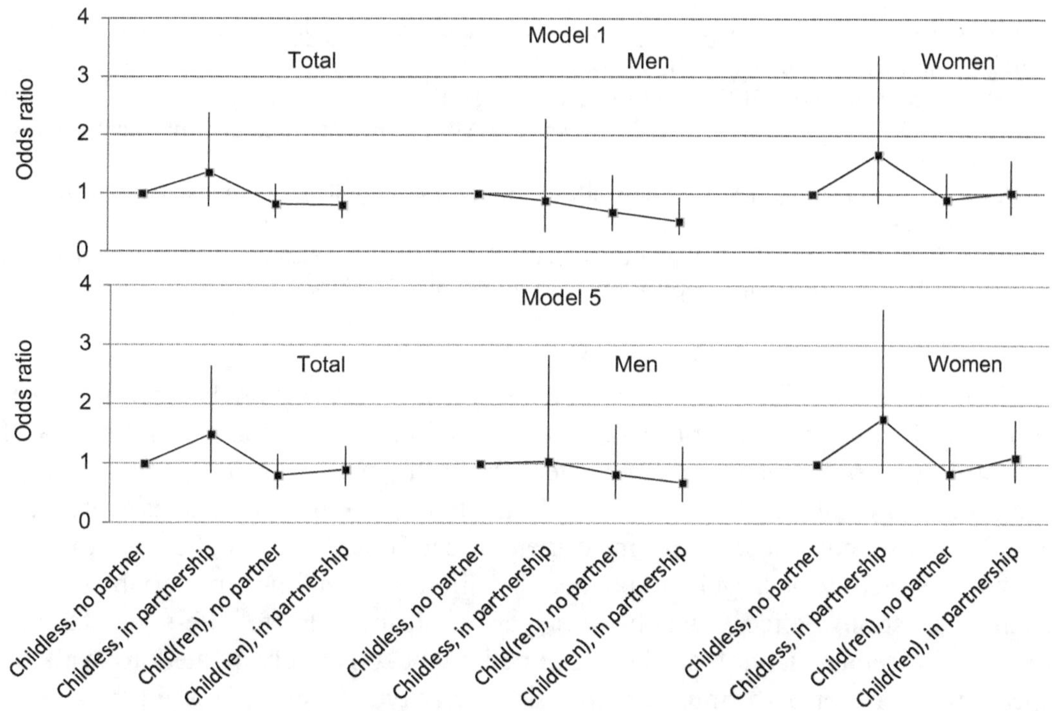

Fig. 3 Odds ratios of the interaction effect between partnership and parenthood in the Level Models: gross-effect (Model 1) and controlled for possible mediators (Model 5)

Table 4 Odds ratios of family situation based on logistic regression models of poor walking speed (Level Models)

	Model 1		Model 2		Model 3		Model 4		Model 5	
Characteristics	OR	*p*-value	OR	*p*-value	OR	*p*-value	OR	*p*-value	OR	*p*-value
Men										
Family situation (ref.: Childless, no partner)										
Childless, in partnership	0.86	0.77	0.98	0.97	1.03	0.96	0.98	0.97	1.04	0.94
Child(ren), no partner	0.68	0.25	0.75	0.40	0.82	0.56	0.77	0.46	0.83	0.60
Child(ren), in partnership	0.52	0.03	0.60	0.08	0.63	0.14	0.64	0.15	0.69	0.25
Not specified	0.27	0.04	0.17	0.02	0.24	0.05	0.19	0.03	0.27	0.09
Women										
Family situation (ref.: Childless, no partner)										
Childless, in partnership	1.67	0.16	1.70	0.14	1.72	0.13	1.74	0.12	1.77	0.12
Child(ren), no partner	0.90	0.59	0.89	0.57	0.88	0.53	0.86	0.47	0.85	0.44
Child(ren), in partnership	1.01	0.96	1.02	0.92	1.05	0.84	1.08	0.73	1.11	0.65
Not specified	0.66	0.21	0.65	0.20	0.62	0.16	0.65	0.21	0.62	0.17

Model 1: family situation, age, design variables

Model 2: family situation, SES, type of residence, age, design variables

Model 3: family situation, SES, type of residence, BMI, alcohol consumption, physical activity, age, design variables

Model 4: family situation, SES, type of residence, number of chronic morbidities, depression, age, design variables

Model 5: family situation, SES, type of residence, BMI, alcohol consumption, physical activity, number of chronic morbidities, depression, age, design variables

To explore the effects of the covariates we turn to the models for both sexes combined (not shown). We observed that women had a significantly higher risk of low walking speed than men, however, this difference was fully explained by life-style and health characteristics. The effects of the other covariates were generally as expected: Those living in residential care units had a higher risk of slow walking, which was largely explained by life-style and health variables. SES exerted a strong effect, which was partly attributable to life-style factors. Light-to-moderate alcohol drinking seemed to be positively related to walking speed; rarely/never performing any physical activity severely increased the risk of slow walking speed. High numbers of chronic morbidities increased the risk of slow walking speed as did signs of depression. As expected, walking speed in the previous wave was a strong predictor of current walking speed.

Turning to the *Change Models*, which explored the risk of a severely declining walking speed, for men we found little effect of living in a partnership, and a

Table 5 Odds ratios of logistic regression main effects models for partnership and children on the risk of poor walking speed (Change Models)

Characteristics	Model 1		Model 5	
	OR	*p*-value	OR	*p*-value
Total[a]				
In partnership (ref.: no partner)	1.01	0.94	1.11	0.40
Child (ref.: childless)	0.83	0.14	0.84	0.16
Men				
In partnership (ref.: no partner)	1.02	0.92	1.00	1.00
Child (ref.: childless)	0.61	0.03	0.64	0.06
Women				
In partnership (ref.: no partner)	1.00	0.98	1.16	0.35
Child (ref.: childless)	0.92	0.60	0.92	0.61

Model 1: controlled for age, design variables
Model 5: controlled for SES, type of residence, BMI, alcohol consumption, physical activity, number of chronic morbidities, depression, age, design variables
[a]Controlled for sex

positive effect of having children (Table 5). This positive effect was not explained by the covariates. For women, the risk of severely declining walking speed was not related to living in a partnership, nor to having children.

The interaction effect between partnership and parenthood (Fig. 4) revealed that for both sexes the *childless, living in a partnership* had the highest risk of a severe decline, however, none of the differences were statistically significant. The presence of children, independent of the form of partnership, tended to be beneficial only for men.

Severe declines in walking speed are predominantly influenced by the characteristics related to poor physical health (Table 6).

Discussion

Among the elderly, the family situation at old age significantly predicts health in terms of slow walking speed; the relationship with changes in health, measured as severe declines in walking speed, is less clear. While much of the relationship is gender specific there are also common patterns. Among both sexes, having no children is related to slow walking speed albeit the effect is only statistically significant for men. In addition, childless persons living in a partnership showed the steepest decline in walking speed. We will return to this later.

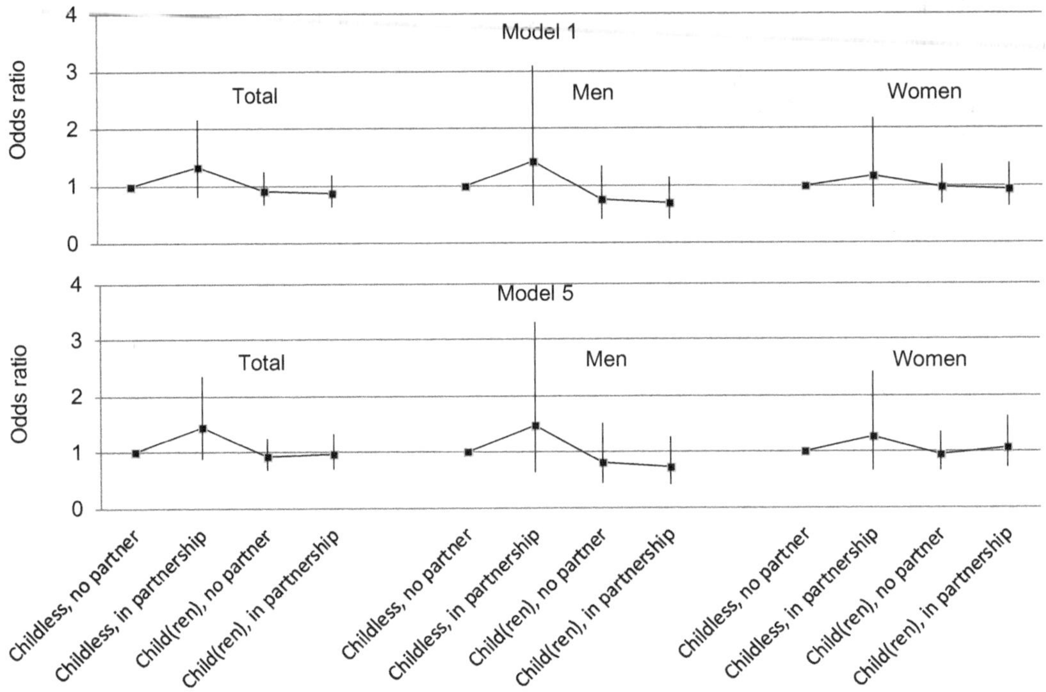

Fig. 4 Odds ratios of the interaction effect between partnership and parenthood in the Change Models: gross-effect (Model 1) and controlled for possible mediators (Model 5)

Using the slowest 25% quartile to define slow walking speed, we found that the pattern of the results did not change and differences by family situation even increased. However, when exploring walking speed in a linear mixed model we found that there was no relationship with family situation (not shown). This suggests that in general walking speed is only loosely related to family situation but that sub-performance and extreme deficiencies in walking speed may be also routed in the family environment.

Living in a partnership tends to be beneficial only for men, for women it may even be detrimental when controlled for life-style and health characteristics. For men there is a clear positive gradient between the amount of family resources and walking speed: the childless living alone have the slowest walking speed, those living in a partnership and who have children have the highest. Life-style factors such as obesity, smoking, and alcohol consumption mediate the advantage of the latter group. This is also true for health related characteristics such as the number of morbidities and signs of depression. For women, no positive gradient exists. On the contrary, living in a partnership exerts a negative effect, both among the childless and among those with children. Thus, for men we can confirm our initial hypothesis that higher amounts of family resources positively influence walking speed, for women we have to reject it; the effect of children appears to be positive, the effect of a partner, however, is negative.

It is difficult to disentangle the effects of health selection and causal factors related to protective or detrimental effects of the current family situation. Both

Table 6 Odds ratios of logistic regression models of the risk of severe decline in walking speed (Change Models)

	Model 1		Model 2		Model 3		Model 4		Model 5	
Characteristics	OR	*p*-value	OR	*p*-value	OR	*p*-value	OR	*p*-value	OR	*p*-value
Men										
Family situation (ref.: Childless, no partner)										
Childless, in partnership	1.43	0.37	1.53	0.29	1.48	0.33	1.53	0.30	1.47	0.36
Child(ren), no partner	0.75	0.34	0.79	0.45	0.78	0.43	0.82	0.53	0.81	0.50
Child(ren), in partnership	0.69	0.16	0.75	0.28	0.73	0.25	0.74	0.29	0.72	0.26
Not specified	0.45	0.21	0.43	0.18	0.44	0.21	0.48	0.25	0.49	0.27
Women										
Family situation (ref.: Childless, no partner)										
Childless, in partnership	1.16	0.64	1.15	0.67	1.18	0.62	1.23	0.52	1.28	0.46
Child(ren), no partner	0.97	0.85	0.94	0.75	0.96	0.82	0.93	0.68	0.95	0.79
Child(ren), in partnership	0.93	0.73	0.93	0.70	0.98	0.93	1.02	0.93	1.08	0.72
Not specified	0.99	0.97	0.98	0.95	0.91	0.75	0.97	0.91	0.90	0.73

Model 1: family situation, age, design variables
Model 2: family situation, SES, type of residence, age, design variables
Model 3: family situation, SES, type of residence, BMI, alcohol consumption, physical activity, age, design variables
Model 4: family situation, SES, type of residence, number of chronic morbidities, depression, age, design variables
Model 5: family situation, SES, type of residence, BMI, alcohol consumption, physical activity, number of chronic morbidities, depression, age, design variables

genders over their whole life course might be strongly health selected into partnership and parenthood. We observed family status at old age, and our categories of current family situation do not necessarily reflect the life-long partnership biography. In particular, those currently living without a partner comprise the never-married, as well as the separated, divorced, or widowed and very different health selection forces have acted on these groups. It is thus highly unlikely that the patterns observed purely reflect these selection processes. On the contrary, for men the strong positive gradient points towards protective effects of having a partner and children who, in addition to their influence on life-style, are also important resources of help and care provision. For elderly women the story is more complex. While living with a partner may be beneficial in terms of emotional support and general resources related to health and well-being, a partner can also be the source of a large burden when his health fails. In Sweden, as in other welfare states with less generous old-age care provision, women are more likely than men to provide personal care in combination with a variety of other caring tasks. Men, on the contrary, are more likely to provide some kind of practical help for a mother or a neighbour/friend (Jegermalm 2006). At the same time Swedish caregivers have worse perceptions concerning self-rated health, psychological wellbeing, and reporting days of poor health in the last month (Berglund et al. 2015). Thus, after the death of a partner, women are released from an immense burden and face a new life situation in which they have to be more self-reliant. As a consequence, they may stay more active, which has a positive impact on their walking speed. However, it was also reported that the well-being of a caregiving spouse was consistently compromised at every stage of the caregiving career, even after the death of the partner (Rafnsson et al. 2015).

Gender specific family roles related to physical fitness may also have detrimental effects on the walking speed of women. Von der Lippe and Rattay found that divorced women were physically more active than married women, and that mothers were the least active, however, little is known whether this also extends into old age. Given the gender specific distribution of unpaid work in families described in the chapter by Oláh, Kotowska and Richter, one would expect that during much of their life course women simply have less time available to spend on physical activity. In addition gender specific preferences of time use have been observed repeatedly: Time use surveys show that elderly men use more of their time for physical activity, while women are more heavily engaged in social activities (Finkel et al. 2016).

While children appear to be associated with faster walking speed among both genders, this effect is not significant for women, while it remains significant for men even after control for life-style and health related variables. Because of the small numbers we were not able to explore the effect by number of children; however, the lack of significance among women may indicate a u-shaped pattern, as found in other studies. Tomassini, Di Gessa, and Egidi describe in their chapter that health is best for mothers of one to two children, and starts to deteriorate for three and more children. This is true in the Italian context of a familialistic welfare state as well as in other countries, such as e.g. the Nordic dual-earner welfare states (for a definition of welfare state see the chapter of Oláh, Kotowska and Richter). The increasing risk posed by a higher number of children is related mainly to cardiovascular disease, as pointed out by Hank and Steinbach in their chapter. On the contrary, for men, the risk of poor health and high mortality decreases continuously with an increasing number of children. Over the life course men's health behavior is less related to the presence of children than is women's (see the chapter of von der Lippe and Rattay), which might be negative in terms of smoking and at risk-alcohol consumption but positive in terms of physical activity. In addition women may face a biological toll of repeated pregnancy (Peters et al. 2016). Children are important care providers for parents of both genders; in case of providing care to fathers they are, however, usually secondary providers, whereas in case of providing care to mothers they often become the primary care provider due to the higher mortality of men at old age. Thus for fathers, children may indeed be an additional care resource, for mothers they may partly take over care work of the partners.

Among both genders, the largest accelerated decline in walking speed was found in the childless living with a partner. In the cohorts observed in this study, childlessness while living in a partnership is a rather rare phenomenon, with only five percent of the elderly belonging to this group at the baseline wave of the SNAC-K. Health selection into childlessness may therefore play an important role and may explain the accelerated speed of health deterioration. This explanation is supported by the fact that neither control for life-style factors nor for physical and mental health can explain the accelerated decline in walking speed.

Hank and Steinbach pointed out in their chapter that current family status was correlated mainly with mental health, while the family biography was related mainly to slowly developing chronic health conditions. In our study we controlled for depression in terms of feelings of sadness and loneliness, in addition to multi-morbidity which attenuated the health advantage of the partnered men with children. This leads us to conclude that current family status, in addition to the family biography, may also be an important predictor of physical health.

It is noteworthy to point out that, at middle ages, women's health is more affected by family status than men's (see the chapters of Doblhammer and Gumà, and Georges, Kreft and Doblhammer) while at old age the opposite is true. At middle ages women not living in a marriage who have children, particularly single mothers, are severely disadvantaged in their subjective health. As Doblhammer and Gumà showed, much of this disadvantage can be explained by financial deprivation. For middle-aged men, differences in their family situation are much smaller and financial deprivation even works the other way; married men with children seem to face financial difficulties more often. At old age men profit from partnership in terms of health, women do not. In our study population financial difficulties cannot explain the differences because the SNAC-K population is highly selected in social terms and generally does not experience financial problems. SES does only account for a small proportion of the health differences by family status.

In our study we cannot disentangle the effect of the partnership biography from the effect of the current family status due to the lack of biographical information in the SNAC-K data. These data also lack information on the health situation of the partner, which prevents us from testing whether the partner's health is an important mediating factor. Another weakness is the highly selected study population in terms of health and social status. This bias may have introduced an underestimation of the effect of the current family situation on health. Because highly educated women may be less dependent on their partners in many ways, including in financial terms, this may also explain the lack of a positive effect of a partner on their health. On the other hand it may also dampen the negative effect of a partner's ill health because older persons with lower education increasingly receive family care, while those with higher education are more likely to purchase and use private services (Szebehely and Trydegard 2012).

Another possible limitation is that non-married people without children may be less likely to survive to participate in the follow-up examination. This may lead to an underestimation of the associations (Koskinen et al. 2007).

Finally, the use of different distances in the test of walking speed may be a potential limitation. However, studies support the view that tests for walking speed are generally considered to be highly reliable, regardless of the distance (Seeman et al. 1994).

The main strength of this study lies in its longitudinal design focused on a large sample of largely community-based elderly. The panel character of the study permitted us to measure the current family situation as a predictor of health which was observed prior to the health outcome, thus avoiding the problem of reverse causation. Moreover, we use an objective measure of walking speed measured by qualified health care professionals, which is also true for the other characteristics related to physical and mental health.

Our study demonstrated that the family situation is an important determinant of the health of individuals. Its influence changes over the life course and differs for men and women. In the future, changing family biographies will also lead to new partnership forms at old age, a phenomenon which so far is only emerging at young and middle-ages. Based on our results we may speculate that living in consensual unions or living together apart may have a negative impact on the health of elderly men because their partners may be less committed to provide care in case of poor health. This, however, may improve the health of elderly women who are released from the burden of providing care. Future studies will tell.

Conclusion

In ageing societies new policies have to be developed to meet the increasing demand for care by expanding the formal care sector in combination with strengthening informal care arrangements. Most importantly, it is necessary to identify those vulnerable groups which need support from both sectors. We have shown that men and women without children may need more support from formal caregivers, not only because of the lack of family members who could provide informal care but also because they suffer from comparably worse health. While partners are important informal care providers to each other, older women living with someone may also have an increased need of societal support. They carry much of the informal care burden at old age, quite often compromising their own health and increasing their own care demand.

References

Atkinson, H. H., Rosano, C., Simonsick, E. M., Williamson, J. D., Davis, C, Ambrosius, W. T., et al. (2007). Cognitive function, gait speed decline, and comorbidities: The health, aging and body composition study. *The Journals of gerontology. Series A, Biological Sciences and Medical Sciences, 62*(8), S. 844–S. 850.

Berglund, E., Lytsy, P., & Westerling, R. (2015). Health and wellbeing in informal caregivers and non-caregivers: A comparative cross-sectional study of the Swedish general population. *Health and Quality of Life Outcomes, 13*, S. 109. https://doi.org/10.1186/s12955-015-0309-2.

Bergman, H., Ferrucci, L., Guralnik, J., Hogan, D. B., Hummel, S., Karunananthan, S., et al. (2007). Frailty: an emerging research and clinical paradigm–issues and controversies. *The Journals of Gerontology. Series A, Biological Sciences and Medical Sciences, 62*(7), S. 731–S. 737.

Bohannon, R. W. (2008). Population representative gait speed and its determinants. *Journal of Geriatric Physical Therapy (2001)* 31 (2), S. 49–S. 52.

Calderon-Larranaga, A., Vetrano, D. L., Onder, G., Gimeno-Feliu, L. A., Coscollar-Santaliestra, C., Carfi, A., et al. (2016). Assessing and measuring chronic multimorbidity in the older population: A proposal for its operationalization. *The Journals of Gerontology. Series A, Biological Sciences and Medical Sciences.* https://doi.org/10.1093/gerona/glw233.

Cooper, R., Strand, B. H., Hardy, R., Patel, K. V., & Kuh, D. (2014). Physical capability in mid-life and survival over 13 years of follow-up: British birth cohort study. *BMJ (Clinical Research Ed.), 348*, g2219. https://doi.org/10.1136/bmj.g2219.

Elbaz, A., Sabia, S., Brunner, E., Shipley, M., Marmot, M., Kivimaki, M., et al. (2013): Association of walking speed in late midlife with mortality: Results from the Whitehall II cohort study. *Age (Dordrecht, Netherlands), 35*(3), S. 943–S. 952. https://doi.org/10.1007/s11357-012-9387-9.

Finkel, D., Andel, R., & Pedersen, N. L. (2016). Gender differences in longitudinal trajectories of change in physical, social, and cognitive/sedentary leisure activities. *The Journals of Gerontology. Series B, Psychological Sciences and Social Sciences.* https://doi.org/10.1093/geronb/gbw116.

Jarvenpaa, T., Rinne, J. O., Koskenvuo, M., Raiha, I., & Kaprio, J. (2005). Binge drinking in midlife and dementia risk. *Epidemiology (Cambridge, Mass.), 16*(6), S. 766–S. 771.

Jegermalm, M. (2006). Informal care in Sweden. A typology of care and caregivers. *International Journal of Social Welfare, 15*(4), S. 332–S. 343. https://doi.org/10.1111/j.1468-2397.2006.00400.x.

Koskinen, S., Joutsenniemi, K., Martelin, T., & Martikainen, P. (2007). Mortality differences according to living arrangements. *International Journal of Epidemiology, 36*(6), S. 1255–S. 1264. https://doi.org/10.1093/ije/dym212.

Lagergren, M., Fratiglioni, L., Hallberg, I. R., Berglund, J., Elmstahl, S., Hagberg, B., et al. (2004). A longitudinal study integrating population, care and social services data. The Swedish National study on Aging and Care (SNAC). In: *Aging Clinical and Experimental Research, 16* (2), S. 158–S. 168.

Launer, L. J., & Harris, T. (1996). Weight, height and body mass index distributions in geographically and ethnically diverse samples of older persons. Ad Hoc committee on the statistics of anthropometry and aging. *Age and Ageing, 25*(4), S. 300–S. 306.

Montgomery, S. A., & Asberg, M. (1979). A new depression scale designed to be sensitive to change. *The British Journal of Psychiatry: The Journal of Mental Science, 134,* S. 382–S. 389.

Peters, S. A., Yang, L., Guo, Y., Chen, Y., Bian, Z., Millwood, I. Y., et al. (2016). Parenthood and the risk of cardiovascular diseases among 0.5 million men and women: Findings from the China Kadoorie Biobank. *International Journal of Epidemiology.* https://doi.org/10.1093/ije/dyw144.

Rafnsson, S. B., Shankar, A., & Steptoe, A. (2015). Informal caregiving transitions, subjective well-being and depressed mood: Findings from the english longitudinal study of ageing. *Aging & Mental Health*, S. 1–S. 9. https://doi.org/10.1080/13607863.2015.1088510.

Revenson, T. A., Griva, K., Luszczynska, A., Morrison, V., Panagopoulou, E., Vilchinsky, N., et al. (2015). Gender and caregiving: The costs of caregiving for women. In T. A. Revenson, K. Griva, A. Luszczynska, V. Morrison, E. Panagopoulou, N. Vilchinsky, & M. Hagedoorn (Eds.), *Caregiving in the illness context* (pp. S. 48–S. 63). Basingstoke: Palgrave Pivot.

Rydwik, E., Welmer, A.-K., Kareholt, I., Angleman, S., Fratiglioni, L., & Wang, H.-X. (2013). Adherence to physical exercise recommendations in people over 65–the SNAC-Kungsholmen study. *European Journal of Public Health, 23*(5), S. 799–S. 804. https://doi.org/10.1093/eurpub/cks150.

Seeman, T. E., Charpentier, P. A., Berkman, L. F., Tinetti, M. E., Guralnik, J. M., Albert, M., et al. (1994). Predicting changes in physical performance in a high-functioning elderly cohort. MacArthur studies of successful aging. *Journal of Gerontology, 49*(3), M97–M108. https://doi.org/10.1093/geronj/49.3.M97.

Studenski, S., Perera, S., Patel, K., Rosano, C., Faulkner, K., Inzitari, M., et al. (2011). Gait speed and survival in older adults. *JAMA, 305*(1), S. 50–S. 58. https://doi.org/10.1001/jama.2010.1923.

Szebehely, M., & Trydegard, G.-B. (2012). Home care for older people in Sweden: a universal model in transition. *Health and Social Care in the Community, 20*(3), S. 300–S. 309. https://doi.org/10.1111/j.1365-2524.2011.01046.x.

Weber, D. (2016). Differences in physical aging measured by walking speed: Evidence from the english longitudinal study of ageing. *BMC Geriatrics, 16*, S. 31. https://doi.org/10.1186/s12877-016-0201-x.

Welmer, A.-K., Kareholt, I., Rydwik, E., Angleman, S., & Wang, H.-X. (2013). Education-related differences in physical performance after age 60: A cross-sectional study assessing variation by age, gender and occupation. *BMC Public Health, 13*, S. 641. https://doi.org/10.1186/1471-2458-13-641.

Welmer, A.-K., Rizzuto, D., Laukka, E. J., Johnell, K., & Fratiglioni, L. (2016). Cognitive and physical function in relation to the risk of injurious falls in older adults: A population-based study. *The Journals of Gerontology. Series A, Biological Sciences and Medical Sciences.* https://doi.org/10.1093/gerona/glw141.

Welmer, A.-K., Rizzuto, D., Qiu, C., Caracciolo, B., & Laukka, E. J. (2014). Walking speed, processing speed, and dementia: A population-based longitudinal study. *The Journals of Gerontology. Series A, Biological Sciences and Medical Sciences, 69*(12), S. 1503–S. 1510. https://doi.org/10.1093/gerona/glu047.

Ziegler, A. (2011). Generalized estimating equations. New York, NY: Springer (Lecture Notes in Statistics, 204). Online verfügbar unter http://dx.doi.org/10.1007/978-1-4614-0499-6.

www.ingramcontent.com/pod-product-compliance
Lightning Source LLC
LaVergne TN
LVHW080031210926
848481LV00011B/3160